FIRE YOUR DOCTOR

Escape the System

Reclaim Your Health

DR. DANIELLE SMITH LOCKWOOD

& RICHARD LOCKWOOD

CONNECT WITH THE AUTHORS

DEDICATION

This book is dedicated to anyone and everyone who suffered loss or took risks by speaking the truth during the COVID-19 pandemic.

DISCLAIMER

The information presented in this book is drawn from my experience and research. It provides insights into the relationship between healthy living, exercise, balance, and overall well-being. This book is not intended for self-diagnosis or treatment of any medical condition, nor does it serve as a substitute for the advice and care of a licensed healthcare provider. Discussing the information in this book with your attending physician is recommended. This book is designed to help you make informed decisions regarding your long-term health goals. If you are experiencing health issues, please consult a qualified physician immediately. Early examination and detection are crucial for the successful treatment of all diseases. The case studies presented in this book are a conglomeration of real patients whose experiences have been blended and anonymized for privacy. All names, identifying information, and specific details have been changed to protect the confidentiality of the individuals involved. While the stories are based on actual cases, they have been generalized and adapted for educational purposes. Any similarities to actual persons, living or dead, are purely coincidental.

Copyright © Dr. Danielle Smith Lockwood, ND, LAC, 2025

CONNECT WITH THE AUTHORS

Visit our website FireYourDr.com for additional content including downloads, podcasts, video interviews, articles, new book releases, speaking engagements and more. We'll also be adding PDF handouts and other supporting documents to the website. The website is also a great way to connect by sending us an email or signing up for updates.

Thanks for connecting with us.

D & R

Visit:

FireYourDr.com

Table Of Contents

CONNECT WITH THE AUTHORS IV

INTRODUCTION VI

CH 1. THE MEDICAL SYSTEM IS FRACTURED 1

CH 2. JUST SAY NO TO ACID BLOCKERS 10

CH 3. THE WAR ON GERMS 37

CH 4. STEROIDS: THE GOOD, BAD & UGLY 60

CH 5. MICROBIOME 101 84

CH 6. MICROBIOME 201 106

CH 7. MICROBIOME 301 126

CH 8. OVERFED, BUT HUNGRY 150

CH 9. YOUR THYROID: THE CANARY IN THE COAL MINE .. 165

CH 10. ADRENALS: REST, SEX AND HORMONES 183

CH 11. YOUR EMOTIONAL BODY 217

CH 12. LIVING IN A TOXIC WORLD 241

CH 13. YOUR GENETIC LANDSCAPE 270

CH 14. BODY FREEDOM: LIVING THE TERRAIN WAY 287

EPILOGUE 311

ACKNOWLEDGEMENTS 313

REFERENCE LIST 318

INTRODUCTION

Cognoscetis Veritatem et Veritas Liberabit Vos

(You will know the truth, and the truth shall set you free)

I'm (finally) publishing this book in the Spring of 2025, after multiple years of writing and rewriting. My husband has been instrumental in my (Dr. Danielle Lockwood) writing and rewriting this book. In editing, we felt that it was best to keep the perspective as first person from my (Dr. Danielle Lockwood's) perspective. Part of the challenge is that the nature of my medical practice has evolved since I began this project. By the time I've finished writing it, I'm sure several aspects of this book will already be somewhat outdated. I personally subscribe to the idea that every great doctor is a great student. I'm not referring to good grades. Rather, I highlight the importance of keeping an insatiable desire to continually learn and innovate. Even still, this book offers crucial insight into what's wrong with medical care and how we might fix it.

The above quote is over 2,000 years old, but in our age of social media, political correctness, and censorship, the message is even more relevant today than when these words were spoken. Over the last few years, doctors, professors, and nurses with decades of experience have been fired and disgraced because they questioned the current narrative. This multitude of professionals was only guilty of telling the truth in public. The truth offers freedom. But when lies have become the norm, the truth can be dangerous. At the height of the COVID-19 Pandemic, even something as unambiguously true as encouraging people to reduce their preventable risk factors was enough to get banned from Facebook®, Google®, and YouTube®. Healthcare workers have long known that losing weight and improving metabolic health helps in several aspects of disease prevention, treatment, and recovery. However, these simple facts became dangerous in the dystopia of post-2020 medicine. The message to doctors was clear:

---

*Do what you're told,
Say what we tell you,
Don't ask questions...
...or else.*

Do what they say or else you'll lose your friends, your job, and your financial security. Adding insult to injury, doctors with decades of respected experience were publicly ridiculed on national news outlets for stating clear facts. In a world where only doctors who follow the narrative remain employed, how can patients trust anything their doctor tells them? It wasn't only doctors who suffered, though. At one point, the situation had deteriorated to the point where people were essentially being told, 'Nothing says freedom like being asked to "show your papers" just to eat at a restaurant in New York City.' In some cases, even family members disowned each other, and marriages ended in bitter divorce. The COVID-19 response revealed something important. Thousands of otherwise brilliant doctors and nurses had their critical thinking completely hijacked; the decades-long 'standard of care' of 2019 was burned out of existence in 2020.

In the post-2020 landscape, even mentioning the previous standard of care was treated like an unforgivable sin by intuitional medicine and corporate news outlets. 2020 confirmed something I've felt for a long time: medicine has sold its soul—but it didn't do so alone. More accurately, our entire culture has gone astray. Belief in God and a moral code has been thrown out in favor of so-called science, reason, and logic. Sadly, it appears that our commitment to objective truth is left along with God and morality. When choosing between telling a dangerous truth or retreating into personal comfort, most doctors choose the personal comfort of saving their careers. If your doctor simply tows the approved party line, what good are they? The simplistic approved narrative is emblazoned all over social media, search engines, and mainstream news. Why pay for propaganda that is so useless that it's given away for free?

Truth be told, I could write an entire book detailing the corruption, lies, and the insidiously organized system that produced the Pandemic, and the response to it. But I'm afraid we don't have time for that now. A better use of our time is to save ourselves from this corrupt medical-industrial complex and then hopefully rescue others. This may sound bleak, but even still, hope springs eternal. Even in these tough circumstances, thousands of doctors, nurses, and others have risked their entire careers to bring hope to dark places. If you're feeling disillusioned with medicine—and the culture that led us here—a good starting point for recovery is to dig as deep as possible to uncover the most profound truths you can find. When you discover a useful truth, it's a clue to keep digging farther in that direction. Let's become more interested in asking why and how. The deeper we can set our foundation of truth, the more we can develop useful solutions that offer actual results.

Let's begin now.

Chapter 1
The Medical System is Fractured

(29+12+6+14+19+5+6+29) / 60 = 2.

Two hours.

The figure was a good enough estimate—it didn't seem necessary to tease out the tedious seconds of eye-rolls and exhales from the front office staff. In any case, it was the total time to see a specialist. My two hours in trade for the specialist's five minutes. Shifting lanes, my wandering thoughts were momentarily sliced by the staccato thump of tires slapping lane departure bumps. Now settled in the less-slow lane, my sardonic psyche resurfaces: "Two hours for five minutes." What sage wisdom did I get in those five minutes? Antacids and 'eat right.' Ten, the doctor spent ten years training to save lives, and the best he could do was prescribe antacids and tell me to generically 'eat right.' *Thanks?*

Twenty-nine minutes in traffic. Twelve minutes finding a spot and guessing the correct parking structure (choose wrong and you're late). Six minutes to find the right suite on the right floor in the right building. Fourteen minutes filling out paperwork and politely letting the staff know I got lost on the sprawling campus. "We get that a lot," came the front desk worker's reply, punctuating the statement with an eye roll and a sigh. *They get that a lot.* Getting lost in the hospital's labyrinthine maze was common.

If getting lost on campus is common, why don't they send new patients a campus map and instructions?

Nineteen minutes alone in an exam room. On the bottom, my buttocks crinkle crunchy paper. One hand holds an iPhone in the middle while the other repeatedly fails to close my open-back gown. On the top, my mind resists the urge to numb itself in phone scrolling as drafts tickle my spine through the impropriety of my gaping gown. All over, I'm chilled by the A/C that has won its war against the sunshine lurking just behind curtains and outside glass. *To be fair,* I quip to myself, *the new gowns are fashionably made of paper.* Still resisting the drafty air, I gingerly tuck the front of the gown deep between my thighs. I torture myself with dark thoughts of paper cuts in tender places. Now it's my turn to sigh and roll my eyes.

Grand finale time: five minutes. The doctor enters the door with a medical assistant and another person they introduce as a "scribe." The doctor fires off a few questions, says he reviewed the labs and that "they look okay." He suggests that my digestive issues are probably heartburn and prescribes an antacid. Forty-five minutes in a crunchy paper gown with no actual physical exam; *what was the gown for?* My takeaway is that I need antacids and to "eat right," whatever that means, I think to myself with wry amusement.

When I ask questions about what caused the acid reflux, he gives me a one-sentence answer of "poor diet" and suggests that I lose some weight. The assistant gives me a generic handout on why weight loss is good. The pamphlet's advice and drawings seem to be from the 1980s. Maybe the drawings are barely 1990s, but they're just after Vanilla Ice and right on time for MC Hammer. So, super old.

The appointment is over now. Then it's six minutes to put my clothes back on and make my way back to the "we get that a lot" lady and her too much makeup. "No," she says, "you don't owe anything today. We'll bill your insurance, and if there's anything left, you'll get notified in a few weeks." Making a polite retreat, I can't tell if she's being patronizing or if that's her normal voice. Retracing my steps, I walk past a hospital cafeteria selling all the foods the don't-be-fat-pamphlet said to avoid. Sadly, it's not even good-tasting junk food, it's hospital cafeteria junk food. Maybe they want people to lose weight by not eating it. *Dear Management, if you're going to serve unhealthy food, at least make it worth it by offering a decent burger.* Another eye-roll. Maybe the hospital needs to read its *don't-be-fat-pamphlet*. Finally, I lock myself away from the strange experience and into the perceived safety of my car.

Twenty-nine minutes on the drive home. I passed the time by diagnosing my frustration. I have a bad case of coming up with the perfect response too late to do any good. If they "get that a lot" how come nobody warned me? Nobody in that giant hospital could be bothered to spare the tiny shred of empathy needed to make a generic email with a campus map and instructions on parking, finding the right building, which elevator to take, and the layout of the dozens of offices once one found the right floor of the right building. They "get that a lot."

Three weeks later, after the inconvenience of the specialist visit was well in the rear-view mirror, I get a not-so-pleasant memento to remind me of my futile ordeal: $397 + $441 = $838. Of course, $397-copay for lab testing and an additional $441- owed as my portion for the specialist visit. The document attempts to console me by stating that the bill would have doubled if insurance hadn't covered a portion, so I should be thankful that I got off easy. To be clear, the prescription antacids help... for a few weeks. But before I finish paying off the $838 medical bill, I begin feeling bloated, gassy, and constipated all over again. Then, my heartburn comes back with a vengeance, and I suspect that I might even be worse off than before. Eight hundred thirty-eight dollars and nothing to show for it... *so much for investing in myself.* Vaguely borrowing a trite pop psychology analogy, I attempt to center myself as a beautiful feminine creature. Unfortunately for myself and my long-suffering husband, I'm now a beautiful and gassy feminine creature. Vapid platitudes and pop psychology failing, maybe it's time to ask Jesus for help.

Don't worry, I tell myself, *they take payments.* As I mentally calculate how to pay the bill, I also consider my insurance premiums. Pay health insurance, pay my primary care doctor, pay a specialist, and finally pay a pharmacist. Altogether, I pay thousands, and all I have to show for it is debt, antacids, and the bloaty gas is back! The so-called specialist just gave me generic advice I could have read online at home for free. On the bright side, I did get to try on a chic paper gown. At this moment, I fully accepted something I had known for a long time.

I'm not the customer; I'm the product.

How does the 3.8 trillion-dollar 4] healthcare industry fail to do any better than a blog article written by a medical student? Is it the doctor's fault? The search for answers led me in circles. Hospitals blame insurance. Insurance blames Big Pharma. Big Pharma blames government regulation. Doctors blame tuition costs and note that universities get manipulated by big-money interests throughout the industry. We all know the system's broken; why isn't it being fixed? Within the government, both political parties blame the other. With each cog in the machine shifting blame on the other, the medical monster collectively dodges all real accountability. Back in 2019, before the pandemic, Americans spent 3.8 trillion on healthcare. Each year the costs go up, while we all get less and less care for our money. The healthcare system is set up to relieve symptoms while failing to address the deeper issues that led to the problem.

We have a major bleed in American healthcare that cannot be fixed with a band-aid. The hospital system is set up for quick turnover to maximize profits and make up for skimpy reimbursements from insurance companies. These quick appointments lead to mistakes and distrust. Rushed doctors misdiagnose and under/over-prescribe. Doctors are unsatisfied and exhausted, while patients are frustrated and desperate. The winners in this scenario are insurance companies, pharmaceutical companies, and institutional hospital conglomerates. The losers are the American public and healthcare workers trapped in a broken system. According to an article published by Stanford Medicine in the spring of 2017, "the United States spends almost 20% of its gross domestic product on health care." 1]

My specialist gave me a short-term solution for my long-term digestive issue. Of course, I got a short-term solution; the doctor only had five minutes to solve it. What else could I expect under such circumstances? I could expect exactly what I got. The many independent parts that make up healthcare become a monster when you zoom out and look at the big picture. Each single patient faces the healthcare monster alone. On the other side, the monster of healthcare has the backing of thousands of employees and a billion-dollar budget.

Individual patients don't stand a chance with those odds. The hydra is a mythical water demon of ancient Greece with many snake heads. It wasn't good enough for Hercules to cut off one of the hydra's heads because another head would take its place. Similarly, just taking on one or two facets of monster healthcare won't defeat the beast. Insurance, big pharma, for-profit research, hospital conglomerates, Medicare, and Medicaid are just a few of this hypothetical hydra's heads.

In the myth, the hydra monster guarded the door to the underworld. Eerily, the hydra of modern medicine stands between life and death for millions of patients. Given the hydra's unfathomable power, how can we defeat the monster of modern medicine and build something better? Let's start by organizing the system's parts. What stands between the patient with the problem and the doctor with the answer? The medical industrial complex is an abominable system that comprises the for-profit medical industry "cooperating" (aka colluding) with the United States Government.

Pharmaceutical companies lobby lawmakers, and taxpayers get burned twice. The first way the public gets burned is that our tax dollars fund government organizations that favor industry. The second way we get burned is by exorbitant drug costs reinforced by government regulations. Pharmaceutical companies get their research subsidized by US taxpayers via grants delivered through the National Institute of Health (NIH). Do taxpayers realize drug cost savings for funding research? Nope; medication costs are higher than ever. Before the COVID-19 pandemic, the NIH had an annual budget of around 40 billion dollars given out through about 50,000 competitive grants. 2]

After COVID-19, Americans saw a jump in the NIH budget to just over 61 billion dollars; pandemics look great for expanding department budgets. We all became very familiar with a branch of the NIH called The National Institute of Allergies and Infectious Disease (NIAID). NIAID is headed by "America's Doctor," Dr. Anthony Fauci. Fauci has been the director of the NIAID since 1984 and has played a significant role in expanding the political and financial influence of the NIH within the medical-industrial complex. So, has Fauci's expansion of NIH power been good for the average person? No. Hospital stays, prescription drugs, health insurance, and disease prevention have gotten much more expensive and also less accessible for the average American. While some may still trust Fauci, both Progressives and Conservatives agree that healthcare costs are out of control. The longest a US President can legally serve is 8 years. In contrast, Fauci has been in charge for almost 40 years. Have things gotten better or worse in the four decades of Fauci's reign? With no term limits and little public attention paid to him for most of his tenure, Fauci became something of a medical dictator during his decades in power. Politically, the US population has a negative view of dictatorships; one leader and his party acolytes ruling for life is a recipe for corruption. Why, then, have we allowed ourselves to be ruled by a medical dictatorship where un-elected officials like Fauci can command NIAID for forty years?

The medical industrial complex includes:
- Insurance companies
- Hospitals
- Colleges & Universities
- Pharmaceutical companies
- Pharmaceutical representatives and Benefit Managers (PBMs)
- Doctors, nurses, and unions
- Nursing homes
- Drug manufacturers
- Real estate and construction businesses
- Health consulting and accounting
- Hospital supply companies
- Medical lobbyists and The American Medical Association (AMA)

The U.S. Government

In the 1970s, the medical industry shifted from smaller practices and grew rapidly into large, consolidated organizations and hospital-based systems. Mom and Pop medicine is out, and Walmart-like hospital empires are in. Over the years, community-based hospitals closed and were gobbled up by large hospital corporations. Nursing homes became more popular as Medicare and Medicaid offered more coverage for the aging population. On the insurance front, the formation of health maintenance organizations (HMOs) and preferred provider organizations (PPOs) led to providers being paid set pre-negotiated rates. Fewer people paid cash as insurance took over health finances. Public outcry led to voters demanding change in healthcare.

But it's illogical for the same lawmakers who opened the door to the hydra of modern medicine to close it. Each phony attempt by lawmakers to fix healthcare offered temporary aid while opening the American public to even more betrayal over time. Healthcare is a big business that uses the government to enforce its monopoly; isn't there a name for autocratic government collusion with big business? Indeed, it's called a Fascist State.

> *"Fascism should rightly be called corporatism, as it is the merger of corporate and government power." — Benito Mussolini 3]*

How did this impact my unfortunate doctor's visit? Simply put, insurance, hospitals, and patients are like two wolves and a sheep negotiating what's for dinner. Let's refocus on insurance. A few massive companies dominate the industry, creating a lack of competition. Now, guess who the real sheep is? Lack of competition created less consumer choice. With less choice and a captive market, costs rose rapidly. Further reducing competition, some healthcare plans were only available to certain companies, employees, and residents of specific states. The insurance market became narrower, more exclusive, expensive, and complicated. The same pattern emerged in hospitals; a few big names control most hospitals and large practices. Larger hospital systems also started their own insurance companies, giving patients preferred care within their facilities. On one hand, this made it so the hospital would no longer be at odds with insurers.

But on the other hand, it strengthened hospital monopolies. Through the mid-late 1990s, the merger of multiple HMOs created more profit and fewer choices in health decisions. Insurance options became narrower; patients had fewer choices. As this pattern emerged, doctor visits also got shorter, and insurance companies put more limits on the care they would pay for. The US Government styles itself as a "neutral regulator" of healthcare. Politicians campaign to fight for the working and middle class. Every new law is heralded as a revolutionary way to help people and improve lives. However, the trajectory of healthcare over time clearly shows that corporations have won, and the people have lost. People get less care while paying more money. Whether through incompetence or bad intentions, the government has favored the bottom line of large corporations over the US taxpayer. Politicians style themselves as heroes fighting the hydra of healthcare, but in reality, lawmakers are just another face of the monster.

The US Government's Role in the Medical Industrial Complex:
- Financing government insurance programs (Medicare and Medicaid)
- Politicians influenced by lobbyists
- Setting pricing for reimbursement based on Medicare coverage
- Making roadblocks to care via expensive licensing and regulation
- Serving insurance through uncapped malpractice premiums
- Failing to break up large hospital monopolies
- Giving taxpayer money to Big Pharma without saving patients money on prescriptions
- Backing Universities via student loans that drastically inflate tuition cost
- Funding for-profit drug research via NIH grants to universities and drug makers
- Funding dangerous "gain-of-function" research using taxpayer dollars

Basically, the US government uses our money to pay drug makers to research new drugs. Then, those same drug companies sell the drugs to the American people at a large profit. Big Pharma is charging taxpayers for drugs that taxpayers paid to develop. When Big Pharma profits from new drugs, they don't pay back the taxpayers who funded the research. Why does this happen? Well, because average citizens don't have a multi-billion-dollar industry to pressure lawmakers.

Spending More, Getting Less

Several entire books have been written about this monster that is modern medicine, and there are a ton of worthwhile topics that I'm skipping over here. There are price-gouging middle-men like Pharmacy Benefit Managers (PBMs), bloated government programs, co-insurances, deductibles, co-pays, cash prices versus insurance prices, teaching hospitals being influenced by big-pharma reps, and more, and more, and more. On top of that, medical school tuition is rising at an alarming rate. The average doctor accrues a debt of $202,453 5], making them slaves to the hospital system. The bottom line is this: America spends more than any other country on its healthcare while getting less actual medication and healthcare for our money.

TLDR: Too Long Didn't Read

I spent a ton of money on health insurance and a primary care doctor co-pay, and then saw a specialist who spent a few measly minutes with me and prescribed an antacid on his way out the door. Obviously, the antacid didn't work, so the book Fire Your Doctor was born. Governments and corporations hide corruption by making the system too complicated to understand. America spends the most on healthcare of any modern nation while also getting the worst medical care of any modern nation. Because the system won't help us, we must learn how to help ourselves. In the next chapter, we'll learn why antacids don't work and what to do about it.

Chapter 2
Just Say No to Acid Blockers

> ...*Fallen is Babylon the Great! She has become a dwelling for demons... The kings of the earth committed adultery with her, and the merchants of the earth grew rich from her excessive luxuries.*
> ...*Come out of her, my people, so that you will not share in her sins, so that you will not receive any of her plagues;'*
> Revelation 18:2-4 NIV 1]

In the last chapter, we stared into the abyss of American healthcare. Healthcare's many faces form a hypothetical hydra: insurance, hospitals, universities, pharmaceuticals, and government. The hydra, with its numerous heads, is a myth. In contrast, the monster that healthcare has become is tragically real. Sadly, the reality of broken healthcare is capable of more damage than any single monster. In the Greek myth, the hydra guarded the gates between life and death. Today, the hydra of healthcare stands guard between life and death via modern medicine. Normally, the healthcare hydra's true form is hidden under the dark waters of boring documents, complex laws, corrupt politicians, and media silence. However, during the COVID-19 pandemic, the people paying attention got a glimpse of the hydra's true power and dark intentions.

Despite the system's corruption, thousands of empathetic healthcare workers do God's work every day. But the greed and authoritarian tone of the healthcare monster are weeding out these compassionate souls one by one. Low morale, stagnant wages, and autocratic policies have made hospital staffing a nightmare. Patients I've spoken to report that today's healthcare staff appear more overworked, stressed, and less compassionate than before COVID. Mentally absorbing the disastrous scale of the healthcare hydra can be disheartening. It's tempting to blame the external world for the state of reality. At times, most of us feel like the problems within healthcare are outside of ourselves and too big to fight. But Soviet gulag survivor Aleksandr Solzhenitsyn knew better: *"The line separating good and evil passes... right through every human heart."* 2] The battle against a corrupt healthcare system begins and ends inside each of us.

Here's the hard truth about defeating the beast. The healthcare hydra feeds on sickness. The way to truly win the fight against Big Pharma, insurance companies, and hospital conglomerates is for each individual to be healthy. We must not be passively healthy; we must be actively healthy. Each of us must take individual ownership of our health. Fundamental decisions that each of us make can drastically reduce our reliance on medical care. Every preventable illness caused by our unhealthy lifestyles makes the healthcare monster stronger. Every small step toward being more naturally healthy undermines healthcare's monopoly on our lives. The quote at the beginning of this chapter predicts a world drunk on greed, luxury, pleasure, and corruption. The decadent dystopia depicted ultimately succumbs to plagues. However, the quote isn't completely hopeless; we're given clear instructions to leave Babylon to avoid sickness. So, how does one leave Babylon? Some see leaving Babylon as moving away, but Babylon feels like more than a place.

My instincts tell me that 'Babylon' is also a set of values, beliefs, and habits. Together, these values, beliefs, and habits form a lifestyle we must leave for our own good. Whether we're living in 'biblical end times' may be debatable, but the stark warnings about societies becoming sick from excessive luxury, hedonism, and corruption are clear to all.

Okay, we've moved out of Babylon, and that's the end of it. But have we come out of the values, habits, and lifestyles of our old ways? Do we still rely on Babylon's healthcare? During the recent pandemic, those dependent on the healthcare system suffered noticeably more than healthier people. Tragically, those with preventable health conditions like obesity, type II diabetes, and poor metabolic health were the more likely to pay the ultimate price. Babylon is more than just a place; it's a way of life we must leave behind.

Leaving Babylon physically may be uncomfortable, but at least the steps are clear: find a new job, sell your house or get a new apartment, pack your belongings, and go. However, the steps to leave Babylon's healthcare behind can be unclear. The system trains us that our bodies are wrong, and a medicine will fix it. However, another way to look at it is that our bodies have lost their ways, and we need to return to a fundamental truth to regain our health. With regard to our physical health, our society is lost. If you're lost, you need a map and compass. Yes, a smartphone GPS would be simpler, but one may also argue that phones pipe Babylon right into our pockets via social media, data harvesting, and distraction. But that's a talk for another day.

The more detailed our map and the more accurate our compass, the better we'll find out where we are and get where we want. This is physically true for lost hikers and metaphorically true for our health. The more honestly and completely we see our current health, the more empowered we are to move to solutions. The better we map out the terrain of our health, the faster and more precisely we can reach our destination. Here's an example; If we define our terrain generally by saying *I'm in pain,* our destination is a cookie-cutter solution: *take a pain-killer.* However, specifically defining the terrain with *I woke up with a stiff neck* is much more useful. Maybe you just need a better pillow, a different mattress, did a new workout, or need to try changing your sleep position? Or you could just keep your old pillow for 20 years and get a truckload of pain pills. Do we take mapping the terrain of our health seriously enough? Too often, a detailed understanding of our health seems too difficult, so we take the easy way out.

Drugs, alcohol, over-reliance on medications, and junk food are all ways that we hide from the true terrain of our bodies. Feel bad? Take a drug. Feel sad? Turn to anti-depressants, over-eating, and addictions. But these dangerous distractions are the opposite of what we really need to do. When confronted with these tough situations, leaning into feeling uncomfortable is how to learn more about our internal terrain. Learning about the terrain of our health can be painful because we're confronted with our lack of willpower and past failures. However, the only way to a better place is to fully accept where we are right now.

Detailed and precise maps increase our ability to get to a desired outcome. Conversely, terrain maps that lack necessary detail and precision can lead to us getting lost even worse than where we started. Because of this, creating more personalized healthcare maps for patients underpins the ethos of my clinic, *Terrain Wellness*. When we better define where we are, we ask better questions. Better questions lead to better answers. In the last chapter, I described my experience with heartburn before pursuing medicine as a career. Let's use this "simple" health condition to create a better map of the terrain.

1. Define the problem in detail.
2. Questioning: What lifestyle habits brought this about?
3. Solutions: Arrive at a solution based on a true understanding of the present condition.

For most people who experience heartburn, it's tempting to breeze through the definition and say:

Heartburn Solution 1:

1. *Define Problem: I have heartburn.*
2. *Questioning: (most people skip this step)*
3. *Solution: Take antacids.*

This is the process most people go through with heartburn. Let's do better. When you say 'I have heartburn', you don't really mean that. What you really mean to say is '*s*tomach acid is getting into my throat where it doesn't belong.' This distinction is crucial. General statements lead to cookie-cutter answers (i.e. take antacids). Being more specific about the condition leads to constructive questions: 'Why is stomach acid getting in my throat?'

Heartburn Solution 2:

1. *Define Problem: Heartburn is when stomach acid gets into my throat where it doesn't belong.*

2. *Questioning: Why is stomach acid getting into my throat?*

3. *Solution: Let's learn & find out!*

Symptoms are warning signs that a deeper problem exists. But since symptoms are painful, most people think that getting rid of symptoms is the same as being healed. **Heartburn Solution 1** is wrong because it only looks at symptom relief. Antacids reduce acid in your throat by reducing acid in your stomach. This is a bad idea because our stomachs need acid to work right. Reduced stomach acid leads to improper digestion of food. Ironically, the painful indigestion caused by low stomach acid leads many people to take even more antacids, creating a vicious circle of worsening GI complaints.

Let's examine **Heartburn Solution 2.** The biggest problem with solution two is that the answer requires mental effort and a doctor to do more than write a prescription. Tough questions can't always be answered immediately. Not knowing is uncomfortable. For me, going to an insurance-based doctor didn't teach me anything, either. Not having an easy answer stinks. But take my word for it—healthy stomach acid that stays where it belongs is worth the effort.

Let's work through **Heartburn Solution 2** in detail now. The word "acid" is culturally associated with hazardous industrial waste, chemical burns, and intense psychedelics. Painful conditions like acid reflux reinforce the idea that acid is bad. For a moment though, set aside acid's negative reputation and ask why we have stomach acid. The answer is that a highly acidic stomach provides several health benefits.

Stomach acid's health benefits are so closely tied to human survival that it's easy to take stomach acid for granted; without stomach acid, you'd die of malnutrition. Everyone knows that stomach acid is crucial to digesting food. However, there's a lot more to this corrosive liquid than *just* sustaining life by making digestion possible. Stomach acid also prevents bacteria, viruses, and other pathogens from invading our bodies. A highly acidic stomach kills off countless invading germs that would otherwise make us sick. Stomach acid is also necessary to absorb specific nutrients for proper hormone balance. Have a thyroid imbalance? Low stomach acid can starve the body of the vitamins and minerals needed for proper thyroid regulation. If stomach acid is vital, why are we working so hard to stop our body's natural processes? Perhaps we believe that our bodies have somehow gone rogue and decided to over-produce stomach acid to make us miserable. Bodies rarely go rogue without cause. Health imbalances generally have several contributing factors involved. Remember, not knowing the cause does not mean there isn't one.

Certain antacids called Proton Pump Inhibitors (PPIs) are in the top ten drugs prescribed in the USA. 3] Prilosec, Prevacid, and Nexium are all PPIs that you've probably heard of. PPIs being common makes sense because 25% of people get heartburn at least once a month. What's troubling about these facts is that PPIs are often prescribed by doctors who perform zero investigation into why heartburn is happening in the first place. Sadly, I fear that doctors who aren't investigating why heartburn happens are paying even less attention to the side effects of antacids. 4] While most doctors and the general public think of PPIs as relatively harmless, mounting evidence shows numerous unwanted side effects.

The harmful side effects of PPIs are well established in the research, even though nobody's talking about them. Side effects of PPIs include decreased absorption of key vitamins and minerals. These deficiencies can increase the risks of contracting multiple disorders, including dementia, malnutrition, cancer, and neurological conditions. Antacids reduce gut function, leading to an overgrowth of unwanted bacteria and yeast in the digestive tract. Prolonged use of antacids can lead to overcompensation with even more acid, creating a harmful condition called Hypergastrinemia. 4] Taking the easy way out is rarely a sustainable long-term solution. In trying to solve heartburn by reducing acid everywhere, the body predictably responds by making even more acid than before. Since becoming a physician, I've seen many patients become trapped in a cycle of increased dependence on antacids and perpetually decreasing health. The current use of PPIs focuses primarily on symptom management rather than addressing treatable factors that have contributed to gastroesophageal reflux, gastritis, peptic ulcers, and even irritable bowel disease. Acid reflux, ulcers, and gastritis are best understood as symptoms, not diseases. Treating GI symptoms with antacids while not considering the negative side effects of these medications just isn't working. Now that we've examined the problem in greater detail, here's how we, as doctors, can do better.

Correct the LOW Stomach Acid

When we explore life's problems, we're often confronted with ideas that initially seem paradoxical or even backward. But, if we want different results, we must be ready to challenge how we think. Learning that we were wrong about something is the first step toward being right! Okay, let's dig a little deeper into the physiology of acid reflux:

The Biomechanics of Acid Reflux:

- Stomach acid can be pushed up into your throat by excess pressure in the gut.
- Excess gut pressure can be caused by gas and bloating.

1. Gas and bloating are often caused by indigestion.
2. Which body fluid is central to the digestion of food?

→ **Stomach Acid!**

- Indigestion signals the body to release more stomach acid.

3. An acid ***Boom/Bust Cycle*** forms where you yo-yo between low acid and indigestion followed by bloating and heartburn.

- **Paradoxically, heartburn can often be solved by increasing stomach acid precisely when and where you need it.**

One recommendation we make in certain cases of acid reflux is temporarily supplementing with betaine HCL, a fancy name for stomach acid. Yes, you read that correctly—one way to reset the *stomach acid response* is to increase stomach acid. It's the exact opposite of what the conventional model suggests. Surprisingly, many people's acid reflux is related to indigestion stemming from low stomach acid in the pattern described above. The gassy indigestion caused by low stomach acid puts pressure on the stomach. This gassy pressure in the abdomen causes the lower flap of the esophagus to open, pushing small amounts of stomach acid up from the stomach, where acid is needed, up into the throat, where acid does not belong.

Taking antacids to address the complex digestive issues above can never resolve the issue and often makes it worse. Many factors contribute to low stomach acid. In turn, low stomach acid causes gas, bloating, and indigestion. Want a gassy volcano of stomach acid to erupt into your throat? Keep taking antacids. Antacids won't solve your problem. Okay, good talk. Even still, we haven't truly gotten to the bottom of acid reflux yet.

What Causes Stomach Acid Disorders?

- Over consumption of the standard American diet
- Taking antacids
- Stress
- Poor posture and tight clothing
- Intestinal infections
- Autoimmune diseases
- Drugs & excess alcohol
- Prescription medications
- Age or injury

Dear America, Your Diet is Killing You

Just Say No to Acid Blockers
Big Food, Big Tobacco & Big Pharma:
Make it cheap and get you hooked.

Far and away, the biggest culprit of imbalanced stomach acid is The Western Diet, also called the standard American diet (SAD). Whether we consciously admit it or not, we all know that SAD is not very healthy. Let's all take in the irony of the Standard American Diet's acronym being SAD. The SAD contains preservatives, refined carbohydrates, sugars, artificial dyes, and hydrogenated oils. Don't get me wrong— the free market is beautiful, but competition at the corporate level also has a dark side. Companies are motivated to make us crave their products while mass-producing them as cheaply as possible. Bring on the additives, preservatives, fillers, and flavor enhancers. Big Food, Big Tobacco, and Big Pharma all have the same goal: make it cheap and get you hooked.

Food additives extend shelf life and enhance flavor, with low cost and good taste being the primary goals. Some processed *"foods"* have strayed so far from their natural form that they are unrecognizable. A typical tactic of processed foods is to create a low-cost, long-lasting product that is addicting. These processed foods lack inherent nutrition, so companies fortify them with cheap synthetic vitamins, which they advertise as nutritional benefits. Can we make junk food healthy by sprinkling vitamins on top? No; it's still junk food.

Deep down, we all know that throwing synthetic vitamins into a batch of processed food is not "just as good" as eating truly nourishing foods like naturally raised meats and vegetables. Nonetheless, vitamin-fortified junk food is business as usual for Big Food. Processed food is never *just as good* as the real thing. Over time, these processed foods negatively affect our digestion. The metabolic burden of fake food slows us down, creating a feeling of bloated sluggishness. The SADdest part is that most people habitually eat so much processed food that they don't even recognize that what they eat is bad and makes them feel bad.

For most Americans, feeling bad becomes normal, and processed foods become habitual. The SAD is not *just as good*. The quote at the beginning of this chapter describes Babylon, a culture where kings and merchants created a tyranny of greed and pleasure-seeking that ended in catastrophic disease. If Big Food had to choose between profit and making people healthier, which would they choose? With a lifestyle maximizing convenience, cost-savings and comfort, compromised health is expected. Artificial ingredients and processed foods are more difficult for the body to break down, resulting in much slower digestion. When digestion slows, our stomach responds by reducing the production of acid in an attempt to give more time for the fake food to digest. Ready or not, eventually the partially digested food must be passed from the stomach to the small intestine.

This occurs even though the food was not properly broken down in the stomach. Making matters worse, the reduced stomach acid fails to kill off the bacteria that are accidentally eaten in small amounts every day. Low acid allows unwanted germs into the terrain of the small intestine. The invading microbes that would normally be killed off in a healthy stomach fester in the gut, leading to an overgrowth of bacteria and fungus. These harmful germs feed off processed, high-carbohydrate food in the intestines. These harmful germs produce waste gas in the gut, which puts bloating pressure on the stomach. The results of the SAD are painfully predictable: gas, bloating, gut infection, indigestion, and heartburn. Sprinkling vitamins to fortify junk food does nothing to address this cascade of negative effects.

Factually Honest, Functionally Misleading

Wait, you argue; my diet crunch snacks say they're healthy on the box. Well, cigarettes used to be marketed as healthy, too. Like Big Tobacco, food conglomerates use their billions to lobby government regulators. Surprise to no one; regulators favor food conglomerates at the expense of public health. Big Food tends to be factually honest but functionally misleading. While the small health benefits advertised on processed food labels may be technically accurate, they're far outweighed by the negatives—allowing manufacturers to exploit the public's lack of knowledge without outright lying. *Diet foods* are often factually low in fat and factually sugar-free. But there's a catch. These highly processed and artificial ingredients are generally more harmful than the non-diet versions they replace. We'll get into the corruption of Big Food and government elsewhere in the book, but it still bears mentioning a deep truth that we've known: there's no free lunch. We'll address nutrition in greater depth elsewhere in this book, but for now, I'll give you a simple, actionable step to improve your food choices. Avoid and reduce your consumption of processed foods whenever possible. What's a processed food? Processed food has been modified beyond its natural state such that you cannot look at it and discern all of its ingredients. Look at commercial dry dog/cat food sometime: can you see the chicken or rice? No, it looks like a weird brown kibble: a processed food. Let's take some examples of snacks you might get from a store.

Example 1: **Peanut-Free Mixed Nuts & an apple.** You can easily see what it's made of. Nuts, salt, and an organic apple (watch out for preservatives, flavor enhancers, and hydrogenated oils on mixed nuts).

Example 2: **Low-Fat Sugar-Free Whole-Grain Cruncher-Crackers.** When you look at things like crackers, chips, and granola bars, you cannot easily understand all the ingredients. Chips, crackers, and granola bars are highly processed, meaning the grains are ground down, vitamin-fortified, preservatives/ binders/stabilizers/sweeteners added, mixed/pressed, cooked, and packaged in plastic.

Let's count the processing steps in example 2. The Low-Fat Cruncher-Crackers have undergone numerous processing steps. My example shows six steps, but in reality, prepared snack foods often undergo dozens of processing steps to turn things like aspartic acid, phenylalanine, and methanol into NutraSweet®. Picture dry dog food in your mind. Now, picture actual chicken and actual rice. One is a processed food, which is not good for you. I know they say Low Fat and Whole Grains on the box, but Big Food is telling you a misleading half-truth. The fact that these foods come in enticing bags and boxes is a clue that Big Food is trying to manipulate you. If you're new to healthy eating, you may need an easy "Yes/No" rule to get started: Yes, to fewer processing steps, No to weird ingredients. An easier example may be orange juice versus actually just eating oranges. At first, the orange juice might seem like a healthy choice. Antioxidants like Vitamin C make fruit seem healthy at first. However, the process of juicing oranges makes the natural sugars enter the bloodstream much faster, creating a much stronger insulin response that has negative health consequences. Foods associated with a high insulin response require the body to take drastic action to maintain normal blood sugar levels. This drastic action can exacerbate insulin resistance, a precursor to diabetes. In this way, the single step of processing oranges into orange juice decreases the dietary fiber in oranges while also making it a much harsher sugar jolt to the system. If a single processing step makes this much difference in changing oranges into orange juice, how much more for soda and snacks that undergo dozens of chemical processes?

Enticing packaging and clever half-truths hide the whole picture: processed foods are a trap. These nutritionally-deficient foods reinforce a vicious cycle of gas, bloating, low stomach acid, and indigestion. Indigestion creates pressure in the belly that pushes what little stomach bile we have left up into our throats. The vicious cycle continues, and stomach acid production reduces further, worsening the unpleasant bloating. Worst of all, this painful symptom cluster leads people to the worst decision of all: antacids. But wait, there's more.

Once the body finally "clears" the poorly digested junk food, the stomach overcompensates by producing too much acid, too late. In this way, patients with heartburn go from too little acid to too much acid in a painful boom-bust cycle. Hello, cough, burning, and spasm. No, there's no silver bullet cure for heartburn. But, with knowledge and change comes healing. Heartburn is a cluster of painful conditions that must be completely dismantled. We must be willing to change our relationship with food completely.

This may require serious changes to our lifestyle and conveniences. Yes, this process can be uncomfortable. However, dismantling heartburn requires a patient ready to truly leave Babylon.

Acid Reflux: The Emotional and Spiritual Dimension

So far, we've learned that acid reflux is more complicated than most realize. But a visit with me wouldn't be complete without a look at your emotional and spiritual health. When we feel negative emotions, we easily turn to junk food. These foods are popular pick-me-ups because they give us a short burst of happy hormones. But there's no free lunch, so what's the catch? Negative emotions medicated by bad food can lead to downward spirals. Even aside from food choices, stress over time hurts digestion. We'll never conquer digestion without making peace with our negative emotions. Maybe negative emotions show up as anxiety, anger, fear, or sadness. No matter how it shows up, we need a way to experience these feelings in a fulfilling and productive way. Let's lump these negative emotions together and call them stress for brevity's sake. It's easy to chalk up stress to external factors like traffic, work, politics, and relationships. However, the common denominator in all these areas is you.

Our spiritual understanding is more than a search for meaning; spiritual health is an important factor in emotional resilience. Without spiritual health, the pleasure and pain of life can leave us empty, unfulfilled, and incapable of properly letting go of stress. Physiologically, stress is manifested as a sympathetic nervous system response. The sympathetic nervous system's fight-or-flight state is associated with immediate life-threatening situations. Since real emergencies require immediate action, fight-or-flight emphasizes short-term decision making and immediate survival and forgets about long-term stability. Properly digesting healthy foods is not part of defending against an attacking wolf pack. Digestion and thoughtful decisions go out the window in high-stress times. In life-and-death disasters, people can become so stressed that they vomit or lose control of their bladder and bowels. This is not an accident; it's the body completely abandoning food digestion and processing waste to focus completely on immediate survival. Your health ten years from now is unimportant when you're trying to survive ten minutes from now.

Unfortunately, modern stress cannot usually be solved by fighting or running. Fighting with your spouse or running from bills and work deadlines worsens everything. High stress causes poor digestion and shuts down long-term decision-making in the brain. This combination leaves a person vulnerable to bad food choices and a gut that can't cope. We really need to move from the sympathetic state to a parasympathetic state (rest and digest). The rest and digest physiological state does exactly what it says: your body repairs, your mind contemplates, and your gut properly digests foods. This "rest and digest" frees the mind to slowly and methodically consider the deep meaning and make stable long-term decisions. The body, free from fear, has the time needed to go through proper digestion to repair tissue and become stronger and healthier.

Even if you make generally healthy food choices, chronic stress is enough to shut down people's digestion and contribute to acid reflux. For the modern working professional, bosses and I'm busy become the norm; burgers and beers become the go-to meal. But it works both ways. Our stress levels influence our digestion, but the reverse is also true. If you've ever been "hangry" then you know that our eating habits also change our stress response. Eating quickly, skipping meals, and choosing easy foods all contribute to a dysfunctional stress response, which turns into a disrupted digestive system. Stress itself has other harmful side effects related to our gut health. One study showed that chronic stress leads to mucosal lining inflammation, making stomach ulcers and gut infections more probable. 5] We all know that we need to get our stress under control. You may say, "Dr. Dani, I've already downloaded a meditation app I never use. Is there anything else I can try?" I could write an entire book on managing stress, but for now, let's keep it simple: get outside, move your body, and get right with God. We can't fight our biology. Humans need time in nature combined with physical activity. Your dog needs a walk, and so do you. Spell dog backward, and things get problematic for many, and I get it. Humans need a higher purpose—ideals and values to strive for. And while much pain has been caused by those who use God to manipulate the good, that need for meaning remains.

A relationship with God provides a moral foundation to stabilize our psyches. As life's seasons change from the pride of victory to the shame of defeat, faith and religion have been a constant force for the entire history of humanity. Go dig up the bones of cultures lost to antiquity, and you'll find the religious artifacts of spiritually connected people. In recent years, we've abandoned faith and replaced it with cell phones, satellites, and central air. Despite these modern luxuries, our society is spiritually homeless. In this brave new world, the idea of God might seem like foolish superstition best left in yesteryear. However, I argue that even if your logical mind has moved past faith in God, thousands of years of our ancestry found spiritual understanding to be absolutely necessary.

The 20th century was humanity's first foray into a truly atheistic culture. Communism under Stalin and Fascism under Hitler were the first two tests of atheism; both failed horribly. The current obsession with so-called Social Justice is the latest attempt to fill the God-shaped hole in society. So far, Social Justice seems to be bringing division and judgment when we truly need healing and forgiveness.

Nietzsche famously said that God is dead. Seeing today's world, I think we need a resurrection. Many people have been hurt by religion. Some carry traumas with them from bad experiences they've had with religious people. Others are angry with God about the cruelty and chaos of the world. Maybe you feel abandoned and suspect that God may not even exist. Well, it's okay to feel that way. No matter where you're at, healing begins with hard conversations. Even if you're angry at God or don't even believe He exists, talk to God anyway. If you're angry, say so. If you doubt the Creator's existence, tell God that, too. For now, you just need to have open, honest communication with the Supreme Being. Aside from our food choices, our spiritual health and how it affects stress management is the next biggest factor in improving digestion. But we're not finished quite yet.

We are a Slumpy Bunch with Pants that are Too Tight

Office jobs, streaming services, and the rise of sedentary lifestyles have also brought dysfunctional posture. On top of nutritionally-deficient processed foods, our collective habit of a slouched posture also makes it more likely for acid reflux to develop. Weight gain, lack of physical movement, pregnancy, and sitting slumped over at a computer all day all contribute to acid reflux. Yes, something as simple as poor posture contorts the gut and puts pressure on the stomach.

The complete picture of this painful pattern is a person who becomes stressed, eats SAD food, and loses track of time slouched over electronic devices. Bad food and lack of movement add up over time, and our pants get too tight. As the belly's outward extension is stopped by clothing, our torso is squeezed like a giant toothpaste tube. The squeezing pressure caused by belly fat and our clothing contributes to acid reflux. The physical discomfort surrounding bad posture, poor diet, and weight gain feeds unpleasant emotions like anxiety, sadness, and even depression. These negative emotions contribute to more poor choices. This pattern can lead to a vicious circle of spiraling health punctuated by weight gain, metabolic issues, and (you guessed it) heartburn. But it doesn't stop there—excessive belly pressure leads to a problem in the stomach called a sliding hiatal hernia. This painful condition is where part of the stomach becomes pinched in the diaphragm. People who have a hiatal hernia will often have the sensation of a "lump in the throat."

They also have the sensation of being full easily, fatigue, non-cardiac chest pain, flatulence, a "tickling cough," regurgitation, a "spare tire bulge," constipation, and anxiety. Some hiatal hernias become so involved that surgical correction is warranted, but most are termed functional hiatal hernias and can be corrected with osteopathic manipulation, massage, and acupuncture. Hiatal hernia due to excess belly fat generally results in heartburn and belly/stomach pain. This belly pain causes a stress response, which halts digestion, further increasing stomach pressure. Regarding heartburn, the hiatal hernia pinching the stomach in the diaphragm releases acid up into the throat. 6]

At our Terrain Wellness office, we use a natural hiatal hernia release technique that involves having the patient lay face up on a flat surface. At the same time, a practitioner performs a specific abdominal massage technique that causes the diaphragm to release the pinched stomach. Our patients are also instructed on specific exercises that help to prevent the hiatal hernia from sliding back under the diaphragm. Most of our patients find relief within the first hiatal release appointment and experience deep pressure relief after 2 to 3 consecutive appointments. This hiatal hernia release technique is not always commonly known, even among functional medicine MDs and naturopathic doctors. I learned this technique from a professor specializing in functional gastroenterology, Dr. Steven Sandberg-Lewis. 7] He adapted the hiatal hernia manipulation technique from Dr. Ralph Failor, a chiropractic and naturopathic doctor who wrote the book *New Era Chiropractic,* which details hiatal hernia syndrome and the corrections my mentors and I have adapted. Although these techniques have been studied, they are not part of the mainstream protocol, so they have been overlooked as a solution to upper gastrointestinal dysfunction. Hiatal hernia release, along with supplements and lifestyle modification, are much safer and more effective long-term than the PPI drugs favored by mainstream medicine. Changes in posture, an exercise plan, and weight loss are also good ideas. With large ad budgets and endorsements from people like Larry the Cable Guy, most Americans seem to prefer popping antacid pills while continuing to eat the foods they love rather than making dietary changes and seeking out integrative gastroenterology.

However, antacids and junk food lead to bad outcomes over time. So, if you're sick of being sick, there's a better way. Slowly but surely, the medical establishment is starting to notice the long-term side effects of acid-blocking drugs. While still commonly prescribed, more doctors are beginning to notice the serious conditions that come from the continued use of antacids. These PPI drugs don't solve the real problem. In fact, in the long run, PPIs make your problems even worse.

Risk Factors for Hiatal Hernia Syndrome
• Chronic constipation • Poor posture • Pregnancy • Tight clothing and belts • Poor form during abdominal workouts • Obesity • Prolonged vomiting or coughing • Smoking • Age 50 & older • Overconsumption of mint and mint-flavored products

Normal is Not Healthy:
Bad Diet, Stress, Poor Posture, Infection and More!

<u>Helicobacter pylori</u> (H. *pylori*) is a type of bacteria that commonly causes infections that result in gastric disorders. This harmful infection suppresses the amount of gastric acid/HCL produced in the stomach. Low stomach acid leads to H. *pylori* infection, but H. *pylori* infection also causes low stomach acid. Since low stomach acid is both a cause and effect of H. *pylori* infection, it is difficult to pinpoint which came first.

H. *pylori* infection also causes stomach ulcers which people improperly treat with antacids. Ironically, going the other way and actually increasing stomach acid can help fight off H. *pylori* infection and solve the underlying problem. It's not just H. *pylori* though; low stomach acid can also cause a number of other infections as well.

When diagnosing digestive issues, it's important to consider underlying infections and imbalances elsewhere in the body, such as SIBO (Small Intestine Bacterial Overgrowth), parasites, or gallbladder and pancreatic insufficiencies—all of which must be addressed for effective treatment. Another key factor is autoimmune gastritis, a common cause of low stomach acid, particularly in individuals with diabetes or Hashimoto's thyroiditis. When autoimmune gastritis occurs alongside these conditions, it can lead to symptoms like anemia, hair loss, and various digestive complaints. Clearly, there is still much more to uncover when it comes to identifying and treating these complex health concerns.

In this harmful autoimmune process, the body begins attacking cells in the stomach called parietal cells. These parietal cells secrete a substance called *intrinsic factor*, which carries vitamin B12 into the small intestine, where the body absorbs it. Poor digestion combines with diabetes and/or thyroid problems to create harmful nutrient deficiencies. In this clinical presentation, we may also see other symptoms like brain fog and numbness in the fingers and hands. People with diabetes and autoimmune thyroid disorders are also at risk for slowed gastric emptying, leading to a decrease in stomach acid production.

Gastritis and low stomach acid are exacerbated by inadequate nutrition and unhealthy eating patterns. Chronic overeating, hydrogenated fats, sugar, and consuming salt in excess will add fuel to the flames of an already dysfunctional digestive process. Low stomach acid (hypochlorhydria) often goes undiagnosed because most people consider their digestion "normal." But in today's fast-food world, **normal is not healthy**. Symptoms of indigestion such as gas, belching, and fullness after small meals, are par for the course for many people. A clinical picture of a middle-aged person with bloating, burping, muscle cramps, soft nails, diffuse hair loss, bad breath, and a white/yellow coated tongue is a picture of someone with chronic low stomach acid. One point that bears repeating is that chronic low stomach acid inhibits the absorption of medications, supplements, and nutrients in food. This leads to many complications when people seek to balance their hormones and gut health.

One study showed improved thyroid hormone markers (TSH) and increased absorption of thyroid medications of up to 95% after eradicating an H. *pylori* infection and restoring normal stomach acid secretion. 8] The medical community really needs to stop treating conditions as if they occurred on their own. Although the above are common complaints in many primary care practices, these symptoms are often misdiagnosed and too many doctors just give patients antacids. When patients present to our office, they frequently have a variety of diagnoses that may be associated with low stomach acid in one form or another.

Diagnoses Associated with Low Stomach Acid
• GERD • Allergies • Chronic Anemia • Gastric cancer • Acne • Eczema • Thyroid dysfunction • Autoimmune conditions • Gallbladder stones • Diabetes • Osteoporosis • Depression • Chronic fatigue

Yes, that's a long and diverse list of health problems that can be caused or worsened by low stomach acid and poor digestion. For this reason, patients may sometimes hear me quip that *it all begins with the gut*.

Age is Only Half the Story

A quick search on Dr. Google® will tell you that "increased age" is a primary reason for a decline in stomach acid. This fact is partly true; but it's also misleading if taken without considering the whole picture. Although we do see a higher prevalence of low stomach acid in patients over age 40, it isn't just because they've been on the earth for several decades. According to a study of "healthy" Americans aged 18 to 94, age had no independent effect on acid output once they adjusted for factors like H. *pylori* infection. What was relevant in the study is that the aged population had a 40% reduction in the production of pepsin. Pepsin is a digestive enzyme that helps the stomach break down proteins. 9] As an aside, researchers also noted that gastric acid was lowered in those who smoked cigarettes. With smoking being more common in previous generations, it could be that smoking is also increasing the prevalence of low stomach acid and, by extension, heartburn.

Ready to leave Babylon? It's time for some tough but necessary truths. To truly regain our health, we must understand our internal landscape.

Over Your Entire Lifetime, Do You Almost Always...

- Avoid processed foods and artificial ingredients
- Drink plenty of clean water (non-chemically treated)
- Avoid pesticides on food and around the home
- Commit and follow through with a weekly exercise program
- Engage in active stress reduction
- Continually improve your spiritual health

Okay, honesty time. I have not done all of the above consistently. Most of my readers haven't either. Let's talk about where our poor decisions have led. By the time most people turn 45, they're on at least 2 to 3 medications. By age 50, many people are on 5 to 10 medications. I had one patient who was 68 and was taking 63 different pharmaceutical medications! This is nearly one medication for every year of his life. Given what we've learned in this chapter, is it surprising that digestive issues are very common? Heartburn doesn't show up randomly. Low stomach acid, undiagnosed gut infections, poor diet, use of acid blockers, reduced digestive function from processed foods, overuse of alcohol, previously prescribed antibiotics, and too many prescription medications can all cause or contribute to acid reflux.

Regardless of age, people frequently have several risk factors for low stomach acid. The underlying health conditions associated with acid reflux aren't just inconvenient; they contribute to potentially fatal conditions like heart disease and increased risk of stroke. Overuse of substances like alcohol, tobacco, and illicit drugs, as well as certain prescriptions, can also cause a cluster of digestive problems. The unpleasant acid reflux that accompanies these destructive personal habits leads many people to take antacids rather than address the deeper issues. Another hard truth is that we unfortunately want easy answers to our health problems. The truth is that most cases of heartburn can be resolved by making better lifestyle changes and food choices. Of course, many readers imagine they're the rare exception whose heartburn is a random fluke and not the result of lifestyle. For those wondering, some serious health conditions can also result in gastritis and heartburn: tumors, physical deformities, radiation exposure, cancer and cancer treatment, surgeries, diverticulitis, Crohn's disease, and ulcerative colitis. We take a thorough health history and complete comprehensive blood panels with all of our patients to check for these serious health conditions. When any of these underlying problems are identified, we are able to connect the dots and identify the culprit of the improper flow of stomach acid and digestive enzymes. Once we better understand a patient's health and biochemistry, we can guide patients toward meaningful recovery.

Case Study: Becky

Let me introduce you to a patient of mine; let's call her Becky. Becky is a 51-year-old mother of two boys, and she came in suffering from persistent abdominal pain. Her health history revealed high levels of stress and anxiety. Both of Becky's parents had deteriorating health conditions and lived far away. Her family had been stuck at home during the pandemic, and her business had slowed down considerably. In the past, she had done well eating a keto-style diet. However, stuck at home during the 2020 lockdown, she slipped back into her old habit of eating the standard American diet along with increased alcohol consumption.

She was putting on weight and "out of nowhere" experienced a sharp pain under her rib cage and the sensation of food getting "stuck" in her stomach. She felt like food was sitting in her stomach for hours without relief from the pressure. When the situation hit a boiling point, Becky went to urgent care and was referred to a gastroenterology specialist. The patient came to our office while she waited for the specialist because she wanted a second opinion. We completed a full physical exam and functional physical testing to narrow down the exact source of the problem. After a full hour of collecting information, listening to her heart and lungs, examining her abdomen, and conducting muscle testing neuro-reflexes related to digestion, our team had a pretty good idea of what was happening. Urgent Care had already referred Becky to a gastroenterologist for an endoscopy so they could visualize what was going on. Still, that appointment was a few weeks away, and she was in pain now. The patient's symptoms were consistent with several diagnoses: gastroesophageal reflux disease (GERD), peptic ulcer, irritable bowel syndrome, and dyspepsia. Further diagnostic work was needed to be sure, but while we waited for imaging, we took action to get her out of pain immediately. Naturopathic doctors trained in soft tissue and spinal manipulation often find that one of the factors in addressing disorders such as GERD, peptic ulcer disease, and irritable bowel disease is resolving hiatal hernia syndrome. This rings especially true in non-emergency cases of dyspepsia and reflux. I explained to Becky that it sounded like she had suffered a hiatal hernia. A painful condition where the top of her stomach had slid up through her diaphragm and had become trapped.

To address this unpleasant state, I performed an in-office hiatal hernia manipulation where very specific physical pressure on the patient's midsection pushes the stomach down out of the diaphragm (don't try it at home). Becky returned the next week, explaining that she felt 80% better and finally began to sleep more comfortably for the first time in over a month. GI imaging confirmed the presence of GERD, a peptic ulcer, and scar tissue near the vocal cords. Sadly, Becky's GI Specialist wanted to solve it by writing up a quadruple dose of a prescription-strength antacid and sending her on her way! Dear Doctors of America: throwing antacids at acid reflux is not a long-term solution. That's one reason we take a different approach at Terrain Wellness—and here's how we helped Becky heal. Instead of prescribing antacids, we ordered a comprehensive GI lab panel to rule out conditions like IBS and SIBO. We then adjusted her nutrition to support healthy gut flora and recommended eliminating alcohol and sugar from her diet

Becky came in weekly to support her stress response through acupuncture, herbs, and emotional release techniques. We also prescribed Betaine HCL and digestive enzymes to address the low stomach acid common in reflux—yes, she needed more acid, not less. The results were remarkable: within weeks, her bowel movements normalized, she began losing weight, her pain disappeared, and her energy returned. With her gut improving, we addressed additional factors like bacterial overgrowth and supported gut lining repair—essential steps for lasting results

We don't stop at symptom relief—our philosophy is focused on full recovery. This holistic approach includes supporting the immune system and restoring healthy neurotransmitter function, a process closely linked to gut health, as many neurotransmitters are produced in the digestive tract. While true healing takes longer than simply addressing surface-level issues, symptom relief often comes much sooner. After completing our 12-week gut repair protocol, Becky returned to her GI specialist for a follow-up. To their surprise, the hiatal hernia and ulcer were gone, and she no longer needed antacids. Her regular doctors were shocked to learn she had achieved this recovery without taking any of the prescribed medications.

Acid Blockers Are a Tool, But Not the Only Tool

The uncomfortable GI symptoms associated with heartburn often signal deeper imbalances in the body that need to be addressed and realigned. These symptoms may be linked to malnutrition, chronic stress, parasitic infections, bacterial overgrowth, or even structural misalignment. When these root issues are properly treated, acid reflux frequently resolves.

Now, I know some of you might be thinking, "But I have Barrett's Esophagus, and it runs in my family." While that may be true, Barrett's Esophagus can still be reversed. I've treated patients with this condition who were able to discontinue their acid reflux medications entirely. Upon re-evaluation, their GI specialists found no signs of ongoing damage. Prescribing acid blockers for more than two weeks is a short-term fix for a long-term issue. We have better, more sustainable tools for treating heartburn—it's time more doctors use them.

TLDR: Too Long Didn't Read

- We need a better map for treating heartburn
- Acid blockers are overprescribed
- Long-term antacid use is dangerous and contributes to severe nutrient absorption issues
- Low stomach acid causes indigestion that creates acid reflux
- Low stomach acid has severe health risks
- The standard American diet (SAD) is terrible for gut health. You need nourishing foods, not antacids.
- Poor posture and hiatal hernia syndrome are two contributors to GERD
- Solving underlying bacterial or parasitic infections in the gut can help resolve GERD
- Autoimmune conditions like thyroid diseases can contribute to GERD
- Age is not necessarily a risk factor for GERD in the true sense

- Find a doctor who knows which tools to use when and for which individuals (NOT antacids or acid-blocking drugs for everyone)

Chapter 3
The War On Germs

Now, when the unclean spirit comes out of a person, it passes through waterless places seeking rest and does not find it. Then it says, 'I will return to my house from which I came'; when it comes, it finds it unoccupied, swept, and put in order. Then it goes and brings seven other spirits more wicked than itself, and they come in and live there, and the last condition of that person becomes worse than the first. - Matthew 12:43-45 NASB 1]

Before we delve into this subject, let's lay out some context. Antibiotics are life-saving medications. I am grateful they exist; these medicines have saved millions of lives. But let's put them in their proper place. We must frame these crucial medications in the right context. Overuse of medicine leads to needless side effects and can make drugs less effective over time. With me so far?

Let's use an analogy to explain what I mean. Crash avoidance and modern airbags have averted many traffic accidents and fatalities. Do airbags and radar-assisted emergency-stopping measures make it okay to drink and drive? Never. Safety features don't make reckless and dangerous okay. Furthermore, no sane human would rely on crash avoidance and airbags to stop the car on their daily commute. Why is this? Crash avoidance and airbags are not perfect; they don't always work and come with consequences. Airbags save lives; they're also an explosive punch that hits you like a body slam. An airbag can save your life but may also break your nose. 2]

Antibiotics can save your life. They also have real health consequences. Airbags aren't soft pillows; they're an explosion in your face. Emergency stops will spill your coffee, interrupt your texting (relax, it's a joke), send your backpack/purse/laptop/groceries flying, and upset your passengers.

Car safety features hit you like an airbag—sudden and impossible to ignore. Antibiotic side effects, on the other hand, are more like a slow burn—subtle at first, but they can build up and have a lasting impact. Antibiotics are indeed miracles of modern medicine. Doctors and patients lean on these miracle drugs too much. Like antacids, we abuse the power and ignore the harm; nothing is free. We fool ourselves into believing that we can wish our problems away with a pill, a shot, or a cut-and-stitch. What's the catch? Find out now.

The quote at the beginning of the chapter describes a person where an evil spirit has been cast out of a person. Medically, an antibiotic does this to all the germs within us. In the quote, the person is described as a house that is left vacant and swept clean. Unfortunately, being left vacant and clean invites something worse to take over. Similarly, antibiotics leave the gut swept clean and vacant, a perfectly open host where all bad germs can quickly and easily take over without any opposition.

"Eating yogurt won't atone for a gut microbiome genocide."
-Dr. Danielle Lockwood

At this point, many people will be aware that antibiotics kill off healthy gut flora. The tired, eye-rolling response from the people who think they know is usually, "I already know antibiotics affect gut health! But it's fine because I take probiotics." If only it were so simple! Eating yogurt won't atone for a gut microbiome genocide. Not all probiotics are the same. It's extremely arrogant to assume you can replace decades of gut microflora development with a few pills and some yogurt from Whole Foods. So, what's the real cost of over-prescribed antibiotics? In some cases, the true cost may be chronic disease, metabolic disorders, and an increased lifetime risk of cancer.

Penicillin: The Miraculous Cure

Anne Sheafe Miller was among the first to receive the new experimental penicillin antibiotic in 1942. She was hospitalized in New Haven, Connecticut, dying of streptococcal pneumonia. There was nothing the doctors could do to save her life using established medicine of the time. Miller's doctors made one last attempt using an experimental treatment called penicillin. Just one injection of this miraculous drug saved her life. Miller's incredible case study ushered in a new era of healing where antibiotics took center stage. Miller's penicillin miracle was one small injection for (wo)man, one giant leap for humanity.

News of the miraculous incident spread like wildfire in professional circles and pop culture. Within a short time, industrial-scale manufacturing of antibiotics took flight. Penicillin production quickly rose from 64 pounds in 1942 to around 156,000 pounds per year of penicillin and a new antibiotic derived from soil fungus called streptomycin. By 1999, the year that Anne Sheafe Miller passed away at age 90, the number of antibiotics produced in the United States was around 60 million pounds per year. Even if you don't personally take antibiotics, keep in mind that 30 million pounds of antibiotics are being used by the livestock and agriculture industry. Like it or not, we've all been exposed to these drugs with or without our consent through environmental and food/water exposure.

From Miracle to Mess

Where do antibiotics go after you take them? What about all the farm animals on antibiotics? These drugs don't just go away; they're released into the environment through urine and feces and thrown away in landfills. Countless whole pills are also flushed down toilets as a means of disposal. In hospitals, millions of pounds of antibiotics are excreted by patients or thrown away as expired yearly. The Pharmaceutical industry wastes millions of pounds annually on expired or damaged antibiotic products. In homes, people throw away untold doses of unused antibiotics and other pharmaceutical drugs. Also, every time a patient on antibiotics uses the bathroom, they're sending active medication directly into the sewage systems and wreaking havoc in our environment. From there, residual antibiotics accumulate in rivers, groundwater, and soil. But the above is not even half the story regarding antibiotics.

The livestock and agriculture industries are the biggest culprits of antibiotic overuse. Factory farms make up over half of all antibiotic use in the US. Like humans, these millions of farm animals excrete antibiotics into the environment whenever they relieve themselves. Farm animal manure is used as a natural fertilizer, meaning residue from drugged animals is used to nourish fruits and vegetables. But that's not all. Industrial farms house thousands of animals so close that they're touching each other and sharing the same air throughout their lives. These cramped living quarters, combined with the copious use of antibiotics, create superbugs that have evolved to resist antibiotics. Factory farms are the main arena for developing superbugs such as methicillin-resistant staphylococcus aureus or MRSA. 3] Later in the book, we'll examine living in a toxic world in greater detail. For now, though, remember that millions of tons of industrially produced antibiotics are being flushed down the toilet and directly excreted by farm animals into the environment, which is a serious problem with global consequences. Even if you've never taken antibiotics or consumed antibiotic-treated animal products, you're still impacted by super-germs—drug-resistant pathogens altered by generations of antibiotic use. These germs are harder for the body to fight and more dangerous. Nearly everyone is affected by the widespread misuse of antibiotics.

Supporters of routine antibiotics often cite clinical studies, but the results depend on what's being measured. For example, a study might show that a drug helped lab mice fight an infection, but that doesn't guarantee it will be effective in broader contexts. After the study, we euthanize the mice, so we never know what long-term effects the drug may have had on them. Then, we try the drug on humans and mass-produce it, often with commercials promoting it on CNN. In these studies, we typically find what we're looking for, but we often overlook the long-term impact of giving millions of doses to people, the potential effects on the population, and the environment. Other studies highlight how antibiotics can increase the risk of various diseases and disorders, revealing that antibiotics are not as selective as we'd like to believe.

Humans are not just one living thing. We're a living petri dish housing untold helpful and harmful microbes living together. Even if a microbe is "bad," eliminating it can have some unintended effects. The microbes in our bodies tend to balance each other out naturally. Tampering with this delicate balance can kill off bacteria that may not be "good" per se and lead to something even worse. Every second of every day, bacteria and fungus fight each other to take over your body. Ideally, these warring microbes will cancel each other out and leave us alone. But, when we tip the scales with antibiotics, we create an open ecological niche where fungal (yeast) infections can run rampant.

Yes, I know that most people hear of yeast infection, they think of women's health and skin rashes. However, drug-resistant fungal infections are a growing concern (bacteria aren't the only super-germs created by human activity). These fungal infections are often misdiagnosed in hospitals and can be exacerbated by antibiotics, primary infections, and other medical treatments. 4]

Making things even more complicated, what about times when the individual effects of a drug might be helpful while the combined societal and environmental effects are negative? A drug may help you recover from illness faster, but using that drug today can contribute to the creation of tomorrow's superbug. Antibiotics are becoming less effective over time as germs adapt in response to how we fight them. By many measures, the germs are winning. Bacteria are gaining antibiotic resistance much faster than new antibiotics are being made. DISCLAIMER: I'm no friend of the World Health Organization (WHO). Nonetheless, a 2020 report from the WHO found the following to be true.

> *"Declining private investment and lack of innovation in developing new antibiotics undermine efforts to combat drug-resistant infections."* 5]

This statement implies that less money is spent on developing antibiotics than other drugs.

Companies have a low incentive to invest in new antibiotics. The report goes on to say that:

> *"Two new reports reveal a weak pipeline for antibiotic agents. The 60 products in development (50 antibiotics and 10 biologics) bring little benefit over existing treatments, and very few target the most critical resistant bacteria (Gram-negative bacteria). While pre-clinical candidates (those in early-stage testing) are more innovative, it will take years to reach patients."* 5]

In plain English, the above means that it looks like the germs are winning. Superbugs are emerging faster than we're making new antibiotics; logically, making new antibiotics will create even more superbugs. We're in deep trouble.

Key Points:

1. The antibiotics we've used in the past have built up as toxins in the environment.

2. Today's drugs are becoming less effective against drug-resistant strains.

3. New antibiotics are NOT being innovated fast enough to keep up with the germs.

We've strayed a long way from the original intent of antibiotics. In their advent, these drugs were only intended for people who had become so ill that their bodies were too weak to overcome an infection. In life-and-death circumstances, antibiotics truly were the best chance for a person's survival. Today, antibiotics are used freely, not only within medicine to treat non-serious diseases like acne but also in the US agriculture system to treat a vast array of meat and dairy products. Additionally, antibacterial agents have become ubiquitous in hand soaps, toothpaste, and other household products. A 2016 study on the use of "low-level" antibiotics in agriculture reported,

> *"It is estimated that 50% to 80% of all antibiotics used are applied in agriculture and the remainder for treating human infections. Since dosing regimens are less controlled in agriculture than in human health care,*

veterinary and environmental microbes are often exposed to sublethal levels of antibiotics." 6]

Most of our antibiotic-resistant germs might be from food and environmental exposure. Numerous studies have corroborated this disturbing finding. Another 2016 study published in Infectious Disease Clinics of North America noted,

"The rapid and ongoing spread of antibiotic resistance seriously threatens global public health. The indiscriminate use of antibiotics in agriculture, human medicine, and increasingly connected societies has fueled the distribution of antibiotic-resistant bacteria. These factors together have led to rising numbers of infections caused by multidrug-resistant and pan-resistant bacteria, with increases in morbidity and mortality." 7]

Patients often come into our office and say, "Well, I haven't taken antibiotics in years, so I am most likely not affected by this." I answer them by stating, "Antibiotics are everywhere."

Antibacterial Soap Makes Germs Stronger

Hospitals, industrial farms, and antimicrobial personal and home-use products all create drug-resistant germs. We're heading for a major infection crisis. Our obsession with killing germs is training the germs to be stronger and more dangerous. Society is delivering a self-inflicted one-two knockout punch. The first blow is delivered by processed foods, sedentary lifestyles, and poor stress management, harming our immune systems. The second punch is that we've unwittingly created a germ boot camp to train tomorrow's pathogens into elite drug-resistant monsters. It may seem trite, but everything from your lunch to your daily hygiene products like soap and deodorants exposes germs to trace amounts of antibiotics, thus training tomorrow's super-germs.

"...there is a direct relationship between the use of antimicrobials and the development of resistance. In addition, one type of antimicrobial could be selected for cross-resistance to another type and/or multidrug resistance." 8]

In 2007, researchers found that antibacterial soaps and household products are responsible for creating bacterial superbugs. Even worse, researchers found that these antibacterial soaps didn't keep people from getting sick. What antibacterial soap used in the home does is create super-bugs while providing no benefit of reduced infection. 8] Over recorded history, the idea that we must wage an extinction-level war on germs is a completely new concept. Are we so prideful to think we know everything better and that our new ideas won't come with consequences we didn't anticipate? Antibacterial soaps are not helpful in a household setting. The widespread use of these products is making the problem worse. This isn't just my opinion. This isn't something controversial. It's just common sense. Millions of households are training germs to resist soap, which won't rid the world of germs; it can only make better germs. But don't take my word for it,

"Soaps containing triclosan within the range of concentrations commonly used in the community setting (0.1%-0.45% wt/vol) were no more effective than plain soap at preventing infectious illness symptoms and reducing bacterial levels on the hands. Several laboratory studies demonstrated evidence of triclosan-adapted cross-resistance to antibiotics among different species of bacteria." 9]

Triclosan is a common mild antibiotic found in hundreds of personal care products, plastics, and even some fabrics. Yes, you might even be wearing triclosan on your skin. There's more to the story regarding antibacterial soap than just creating superbugs. A Swedish study compared 36 nursing mothers in Sweden using triclosan household products to mothers without known exposure to the compound. The results of the study were disturbing. Breast milk from both mothers in the study had measurable levels of triclosan in both the antibacterial soap group and the group with none. Not surprisingly, mothers using triclosan hand soap had higher concentrations overall. The blood plasma levels of the drug were even higher than the breast milk, demonstrating that the moms themselves were getting an even higher level of exposure than they were giving their babies through nursing. 10] Even people firmly on the pro-antibacterial soap side would not want their healthy baby drinking triclosan-laced breast milk. Is it wise to allow ourselves to swim in antibacterial compounds from cradle to grave?

The easiest solution to antibacterial soap is to switch back to normal, regular soap. Good old-fashioned soap and water do the trick without creating super-germs. Multiple clinical trials have found that handwashing with proper technique using normal soap and water works just as well as washing with antibacterial products. A 2005 study separated people in a remote village into three groups. One group of residents was given regular soap and asked to wash their hands and bathe with the soap daily. The second group was given an antibacterial soap and instructed to do the same. The third group was not directed to do anything and presumably didn't use soap. This study found that both soaps improved health outcomes, and they were not different.

> *"Handwashing with soap prevents the two clinical syndromes that cause the largest number of childhood deaths globally. Namely, diarrhea and acute lower respiratory infections. Handwashing with daily bathing also prevents impetigo."* 11]

This means that soap works, but antibacterial soap has no benefit. Given this information, why risk creating multidrug-resistant germs? If we overuse antibacterial chemicals, we risk having antibiotics not work when we really need them.

Good practices of prescribing antibiotics, limiting the use of antibiotics in our food, and limiting antibacterial additives in household and personal care products are all simple steps most people can agree on.

Two Steps Forward, Three Steps Back

In 2016, triclosan was banned by the FDA after a nearly four-decade battle to have it removed. But, when the Pandemic started, regulators bowed to pressure from manufacturers and brought it back. From 1978 to 2016, industry watchdogs and whistle-blowers fought this harmful ingredient and finally achieved their goal after 38 years. But it only took 4 years for industry lobbyists to bring it back. To be clear, the FDA's former limit on triclosan still allowed it to be used in institutional settings like commercial food preparation and hospitals, just not in consumer products for household use.

Unfortunately, triclosan is just one of many low-dose antibacterial products added to soaps, fabrics, and plastics. The story doesn't end with triclosan. Compounds such as benzalkonium chloride, benzethonium chloride, and chloroxylenol are now used alongside triclosan, although they were intended as replacements. The real question is, why are we exposing millions of people to artificial chemicals that harm us? These compounds are ineffective at the individual level; at the societal level, antibacterials strengthen germs. It's a double-fail on a global scale. As the Covid pandemic powerfully illustrated, super-germs are one of humanity's deepest fears. I've built a strong case that compounds like triclosan contribute to stronger germs over time.

The industrial-scale stupidity surrounding antibacterial household products is not a secret either. An FDA official was quoted as follows,

> *"No data demonstrates that these drugs provide additional protection from diseases and infections. Using these products might give people a false sense of security," Michele says. "If you use these products because you think they protect you more than soap and water, that's incorrect. If you use them because of how they feel, many other products have similar formulations but won't expose your family to unnecessary chemicals. And some manufacturers have begun to revise these products to remove these ingredients."* 12]

Like it or not, we're primal creatures led largely by unconscious desires and fears. Maybe it's marketing; people want to feel like they're doing something. Whatever it is, Big Tech and manufacturing conglomerates tap into people's desires and fears. Human logic is abandoned when huge companies collude with governments to market products that play on people's fears. We can't see germs, so they've become this invisible ghost that could be lurking anywhere and everywhere. Antibacterial products have become an idol for some, a magic talisman to ward off the specter of killer germs that could be lurking in every home.

Even more strange is that the FDA acknowledges that science doesn't fully understand how triclosan may affect people over time. They're quoted stating that "more research is needed" to determine how triclosan affects us. More research is needed. Really? So, we have put chemical soap beside every sink in America for several decades, and our scientists still don't really understand what the side effects might be. A quick online search on "triclosan and human health" reveals over 700 published articles at the time of writing, none of which hold a positive view of triclosan. At best, it's useless. At worst, it's training super-germs and harming us individually in ways we don't yet know.

It Gets Worse

Certain antibiotics might increase the risk of numerous types of cancer. Multiple studies link antibiotics to the development of cancer. Adding insult to injury, you'll never guess what type of cancer some experts find associated with these drugs. Not just any cancer; it may be rectal cancer. In general, researchers find the link to cancer especially relevant when these drugs are used in multiple rounds or for long periods. A 2019 systematic review of multiple studies found that

"There is moderate evidence that excessive or prolonged use of antibiotics during a person's life is associated with a slightly increased risk of various cancers. The message is potentially important for public health policies because minimizing improper antibiotic use within an antibiotic stewardship program could also reduce cancer incidence." 13]

Prolonged exposure to antibiotics increases cancer risk over a lifetime. Let's recall that antibiotics are in our food and environment, and antibacterial agents are added to several household products. Whether prescribed or not, we end up taking them, whether we want to or not. This fact raises serious concerns about informed consent. I may have asked for a chicken sandwich, but didn't ask them to add antibiotics. Given the pros and cons of these drugs, you'd think that we'd reserve them for serious cases of life-threatening infections. But actually, it's quite the opposite: we use antibiotics everywhere.

Using antibiotics sparingly isn't the only purview of the natural and functional medicine community; plenty of conventional medical doctors agree. We must stop overusing and abusing antibiotics. During a 2018 symposium for gastroenterology held in Rome, Italy, it was noted,

"Besides the known beneficial effect of antibiotics in treating infectious diseases, these drugs have shown detrimental effects on gut microbiota which, in turn, might have long-term consequences on the host." 14]

It turns out that many cancers, especially colorectal cancers, are more likely to occur in digestive systems where the person has been exposed to antibiotics. Why is this? Taking antibiotics kills off normal gut flora. Pathogenic "bad" bacteria and fungi can take over when the normal gut flora is killed off. Research has identified one such bad bacteria known as Fusobacterium. This type of bacteria has been linked to a higher incidence of colorectal cancer. Here's the proverbial smoking gun; Fusobacterium was found in tumors removed from patients with colorectal cancer. 15] I have much more to say about the gut microbiome and how it is crucial in helping your body fight cancer later in the book.

For now, please understand that there's no free lunch in medicine. Everything good comes with costs and side effects. The harm to gut health goes beyond just cancer. Healthy gut bacteria, which are essential for proper digestion, play a significant role in how we process food. Disruptions in digestion can impact nutrient absorption, metabolic health, and even contribute to unwanted weight gain. It's no surprise then, that antibiotics have been linked to other disorders, including diabetes. A 2015 study stated,

"Our results could support the possibility that antibiotic exposure increases type 2 diabetes risk. However, the findings may also represent an increased demand for antibiotics from the increased risk of infections in patients with yet-undiagnosed diabetes" 16]

This statement points toward an interesting dilemma. It seems that antibiotics may put people at risk for developing type 2 diabetes. This makes sense, given that poor gut health affects metabolic health. However, the researchers also noticed that a person who already has diabetes is more likely to get infected and need an antibiotic.

I propose that what we see here is a vicious circle:
- Antibiotics cause poor gut health
- Improper food choices reinforce poor gut health
- Poor gut health results in poor digestion
- Poor digestion causes/worsens diabetes
- Diabetes leads to more infections
- More infections lead to more antibiotics
- The cycle repeats

Diabetes is About More Than Blood Sugar

Diabetes affects more than just blood sugar; it also weakens the immune system. It's common knowledge that people with diabetes are more susceptible to infections. Weakened immune systems in people with diabetes are such a huge issue that it's not uncommon for simple things like toenail infections to escalate dangerously. Simple cuts and skin tears can become serious healthcare situations that may even require amputation in extreme cases. Studies show that people with diabetes are at one of the highest risk levels for poor outcomes of COVID-19. Health issues like obesity and diabetes are not an issue of vanity. These health conditions contribute to premature deaths. Often, these premature deaths are slow and involve a lot of suffering. The ongoing saga of antibiotics and diabetes clearly shows the need for drastic individual and societal change. The vicious cycle of poor food choices, abuse of antibiotics, rising diabetes, and lowering immune systems was on full display during the COVID-19 pandemic. A retrospective multicenter study with over 7,000 cases showed the following:

"*…subjects with T2D (type 2 diabetes) required more medical interventions and had significantly higher mortality (7.8% versus 2.7%; adjusted hazard ratio [HR], 1.49) and multiple organ injury than the non-diabetic individuals. Further, we found that well-controlled BG [blood glucose] (glycemic variability within 3.9 to 10.0 mmol/L) was associated with markedly lower mortality compared to individuals with poorly controlled BG (upper limit of glycemic variability exceeding 10.0 mmol/L) (adjusted HR, 0.14) during hospitalization.*" 17]

Put in simple terms, type 2 diabetes tripled the chances that someone would die with COVID-19. The use of antibiotics, especially early in life, has been shown to set a person up for both obesity and diabetes later in life. This is especially disturbing, as kids are treated frequently with antibiotics for simple ear and throat infections. Is it wise to expose kids to numerous rounds of antibiotics before they hit their teenage years? You might still be asking yourself, can gut bacteria imbalance *really* make you fat and lead to diabetes? Yes, it can. And I've brought the receipts to prove it.

> "...the intestinal microbiota can influence host metabolism. When given early in life, agents that disrupt microbiota composition and consequently its metabolic activity can influence body mass of the host by either promoting weight gain or stunting growth, which is consistent with effects of the microbiota on development." 18]

This same research later determined that the use of antibiotics at an early age killed off healthy gut bacteria and led to the development of serious metabolic conditions later in life. 19] Both the research and I recognize that antibiotics save lives. But our current overuse of antibiotics is killing people. The destruction of the healthy microbiome increases the risk of obesity, cancer, and diabetes. Isn't this enough to push us toward alternative options when treating non-life-threatening childhood illnesses?

What You Don't Know Can Hurt You

Disruption of healthy gut bacteria has several downstream negative effects on immune function. Ironically, antibiotics both help and harm your immune system; this fact is not widely understood in conventional medicine. Here's a simple way to think about it. You take an antibiotic that kills off both good and bad bacteria in your body. Gut microbial die-off leaves a desolate environment open to invasion by whatever can get there first. Bad fungi and bacteria inevitably take over the gut, and our digestion, nutrient absorption, and metabolic health suffer. Logically, the overload of bad gut microbes must put at least some additional strain on our immune systems. This additional burden on the immune system lowers our ability to fight other infections. But that's not all; the body being forced to wage an unnatural germ war inside the gut could be a major factor in developing autoimmune conditions.

A 2017 research program studied mice infected with E. *Coli* bacteria. The mice were treated with antibiotics while immune system markers were tracked. The researchers found that the mice treated with antibiotics also experienced negative effects on their immune systems. The ability of white blood cells to envelope and destroy pathogens was particularly harmed by antibiotics. In addition, the research noted severe damage to cell mitochondria; these are the body's microscopic "powerhouses" that turn glycogen into actual energy. 20] Reduced mitochondrial function results in cells that cannot efficiently perform work like physical movement, internal repair, brain function, and waste removal. Mitochondrial dysfunction is now linked to many illnesses, including epilepsy, heart disease, stroke, diabetes, chronic fatigue syndrome, and various muscle disorders. Science is in the early stages of understanding how antibiotics damage mitochondria. Researchers know even less about all the illnesses connected to mitochondrial dysfunction. The potential that antibiotics may harm mitochondria is made doubly alarming by how little we know and how late we find it out. Antibiotics have been used for almost 100 years, and we're only now realizing the real costs. Our clinic doesn't have the luxury of waiting until the science is settled before treating patients. There are long-term complications to antibiotics, and our patient base's symptoms match the ailments that the research predicts. For this reason, our strategy usually centers on bolstering mitochondrial health when we have patients with chronic fatigue and other long-standing illnesses.

Published data is catching up to our clinical practice, as this chapter describes in detail. While we're here, though, it's worth mentioning that clinical practice is supposed to come before research. Doctors treating real patients out in the community are supposed to innovate and then report their direct experiences and outcomes with patients. Then, researchers are supposed to create studies to test and flesh out the reported clinical findings. Unfortunately, the COVID-19 pandemic saw a reversal of this relationship, where public health officials commanded doctors to be obedient and stifled doctors' clinical practices. When reports from doctors showed problems with the government response, those doctors were sanctioned, fired, and banned from social media. Public health policy should not stifle dissenting doctors, especially when those doctors are reporting their direct clinical experience. Quite the opposite; clinical practice must inform public policy if we want healthcare that can adapt and grow. Clinical experience aside, new studies support a growing body of evidence that antibiotics may damage or destroy our cells' mitochondria and genetic material. In 2017, the research highlighted how antibiotics increased the chances of DNA damage within cells, which puts the patient at risk for numerous negative health outcomes. 21]

Together, the research supports three conclusions about antibiotic use:

- These medications harm the gut microbiome
- Cells within the body may be damaged
- Cell damage increases the risk of negative health outcomes

Case Study: Lilly

Lilly is a 32-year-old female with a lifetime history of digestive problems, eczema, and ADD (attention deficit disorder). She's had decades of what she calls "bad belly." These uncomfortable symptoms started when she was a baby and have been an unwelcome companion for her entire life. Her mother reported that she had ongoing colic as an infant and would scream for hours from frequent excessive gas and belly pain. At one point, her pediatrician had recommended her mom place her on an antacid to help with the suspected heartburn. Of course, we've already learned about antacids, yikes! But, no matter what they tried, nothing worked, even though they followed the pediatrician's suggestions closely. As part of the detailed patient interview that we do with all new patients, we found that Lilly was born via a scheduled C-section and formula-fed from birth. At the time, her mom was told that formula was "better" for babies than breast milk, so she obediently followed the science of the time.

By age 2, Lilly had already had multiple rounds of antibiotics due to chronic throat and ear infections that would persist no matter what her mom tried. By age three, she had "tubes" placed in her ears, which helped for a few years, but then had to be replaced a few years later at age 5. She also began using prescribed steroid creams at age 2 for small patchy skin rashes that her pediatrician diagnosed as eczema. The rash would go away for a few months but return worse than before (we'll learn about steroids in the next chapter).

By the time Lilly was in her teens, the rashes were around her eyes and face, and the steroids didn't help much at all. At 16, she was diagnosed with ADD and placed on a stimulant drug that seemed to help her concentrate better but left her feeling exhausted and shaky all of the time. She began to lose weight, had no appetite, and complained that food just "didn't feel good in her stomach." By the time Lilly came to visit us at Terrain Wellness as an adult, she'd seen multiple specialists who dismissed her digestive complaints of constant gas, bloating, abdominal pain, and mixed constipation and diarrhea as irritable bowel syndrome.

The specialists offered her both laxatives and anti-diarrhea medicine to take as needed for her symptoms. At this point, her eczema was being "controlled" by a TNF-blocking injection every 1-2 months. She had dark, almost purple circles under her eyes and was severely underweight. Her health had declined to the point that she was frequently missing months of her menstrual cycle. She'd been taking birth control pills since she was 16 to help with the iron deficiency and cramping when she did have periods. But by the time she came to our clinic, she had completely ceased bleeding during menstrual cycles. Lilly was anxious, depressed, and feeling like this was her last hope to feel better again. Our care team began by running basic blood labs to check her cholesterol, blood, liver, and kidney function. We added tests for anemia and a full thyroid panel, which included thyroid antibodies. We had her take a salivary adrenal stress test and a comprehensive digestive health panel.

Side note: better labs lead to better outcomes; your lab tests aren't good enough.

Once our enhanced test panels returned, we identified that she had a digestive condition called Small Intestinal Bacterial Overgrowth (SIBO) and was highly stressed. She had a low-functioning thyroid, but thankfully, we caught it soon enough that there were no signs of an autoimmune thyroid process. However, she was severely anemic and was having major problems absorbing her b vitamins. We had her take a gluten and celiac allergy blood test, which returned positive for sensitivities to wheat and gluten, the protein found in wheat-containing products. When we treat patients, we don't just hand out supplements and prescriptions; we build a comprehensive care plan that lays out the steps needed for the patient's desired outcome. We call this care plan a roadmap.

Follow the map to get to the goal. Our initial roadmap focused on killing off parasites that lead to imbalanced gut flora and the overgrowth of unwanted gut bacteria that lead to SIBO. Once we cleared out the unwanted parasites, we added herbs and specific probiotics to support a healthier re-population of the digestive landscape. We also removed allergen foods, especially wheat, corn, and dairy, so that we could measure the patient's response. Then, we developed a customized nutrition plan along with practical and convenient meals, as well as recipes she'd like. Concurrently, we prescribed a series of custom IV nutrition replacement formulas to give her iron, B vitamins, vitamin C, and trace minerals that she severely lacked. IV nutrition was important because it bypassed her damaged digestive system, which was not properly absorbing vitamins, and gave her the much-needed co-factors her body could use to repair the damage.

But there's more to the story. I'm sure anyone reading Lilly's story can imagine what it must have been like to be a teen girl growing up with facial rashes, excessive gas, and recurrent bouts of diarrhea and constipation. This lifetime of ongoing illness was also an ocean of emotional pain. Our roadmap addressed this via Neuro-Emotional Technique (NET) to help her process the trauma surrounding her health. Her trauma was entangled in a deep sadness. The emotional pain accompanied her illness and contributed to her persistent physical stomach pain. Being in a constant state of stress was somatically linked to her stomach.

Lilly reported feeling constant thoughts of inadequacy; she confided that she lacked a sense of grounding. Using a combination of spinal manipulation, 5-element acupuncture, and homeopathy, we reset her nervous system responses to stress one layer at a time. After a few weeks of treatment, we got our first win. Lilly began to have regular bowel movements every day without straining. Her sleep became more consistent, and she woke up less at night to use the bathroom. She also became more self-aware, recognizing how and when her body was not feeling well. For example, Lilly realized that she was using her physical symptoms like headaches as excuses in her relationships. Realizing this, she began to place healthy personal boundaries. One of the things we encouraged her to start doing was to cultivate healthy boundaries before her body forced her to do so. In time, she recognized that her emotional pattern of using physical symptoms as excuses instead of setting proper boundaries was an unhealthy coping strategy.

But, once she saw how she didn't need a headache to say "no," she began to gain confidence in her relationships and made huge progress in her physical health. Her physical health could not fully heal without addressing her emotional health. After completing a few rounds of herbs to kill off unwanted parasites related to SIBO, we restored proper gut microbes by repopulating her gut with very specific probiotics. These new probiotics were selected to prevent additional gas in her digestive tract. Once we repaired her digestive health, her eczema began to improve. Although her complexion was the last to show improvement, her mood lifted much sooner. The severe mood swings around her periods subsided, and regular menstruation resumed.

Around this time, she began to see her energy levels to gradually increase. Lilly told us that she could "finally concentrate better." Her anemia stabilized, she no longer had frequent headaches, and the bloating and "bad belly" became a thing of the past. As a bonus, she developed much healthier relationship boundaries with the people in her life. Finally empowered to say "no" without the excuses of her poor health, she felt confident enough to try dating again. Lilly also began to wean herself off the stimulant ADD medication. Finally, after about a year, felt safe enough to discontinue the steroid injections for her skin. To her surprise, there was no flare in her skin rashes. Once she was able to lower her stimulant medication for ADD, she was able to sleep much better, and her appetite returned.

What's the way out?

Lilly's story emphasizes the importance of building a strong foundation of health before making any changes to medications. Many patients discover that quitting prescription medications cold turkey doesn't work, as their symptoms often persist. This leads to frustration and discouragement, causing them to give up on making further changes and return to their medications, ultimately ending up where they started.

For Lilly, her lifetime dependence on medications to manage basic bodily functions had disrupted her body's natural hormonal processes. As we've discussed, many commonly prescribed medications also contribute to significant nutrient deficiencies. Nutrients like vitamins, minerals, balanced fats, proteins, and carbohydrates are essential for the body's proper function. Without these foundational nutrients, healing becomes impossible. Discontinuing prescriptions isn't as simple as it may seem.

For this reason, many people who come to our office have tried to navigate their health using "Dr. Internet Search" with mixed results. If you're already healthy and have a few simple questions, you could do your research. But, for people with complex cases and multiple health conditions at the same time, it's not so simple. For these complex cases, patients find that working with our team and following our customized *roadmap to health* is the most efficient path to optimal wellness. In our practice, we like to go deeper and get to the heart of the matter. Or should I say, we like to get to the guts of the matter (I couldn't help it; docs love body-related puns)? Repairing the digestive system is the most significant factor in reversing autoimmune diseases. Studies have supported using probiotics in preventing allergy-related diseases, especially eczema. A 2015 systematic review of studies using probiotics to prevent atopic/allergic disorders found that.

> *"Growing evidence underlines the pivotal role of infant gut colonization in developing the immune system. Modifying gut colonization through probiotic supplementation in childhood might prevent atopic diseases."* 22]

In this review, the research showed that giving pregnant mothers and their infants a multi-strain probiotic significantly reduced the baby's risk of skin issues like eczema. Antibiotic use damages the human microbiome, causing an overgrowth of pathogenic bacteria, leading to various disorders.

The skin is a major detoxification organ in the body. The skin eliminates wastes and even bacteria through the sweat glands. Emerging evidence supports what naturopathic physicians have known for years:

to clear the skin, you must clear the burden from organs in charge of waste elimination. This means that the digestive system and all of the supportive players, such as the liver, lymph tissue, lungs, and kidneys, need to be in working order to effectively eliminate waste so that the elimination does not happen through the skin. Comprehensive research on the gut microbiome published in 2019 supports this connection.

> *"Until recently, diet and psychological stress were thought to have little relevance to the pathophysiology of acne. However, with the understanding that the brain-gut–skin axis exists, it is clear that intestinal microbes significantly affect acne."* 23]

Diet, gut health, and mental and spiritual well-being all play a big role. And, of course, avoiding antibiotics when they're not needed is key. Another great tool for restoring gut health is botanical medicine.

Herbs are a fantastic way to eliminate unwanted bacteria, parasites, and yeast while creating an environment for desirable microbes to live and thrive. Certain herbs and herbal combinations are an effective way to clean up the gut and the skin to make ailments like acne a thing of the past. Herbs like berberis (Oregon grape) used in an alcohol tincture or as water-based topicals are fantastic at soothing inflamed skin. Ear infections are one of the most common reasons for childhood antibiotic prescriptions. Instead, why not utilize the potent antibacterial properties of medicinal herbs like garlic? At Terrain Wellness, we often prescribe a simple recipe that is effective against some common bacteria responsible for ear infections. These common germs include Haemophilus influenzae and Staphylococcus pneumoniae, as well as others, all frequently respond to treatment with garlic-containing compounds. This herbal solution is called Garlic Ear Oil. It combines Garlic, olive oil, and either mullein tincture or eucalyptus essential oil.

You can download this simple recipe as a PDF at FireYourDr.com. You can also find the blend online or at most health food stores. Either way, it's easy to make and use at home. Just a few drops of this powerful herbal antimicrobial, given several times a day, can clear up most ear infections, relieve pain, and help patients feel better fast. What makes these herbal remedies especially valuable is that they don't typically damage the digestive system the way antibiotics can. When the gut is harmed, the immune system suffers too. Herbal treatments support the body while also tackling the infection—what could be better than that?

Closing

Antibiotics like penicillin are rightly respected as wonder drugs that have saved millions of lives over the last century. Nonetheless, miracles must be respected. Those of us who believe in miracles know that repeatedly asking God for miracles while we stubbornly continue in bad behavior is risky. But even for the non-religious, the analogy holds. It's common knowledge that the overuse of antibiotics and widespread home use of antimicrobial products are creating super-germs. Remember, we're not making new antibiotics fast enough to keep up with the biological arms race. But, even if we had plenty of new highly effective antibiotics coming on the market, would we want to use them?

Antibiotics kill off our healthy gut microbiome and leave behind a dangerously vacant "windswept house" left open for parasites, nasty germs, and fungus to run amuck. In closing, I believe in antibiotics and support their responsible use in serious healthcare situations. Respecting the power of antibiotics means that we must reserve our most potent weapons for when these medications are truly necessary. Unless we use them sparingly, they won't work when needed.

TLDR: Too Long Didn't Read

Antibiotics burst onto the scene at the beginning of the last century and have saved countless lives. Once the lifesaving power of antibiotics became widely known, antibiotics were put in everything and given to everyone at least once in their lifetime. Over the years, modern medicine has come to rely on antibiotics too much. This pattern is training germs to become much more dangerous. Even worse, antibiotic products have become ubiquitous in the home and our food supply. Given this pattern, germs will outpace new antibiotic production and development, which might leave us worse off than before. This over-reliance on antibiotics has killed off many people's healthy gut microbiome, resulting in numerous negative health consequences. Most people never connect these long-term problems to antibiotics because the harmful side effects may not show up until years later.

Chapter 4
Steroids: The Good, Bad & Ugly

"Thus, it is, that we pay dearly for chasing after what is cheap." - Aleksandr Solzhenitsyn (The Gulag Archipelago 1918-1956)

For this chapter, let's first disambiguate between corticosteroids and anabolic steroids. Anabolic steroids generally refer to hormones that increase testosterone and are commonly (ab)used by bodybuilders and professional athletes. Falling under the umbrella of Performance Enhancing Drugs (PEDs), anabolic steroids increase muscle mass and bone density, but come with significant health risks too. Abuse of anabolic steroids has given this class of drugs a generally negative public image, even though commonly prescribed corticosteroids have vastly different effects on the body. The source of much public fear of steroids may be a bit misguided. Even still, trepidation is still warranted, but for different reasons.

In pop culture, people almost universally mean PEDs when they talk about steroids, even though not all PEDs are technically steroids. Environmental toxins, diet, and lifestyle all contribute to depressed testosterone levels, so there are legitimate situations for TRT (testosterone replacement therapy). However, at the moment, we're talking about the other steroids. Where anabolic steroids affect testosterone, corticosteroids artificially mimic cortisol. Cortisol is a hormone made by the adrenal gland with powerful anti-inflammatory properties. For this chapter, I'm referring to corticosteroids when I say steroids. Inflammation is closely associated with severe injury, stress, exposure to toxins, and trauma. In emergency rooms across the world, inflammatory responses are known to be dangerous and potentially fatal conditions. For life-threatening inflammation reactions, steroids are, in fact, a miracle drug. Even for nonlethal inflammation, the judicious use of steroid medications can be helpful. But as with anything else, the ubiquitous use of complex chemical compounds comes at a cost that we may not realize. Steroid medications include asthma medications, arthritis drugs, and some treatments for allergic reactions.

If you're having an asthma attack, allergic reaction or you're in the emergency room, corticosteroids can save your life. Even as an outpatient, there may be narrow and temporary circumstances where a corticosteroid is the best option for the patient. Classifying drugs as good or bad is complicated. Even life-saving medicines can and do have real side effects worth considering. Short-term good must be weighed against long-term risk. In life, things that seem beneficial in the current moment can have negative outcomes in the future. Let's use debt as an example. A credit card can bail us out in a financial emergency, but debt is also a trap. There's profound wisdom in the quote at the beginning of the chapter; chasing convenient quick fixes can cost us dearly in the long run.

To be clear, steroids are powerful life-saving tools. It's also true that the medical establishment and the public tend to downplay the side effects of treatments. This is not to say that steroids are good or bad. In fact, during the pandemic, I found myself prescribing more steroids than I ever thought I'd ever need to. Like debt, bad choices (even other people's bad choices) may force us to make more bad choices.

Irony

Here I am writing a chapter on why steroids are over-prescribed, but the hard truth is that I've also prescribed more steroid medications over the past few years than I ever thought possible. But don't worry, I'll land this plane and it'll make sense.

I don't need a cure, I just need to buy time

During the height of the delta wave of the COVID-19 Pandemic, many patients experienced flu-like symptoms for about a week, then felt better for a few days. But "feeling better" was often just the calm before the storm. Some at-risk patients who thought they had recovered from COVID would then crash into serious respiratory and inflammatory symptoms. These symptoms would cause noticeable decreases in blood oxygen saturation (SpO2). Below 90-95% SpO2, a physician will prescribe supplemental pure oxygen. If the patient doesn't rise above 95% SpO2 using supplemental oxygen, then the patient is hospitalized. Alarmingly, hospitals were sending COVID patients with 80% SpO2 home without supplemental oxygen. Just giving these low-SpO2 patients home oxygen concentrators would have saved many lives. In response to this gross incompetence (or malice) by the hospitals, my clinic stockpiled oxygen concentrators to meet the demand.

People who turned on the news got beaten over the head with the mantra that there's no "cure" for COVID. Even though this is technically true, it's misleading. We can't "cure" many diseases, but we can still effectively treat them. COVID is no different. All I needed to do was keep patients alive long enough to beat the disease. No, I can't cure COVID. Deaths of COVID were caused by things like inflammation, blood clots, and lack of oxygen. Even if we doctors can't cure the virus, we can certainly treat systemic inflammation, prescribe supplemental oxygen, reduce blood clot risk, and treat the acute asthma-like symptoms that many patients present with. There's still no perfect cure for COVID, but there are effective treatments.

Sit down, Fauci; I'm not talking about Pfizer and Moderna.

The main threats in late-stage delta-variant COVID are lack of oxygen, blood clots and inflammation. When systemic and life-threatening inflammation reactions become a lethal cytokine storm, we treat the cytokine storm. As a physician, I took active measures to monitor SpO2 levels and prescribe medications to minimize inflammatory reactions. Cytokine storm is a potentially lethal condition where the immune system overreacts to a pathogen. 1] When the body destroys a COVID-19-infected cell, the viral debris of that destroyed cell is still physically inside the body. These viral remnant particles (spike proteins) of the destroyed COVID-19 virus became dangerous toxins floating in the patient's bloodstream and tissues. In my clinical experience, viral remnant particles common to late-stage COVID were strongly associated with blood clots, reduced SpO2, and inflammation reactions. The body knew that these viral remnants were dangerous. However, eliminating viral debris is a harmful inflammatory process.

This created a dangerous Catch-22 where the body removing a dangerous toxin resulted in increased inflammation.

Patients' blood was compromised as they were starved for oxygen. In most but not all circumstances, when a person is hypoxic (lacking oxygen), there is a deep sense of panic. One of the many things about COVID that was diabolically unique was that patients would have dangerously low oxygen levels without even knowing it. In patients experiencing severe "late-stage COVID," I realized that I wasn't fighting a virus so much as a runaway allergic and clotting reaction to viral remnants, likely including the famous "spike protein." Given long enough, the body would eventually fight off the virus. People just needed to buy time so their body could handle the late-stage inflammation.

The problem with COVID was that people were succumbing to complications faster than their bodies could recover. All of the life-threatening COVID cases I treated involved flare-ups of uncontrolled inflammatory processes in the body. I didn't need to cure COVID; I just needed to buy time. Given more time, my patients safely weathered the storm of late-stage inflammation, blood clots, and SpO2. During the height of the "Delta wave" of the pandemic, things like asthma, low SpO2, blood clots, allergic inflammation, and cytokine reactions spread like glowing embers thrown on dry grass. For patients with severe cases, the latter stages of COVID-19 infection became a battlefield. Why did this happen? My clinical experience clearly showed that COVID-19 is a multi-stage illness.

Stages of COVID-19 2]

1. **Viral replication:** In this stage, people felt normal but were already deeply compromised. Patients became walking biohazards that exponentially multiplied the virus in secret. Rapid viral replication in asymptomatic patients escalated public fears early in the pandemic.

2. **Symptomatic Infection:** Patients presented with symptoms, but many still didn't test positive for COVID-19. Some patients had severe flu-like symptoms, while others experienced less severe Cold

symptoms. Luck was involved, but older and less healthy patients were more likely to suffer during this stage.

3. **Intermission:** After about a week of symptomatic infection, patients began to feel better. On day 7, patients would call in and say they wanted to discontinue medications and "go for a jog." For many younger and generally healthy patients, this intermission was the end of it. But...

4. **Inflammation:** After a few days of feeling better, certain patients would fall into severe late-stage COVID-19. Life-threatening inflammation, autoimmune symptoms, allergies, blood clots, and lack of oxygen typified this late stage. Particularly in older, obese, and diabetic patients, these symptoms had the possibility of coming on with a vengeance.

While the above disease progression was frequently described, the mainstream pandemic response ignored these treatable but life-threatening symptoms until it was too late. The hospitals gave late inflammation phase COVID patients a drug called Remdesivir.

Let's take a minute and learn about this medication. Remdesivir's only possible benefits are that it reduces stage 1 viral replication and that it's extremely expensive, which helps Big Pharma's stock value. 3] This means that the only possible time that Remdesivir might have helped would have been at the first sign of infection. Fighting viral replication during the late inflammation stage was a waste of time, and any doctor who had thought about it carefully should have seen it. The hospitals were treating stage 1 COVID when patients were in stage 4.

Remdesivir destroys kidneys

So why didn't the hospital give everyone Remdesivir right at the start? Doctors couldn't prescribe Remdesivir in stage 1 viral replication because the drug is fundamentally dangerous. Remdesivir causes lifelong damage to the kidneys. Doctors should have been using time-tested and affordable anti-inflammatory steroid medications, providing cheap and easy supplemental oxygen and monitoring for blood clots. The above is basic, easy stuff that should be a core hospital care competency. Instead, doctors in hospitals were using a horrifically expensive drug whose most notable effect was destroying kidneys. 4] In plain English, getting prescribed Remdesivir in the hospital was close to a death sentence.

Yes, I'm aware that I'm irony personified: I'm a naturopathic primary care doctor arguing in favor of steroids. Thank God it's impossible to suffocate on irony because I'd have long passed away. To be clear, I never once cured COVID. However, in an acute infection, you don't need a final cure; you need to buy time and get the patient through the disaster alive. Before COVID-19, every hospital in the country knew how to treat blood clots, runaway inflammation, and crashing SpO2. I got excellent results in my clinical practice using affordable treatments like oxygen concentrators and steroid medications. Other simple precautions like monitoring patients for Pulmonary Embolism and Deep Vein Thrombosis were fundamental in helping the dozens of patients I successfully treated.

Let's do an exercise together.
Say the following out loud with me:
"In the COVID pandemic, most doctors ignored basics like steroids & oxygen."
Now, look at the cover of this book; what does it say? It says to "Fire Your Doctor."
Act accordingly

Okay, good talk. The fact that so many doctors remained silent about all of the above is more than enough to not only fire your doctor but also to tear down the entire Medical Industrial Complex and its corrupt government propaganda agency that we know as the FDA. We got a letter from the State Licensing Board threatening that any doctor who didn't toe the party line would have their license revoked, so we had to work silently. Political activists in the community (who weren't even patients) filed malpractice complaints against us for telling the truth about the disease. On a societal scale, the media and public health officials made treating the virus a political, moral virtue signal. Under this intense pressure, most doctors chickened out and let patients die even though everyone should have known better.

People became emotionally invested in the official narrative and reacted with disgust and hostility to those questioning the government talking points. In this fraught environment, telling the hard truth to the wrong patient could have shut our clinic down. With gravely ill patients and scared loved ones calling in almost daily, the clinic getting shut down would have cost many lives. To be clear, there is nothing abnormal, unethical, or illegal about a doctor prescribing medications off-label. But, during the COVID panic, the law didn't matter. Treating COVID caused "vaccine hesitancy," and causing vaccine hesitancy would get you shut down. What developed was a system where we'd have to determine whether the patient (or their family) would turn us in to the authorities if we told them the truth. If we trusted the wrong person, we'd get shut down, be unable to help future patients, and suffer absolute financial ruin. But wait, there's more. Don't forget about the social media mob and mainstream news permanently destroying your career. I lost a best friend and had family members rudely denounce me. During former President Biden's completely unnecessary winter of sickness and death (5), the only thing that got me out of bed in the morning was my faith in God and the somewhat dark humor of my husband, Richard.

It's hard to answer when people ask what my husband does because he does everything. One of his many duties was helping the clinic with COVID-19 patient interviews because we couldn't trust our staff at the time to not to turn us in. The stress of deathly ill patients and the threat of legal action against me led me to tears on multiple occasions. Dawn ended one of the countless nights of bad sleep and early mornings. "What if I lose my license?" I exclaimed between sobs. I hung onto my blankets while my emotions let loose. Richard, my husband, sat up in bed with a somewhat sour expression that I knew by then not to take personally. He took a deep sip of black coffee that had long since gone cold on the nightstand. Then, he held me in a close embrace and dryly remarked, "Ride or die." Side note: one of my guilty pleasures is 90s and early 2000s hip-hop music. We both laughed through what felt like the weight of the entire world bearing down on us.

Laugh.
Cry.
Check the secure messaging app on my phone.

The ICU nurse we hired was fired from the hospital for her dissent gave us her morning report. The steroids I'd prescribed were working, and the deathly ill patient that the hospital had turned away was beginning to improve. I went back to the clinic for my day job. Patients or their loved ones would frantically call the clinic, and the story was always the same. They had COVID, they were scared. Could I help them? At this point, state medical boards, federal officials, and social media were forcefully pushing the message:

There's nothing you can do. Go home, do nothing, and self-isolate.
Call 911 when your life's in danger.
Then, close your eyes one last time while
your family watches you die alone over a video call.

The newscaster solemnly announces the latest COVID death, and we're all supposed to be comforted that the vaccine is safe and effective. So went the approved messaging. Say anything different, and you'd get hypothetically nuked from space by the entire force of the establishment. Various authorities corporations still censor true information about COVID-19, so doctors had to make do. Doctors who shared their actual clinical experience of treating COVID were censored, fired, and ostracized. Early on, a doctor in New York City spoke up about the COVID response. He said that ventilators were killing patients. He was fired. His social media accounts were blocked. His videos were taken off YouTube®. The death toll climbed to dizzying heights, and CNN kept an hourly death count like some macabre election-day tally.

As a human, in those first days, I was scared about what the disease would do to me and my loved ones. As a doctor, I was terrified. We physicians were trapped in a brutal vice of treating patients and risking our careers on one side, or doing nothing and watching people die on the other. Months later, the authorities stopped talking about ventilators. Later on, they stopped talking about Remdesivir. There was no apology, no real transparency. A doctor with a distinguished track record had been destroyed for telling the truth a few months too soon. Doctors were being fired for doing what we swore an oath to do. The strangest part of the COVID tale is that critical care medicine has traditionally been really good at treating inflammatory reactions using drugs like steroids. While steroids have a bad name in the public eye, they're a staple of Western medicine. During COVID, steroids were one of the drugs I prescribed to very ill patients, and I achieved excellent clinical results. That said, my main focus is naturopathic medicine, so my Naturopath brain also has a lot to say about steroids. Let's take a moment to learn more about these fascinating compounds and how they interact with our biochemistry.

Steroids, like most medicines, are complicated. For acute conditions, they can be wonder drugs. However, relying on them as continuing treatments for chronic conditions masks more complicated issues, and in some cases, they can even make the real problem worse over time. Steroids are fat-soluble hormones that influence the body in profound ways. As I said earlier in the chapter, corticosteroids interact with our cortisol response. Let's back up a minute and learn about cortisol and its importance. While corticosteroids were routinely ignored by the establishment during the pandemic, in normal times, doctors and hospitals hand them out routinely. Examples of corticosteroids are cortisone, prednisone, dexamethasone, deflazacort, and hydrocortisone, to name a few.

Many patients talk about taking a "round of steroids" or a "quick cortisone shot for pain" like it's a typical solution to common problems. The typical reasoning:

I have joint pain→ I'll get a cortisone shot

People often view corticosteroids as no big deal. Steroids are serious medications, and overuse can cause more harm than benefit. For many chronic conditions, safer natural alternatives are often available. Corticosteroids are made naturally by your body to help reduce inflammation after an injury. Inflammation and heightened immune response immediately up-regulate after an injury or illness. But the body also needs a way to naturally slowdown that inflammation and a heightened immune response after the emergency. Your body can't recover if your body stays in the emergency inflammation phase. Corticosteroids (natural and artificial) are useful in reducing that inflammatory response. They're also used to modulate stress both physically and psychologically. Biologically, emotional stress, physical injuries, or illness are all tied together by cortisol. Stress, anxiety, anger, and proximity to danger all cause the body to release adrenaline. Adrenaline puts you in a heightened fight-or-flight state where you're hyper-alert, extra-strong, and ready to defend or attack. But what goes up must come down.

Your body uses cortisol to recover from adrenaline. Cortisol is instrumental in the body's response to injury and managing stress. So, cortisol is good, right? Well, not so much. Too much cortisol over time produces symptoms like bone loss, type 2 diabetes, and weight gain. Patients may develop symptoms of Cushing's Disease. Patients with too much cortisol have thin arms and legs, weight gain on the abdomen and around the genitals, and fat on the upper back between the shoulders. You may also see stretch marks, flushed or red cheeks, and easy bruising. Early signs of elevated cortisol levels may include difficulty losing belly fat and a noticeable loss of muscle in the arms and legs. These symptoms can result from a variety of factors, including chronic stress, poor dietary choices, and the use of steroid medications. While it's easy to view these changes through the lens of societal beauty standards, they also point to real and lasting harm to our long-term health. Thankfully, the body has natural inhibitory responses to help mitigate the negative effects of too much cortisol. Even still, long-term stress and lifestyle choices can lead to these and more negative effects. In contrast to naturally occurring steroids, steroid medications are much more potent in the body. This potency is good when treating a serious acute allergic reaction. But this power comes at a cost. Steroid medications act outside of the body's inhibitory signals that reduce the potential for natural cortisol to cause harm. Essentially, steroid medications come with faster benefits but bypass the body's natural defenses against the side effects of cortisol.

Steroids are commonly prescribed for issues such as asthma, allergies, acne, and other skin disorders. While temporary use of steroids for many of these issues can provide short-term relief, they don't dismantle the issues that caused the original problem. In this way, steroids become a mask that covers up painful symptoms while not addressing the actual harm that is taking place underneath. Because steroids mask symptoms, there are two levels of risk to be considered. First, there are the primary side effects of the steroid. Second, there's the inconvenient fact that whatever underlying injury or disease process causing discomfort has been covered up but not resolved. Rashy skin, acne, asthma, and allergies are best viewed as symptoms, not diseases. What caused the rash? "It's an autoimmune condition" is the usual response. Not so fast. Why did the body randomly decide to start attacking itself?

When doctors prescribe a steroid, they frequently trot out vague platitudes about how autoimmune conditions are the body randomly attacking itself because of genetics or just because. Let's get some context for a moment. Our ancestors survived and thrived through war, plague, famine, mass starvation, saber-tooth cat attacks, brutally cold winters, and scorching hot summers. Our ancestors didn't have access to the best genetics; they only had their local area's woefully small gene pool. If genetics were just killing off large swaths of the population due to autoimmune conditions, then how would we have ever survived this long? We come from untold generations of people who spent their entire lives in a ruthless environment that was trying to kill them. Now we're here in climate-controlled comfort surrounded by the most abundant food and luxuries ever known in recorded history, and we passively accept that our bodies are destroying themselves just because.

The previous paragraph hints at what may bring about this historically significant lack of health. Humans thrived in harsh conditions, yet we're struggling when given luxuries like plenty of food and shelter. Could industrially processed food, household chemicals, indoor air filtration, and technology devices like smartphones influence our health negatively? As a matter of fact, yes. Diet, emotional stress, and long-term digestive dysfunction are closely tied to allergic and inflammatory conditions. Fried food, sugar, corn syrup, artificial sweeteners, excessive alcohol, refined carbohydrates, and industrially processed fats all contribute to inflammation in the body. 6] A poor diet and a sedentary lifestyle typified by "screen time," create an inflammation combination.

Our screens and social media sites distract us, leading to emotional stress that worsens the inflammation from our poor diet and low activity. Adding steroids into the mix of a sedentary lifestyle and poor food choices won't solve the problem. Those steroids will only accelerate your progress toward Cushing's Disease and its swollen midsection and weak arms and legs. Steroids only treat the symptoms; they don't cure disease. Don't get me wrong, steroids have their place and can be life-saving in certain serious situations like late-stage COVID-19 inflammation. Steroids have their place, but they also need to become less of a knee-jerk (pun intended) response to pain and common skin conditions. In most people, most of the time, short-term steroid use is relatively safe and seems to address symptoms. Even still, the long-term effects and damage need to be considered before we pretend that steroids are a permanent solution. Frequently, the negative effects of steroids occur much later, sometimes even after steroid therapy has stopped. The distance between the treatment and the harm means it's tempting to ignore the negatives as a strange coincidence. The negative effects may go beyond what we've covered so far. A 2001 systematic review of research on oral steroid therapy and mood disorders revealed the following:

> *"Symptoms of hypomania, mania, depression, and psychosis occur during corticosteroid therapy, as do cognitive changes, particularly deficits in verbal or declarative memory. Psychiatric symptoms appear to be dose-dependent and generally occur during the first few weeks of therapy. Patients who must remain on corticosteroids may benefit from pharmacotherapeutic approaches, such as lithium and the new antipsychotic medications."*

This is a common example of trading one health condition for another. For my patients who need a little humor in their lives, sometimes I'll joke that this is the "whack a mole" system of medicine. Do you remember the game "Whack-a-Mole?" Whack a Mole is an arcade game where you're given a giant cushioned hammer, and the goal is to smack fake mechanical moles as they animatronically pop out of their synthetic mole holes. As soon as you hit a mole, another one pops up. As the game progresses, the moles begin to pop up faster and faster until you're overwhelmed and can't hit them fast enough. Hitting mechanical moles between their beady eyes is fun as a child's game (sorry, PETA), but it's not an allegory for good medicine. In this analogy, conventional medical doctors use drugs and surgery as the hammer, and your symptoms are the moles that pop up faster and faster. The funny analogy breaks down a bit, but the better solution is to stop whacking moles and start creating conditions where moles don't want to live.

Steroids & Joint Pain

Steroids are commonly prescribed for painful joint conditions like arthritis. Of course, over-the-counter pain relievers called non-steroidal anti-inflammatory drugs (NSAIDs), such as ibuprofen or naproxen, come before steroids. But guess what? NSAIDs are also bad news. Because NSAIDs are part of the standard of care for arthritis, they're worth mentioning here—even though they aren't steroids. Many people are now aware that NSAIDs can harm the kidneys and digestive system. What's less commonly known is that their anti-inflammatory effects may actually damage joints over time, since inflammation plays a key role in the body's healing process. Yes, in emergencies, inflammation can lead to life-threatening shock. Rashy inflamed tissue is also uncomfortable. However, inflammation is a natural part of the body's healing process. Maybe we should ask more questions before we spend decades taking NSAID meds that stop this natural process. Culturally, NSAIDs and joint pain go hand in hand. Military veterans joke about prescription strength 800mg ibuprofen by calling it "ranger candy." The harsh conditions of boot camp and the battlefield, combined with the fact that NSAIDs are commonplace, lead these medications to be used almost habitually. Similarly, in many civilian professions, daily NSAID use has become as common to many daily routines as a morning coffee. As a society and as individuals, we're beginning to see the dark side of NSAIDs coming up in the research.

> *"Growing evidence suggests that nonsteroidal anti-inflammatory drugs (NSAIDs), while able to alleviate inflammation, may damage articular cartilage"* [7]

This growing body of evidence corroborates the experience of patients worldwide. People have joint pain, so they use ibuprofen to get through the day. Consequently, over the years, the joint pain gets worse, and they have to use even more NSAIDs, creating a vicious cycle. We all know this familiar pattern when it comes to illicit drug use. Someone starts dabbling with a substance and gets a positive result. Then, the person starts using the drug more often and feels even better. Soon, the person is using the drug daily. After a while, the drug doesn't work as well as it used to, so the person takes progressively higher doses more often. In the end, the drug takes over, and the person is left in a much worse condition than before. Similarly, NSAIDs relieve pain and inflammation, but over time, the medication harms joints, leading the NSAID user to take even more NSAIDs, creating a downward spiral.

Enter Cortisone

How does this NSAID joint pain spiral relate to steroids? Meet our old friend cortisone. Before I say what I'm about to say, please realize that I understand that cortisone shots are the only relief that many patients have received from joint pain for many years. I understand it's a sensitive subject because anything that provides relief is welcome after years of suffering. You know what's coming, but don't worry; by the end of this chapter, I'll lead us to new solutions that relieve pain and help with long-term healing. Anyway, here goes.

The only medical treatment worse for joints than NSAIDs might be cortisone injections. Also, this isn't just my outlying opinion as a doctor on the fringe. The latest research shows that cortisone shots cause joint damage over time. 8] Joints are naturally very slow to heal because these tissues lack blood vessels. Joints need inflammation to heal because they lack blood vessels. Inflammation brings in additional resources that are used by cells in the joint repair process. If you stop inflammation, you stop healing. In this way, reducing inflammation via NSAIDs or injected steroids speeds up cartilage loss. Research studies corroborate the finding that cortisone ruins cartilage, but you'll also see hints of the truth surfacing in normal doctor's visits. The guidelines by which cortisone shots are administered provide another data point worth considering. Currently, doctors mitigate the damage done by cortisone injections by limiting patient exposure. The first tacit admission came with doctors limiting the number of cortisone injections a patient can get yearly. 9] But the concern goes even further—more and more physicians are now placing lifetime limits on the number of injections they'll give a patient, due to legitimate fears of worsening joint damage.

If you ask people who have suffered from joint pain for multiple decades about their progression, a pattern begins to emerge. They started managing their painful joints with occasional NSAID use. Occasional NSAIDs escalated to daily use. At some point, NSAIDs progressed to corticosteroid injections, which offered miraculous relief from pain, but the relief didn't last. Eventually, we all know what happens next: surgery. Then, more surgery. Rinse and repeat.

Yes, we're indeed all fighting a losing battle against the time God has given us. But as both physicians and humans with joints, perhaps we should question this inevitable progression of joint pain and reliance on medication and surgery. Can we use the brains we've been given to better care for the joints we've been given? By the end of this chapter, I intend to prove that the answer is yes. The story of the damaging effects of NSAIDs and cortisone isn't just my medical opinion; the latest research clearly supports it. In a recent study over two years, cortisone injections provided no long-term improvement for patients. More than that, the research shows that cortisone sped up cartilage loss in patients with knee osteoarthritis. Cortisone shots are a deal with the devil: feel good now, feel bad later. This isn't just some obscure paper either; it is real data finally coming from our old NIH friends.

> *"Among people with osteoarthritic knees, repeated steroid injections over two years brought no long-term improvement in reducing pain, according to a study funded partly by the NIH's National Institute of Arthritis and Musculoskeletal and Skin Diseases (NIAMS). Rather than showing any benefit, the results revealed that the injections sped the loss of the cartilage that cushions the knee joint"* 8]

One of the serious side effects of cortisone injections is reduced bone density—an especially troubling risk given the prevalence of osteoporosis. Repeated cortisone shots may offer short-term relief, but over time, they can lead to weakened bones and deteriorating joints. The bottom line is that cortisone, much like NSAIDs, makes the problem worse in the long run. In summary, I do not recommend NSAIDs and cortisone. If you've been a long-time user of NSAIDs and cortisone, it's okay. I forgive you, and I still accept you. The goal isn't to browbeat anyone; I'm here to save your joints. Wherever we've come from, we know better now, so let's do better together.

A Better Way

At this point, you may think I've taken away the only things that allowed you to lead a normal, productive life. But with the old way cast aside, now we can talk about a better way. Instead of NSAIDs and steroids that interrupt cartilage repair, what if there were treatments that could actually stop cartilage loss? Even more, what if we could even cause cartilage to regrow? The answer is that, in most cases, we can stop the loss and even regrow cartilage through treatment.

Okay, it's disclaimer time. In this section, we're narrowly focusing on regenerative injection therapy, but there's also a strong correlation between joint health, the foods we eat, and the life we lead. Inflammatory foods, alcohol use, obesity, uncontrolled blood sugar, and a condition called "leaky gut" all profoundly impact joint health. Regenerative injection therapy is highly effective, but if your foundational health is lacking in any of the above areas, then your joints will suffer.

To understand how to heal joints, we need to take a minute and review some basic biology. Joints are avascular, meaning they don't have blood vessels. In comparison, muscles have a lot of blood vessels. Muscles heal quickly and can grow stronger because blood vessels supply oxygen and nutrients. Joints heal much more slowly because they must survive and rebuild using only what little material leaks into them. When a joint injury occurs, the area experiences severe pain and swelling. Historically, the swelling was considered a side effect of the injury that needed to be eliminated. Swelling goes down, pain goes down.

The common medical advice is to take ibuprofen and apply ice to reduce as much swelling as possible. But why do we assume that swelling and inflammation are always bad? To be clear, systemic inflammation due to eating historically unprecedented levels of sugars and industrially-produced fats and carbs is bad. However, swelling when injured is part of the healing process. Swelling after a joint injury has existed throughout human history, and we survived and thrived. All of a sudden, in the last few generations, we've magically decided that the body's response to joint injury is wrong, and we're the ones to fix it. Swelling and inflammation aren't always a side-effect of an injury; sometimes inflammation is a constructive response to an injury. Modern medicine's obsession with reducing pain and inflammation is part of why we have so many joint problems. The immediate swelling of an injured joint brings a rush of much-needed nutrients and white blood cells into the affected area. Since joints don't get direct blood flow, the material brought in by the swelling is just about all the joints have to repair themselves with. By arresting the swelling of injured joints, we're stopping the flow of extra nutrients and white blood cells into the area. This mistake in treatment stops the healing process dead in its tracks. The symptom is not the disease.

The vicious circle of joint injuries:

1. Injured joint swells up

2. Take meds/treatment to reduce swelling

3. Reduced swelling leaves joints without nutrients to heal

4. Incomplete healing makes repeat injury more likely

5. Cycle repeats

For this reason, my preferred technique for joint repair is **prolotherapy**, or **prolo** for short. In this procedure, a liquid mixture—typically a pain reliever combined with a *proliferant agent*—is injected into the soft tissues in or around a joint. The proliferant (often a dextrose solution) is a non-toxic substance that triggers the body's natural healing response. It works by mimicking the signals your body sends when tissue is injured, essentially encouraging self-repair.

The way prolotherapy promotes healing is both complex and elegantly simple. When tissue is damaged, cells rupture and spill their contents into the surrounding area. We see this externally as bruising or swelling, but internally, it's a powerful call to action. These released cell contents act as biochemical signals, telling the immune system and repair mechanisms to show up. White blood cells, growth factors, and other healing agents rush to the site, reducing infection risk and rebuilding damaged tissue. Prolotherapy leverages this process—by carefully injecting the proliferant agent, we simulate injury without causing real harm, repeatedly triggering this healing cascade.

Platelet-rich plasma (PRP) is another highly effective therapy used in a similar way. With PRP, we draw the patient's own blood, spin it in a centrifuge to concentrate the platelets and growth factors, then re-inject that potent mixture into injured joints or tissues. This natural, regenerative therapy has the added benefit of being useful not only for joint and soft tissue repair, but also for cosmetic concerns—PRP is commonly used to stimulate hair regrowth and to reduce wrinkles.

To further enhance both prolotherapy and PRP, we often incorporate ozone therapy through a technique known as Prolozone®. Prolozone® not only accelerates tissue healing but also disinfects the injured area, adding an antimicrobial effect while boosting the body's natural repair mechanisms.

It's important to understand that swelling is not the enemy—it's an essential part of the healing process. Swelling signals injury and initiates the body's repair response. So instead of suppressing these natural signals with NSAIDs or cortisone—which may reduce pain in the short term but impair long-term healing—wouldn't it make more sense to work with the body, not against it?

That's the power of regenerative therapies like prolotherapy, PRP, and Prolozone®: they don't just mask symptoms—they help the body truly heal.

Case Study: Carina

Carina, a 56-year-old grandmother of five who loves gardening and walking in nature, was sidelined by constant pain. Diagnosed with osteoarthritis in her hands and knees, gripping objects became difficult, and numbness lingered in her hand from a past carpal tunnel surgery. Pain and instability in her knees made it hard to get up from her garden, and keeping up with her grandkids became a challenge. Over the years, she'd had three rounds of corticosteroid injections.

The first cortisone shot offered relief for a while. But, during subsequent treatments, the cortisone shots stopped having any positive effect, temporary or not. It had been a year since her last cortisone shot, and that didn't work. The best her old doctor could offer was to have her start taking high doses of over-the-counter pain relievers. The final straw was when that doctor told her that, eventually, she'd need full knee replacements on both knees. That's when Terrain Wellness joined the picture. The first goal of treatment was to reduce her systemic inflammation by improving her digestion and eliminating potential allergens from her foods. Concurrently, we also spent time working with her to manage her emotional stressors better. Dietary choices and emotional health greatly influence cortisol levels and inflammation. Excess cortisol, over time, damages joints, among many other things. While my team continued to work with the patient on these supporting treatments, we also told her about prolotherapy. Carina agreed to try a few rounds of prolo because, at this point, she was in so much pain that double knee replacements seemed like the only other option.

Our short-term goals with prolotherapy were pain relief, and our medium-term goal was to improve joint stabilization. After the first round of prolo, she noted that her pain had been reduced to half. She felt like both knees were "stronger and more stable" than before. She felt so good that she wondered if we could treat one of her hands to see if it would make a difference. After the second round of prolotherapy, she again had a significant pain reduction to the point where she "wanted to try and take a run." We advised her to wait, start walking, and see how it went. We agreed to treat her hand as well, and sure enough, Carina began to notice an increased range of motion and significantly less pain. She also mentioned that she started reducing her pain medication by over half.

Given Carina's extensive history with cortisone, NSAIDs, and scarring from previous surgery, we were still determining if she'd experience the full benefits of prolo and comprehensive treatment. But I'm glad to report that Carina became one of our best cases. After a few rounds of treatments over six months, Carina is now back to pain-free gardening with the occasional run in nature, without surgery. We achieved these results by holistically reducing inflammation in her diet, managing her biological stress response, and carefully applying prolotherapy to stimulate her joint's natural healing response.

The (Other) Problem with Steroids

As we discussed earlier, in emergencies and very specific short-term situations, steroids are wonder drugs. But, their miraculous properties come at a cost. Among many other side effects, steroids down-regulate the immune system. This lowering of the body's ability to fight infection can become a significant risk over time. As we learned previously, steroids drastically inhibit inflammation, shutting off signals that normally let the immune system know there's an infection. Numerous studies have highlighted the increased risk of infection that accompanies steroids. As if we needed one more reason to avoid these drugs, bacterial and fungal infections increase in people on steroids. Steroids are the standard modern medicine treatment for autoimmune conditions like eczema, psoriasis, Crohn's disease, and rheumatoid arthritis. Of course, steroids come with all of the unpleasant weight gain and muscle and bone loss common to excessive cortisol in the body.

It should be noted that a new class of drugs known as anti-TNF agents promise more targeted relief from autoimmune conditions. TNF stands for Tumor Necrotic Factor. As the name implies, TNF helps us get rid of tumors naturally by using inflammation. Anti-TNF drugs do lower inflammation, but they also suppress your immune system, making you vulnerable to bacteria and fungus. Your body's natural TNF is also useful for killing off tumors before they become cancer, which is also pretty useful. With steroids or anti-TNF drugs suppressing the immune system, otherwise harmless germs can quickly become aggressive infections. 12]

Concurrent conditions such as diabetes, obesity, or alcoholism further increase the risk of getting opportunistic infections while on steroids. Nutrition deficiencies and improper nutrient absorption are common in people with chronic diseases. This malnourished state increases the risk of succumbing to an opportunistic infection. Like many health conditions, these factors can combine into a vicious cycle that self-reinforces a cluster of serious health issues. 13] 14]

The evidence is clear that infectious complications occur more often in people with exposure to steroids. The likelihood of infection is influenced by how long steroids are taken and what other health conditions the person has. One study found that people with underlying neurological conditions were among the highest risk of getting an infection while taking steroids. 15]

Another study found a disturbing connection among people with diagnosed Systemic Lupus Erythematosus (SLE) who took steroids and antibiotics. The study linked this combination of Lupus, steroids, and antibiotics to Invasive Fungal Infection (IFI). IFI is commonly found in the lungs and the nervous system. FYI, IFI is a bad kind of fungal infection. We're all familiar with fungal infections like yeast and athletes' feet. While those are unpleasant, Invasive Fungal Infections are where things like the heart, blood, brain, and bones are attacked. Particularly when combined with antibiotics, steroids put patients at high risk for infection. 16] Much like our talk about antibiotics, we again see a pattern of over-prescribing medications with little care given to the side effects.

While many may shrug off increased infection risk, a compromised immune system is a serious problem. Trapped between autoimmune diseases and serious infections, it's time to address autoimmune conditions from the ground up. Modern medicine needs to stop using whack-a-mole medicine to try and prescribe our way to better health. For some people with autoimmune conditions, steroids (and anti-TNF agents) are a game changer. Some patients find tremendous relief in the beginning when they use these immune-suppressing drugs. According to one study published in 2003, autoimmune disease is one of the leading causes of death in middle-aged women in the United States. 17] Across a host of ethnic, age, and gender demographics, autoimmune conditions are rising. 18] Autoimmune conditions are even on the rise among teenagers. 19]

Evidence for increasing rates and various groups affected by autoimmune disease is significantly increasing. With opportunistic infections climbing as we prescribe steroids and anti-TNF agents, we've got to find a better way. There's one more elephant in the room: drug costs. Prescription steroids, especially tumor necrosis factor (TNF) blocking drugs, are very expensive. In 2014, researchers found that the average yearly cost of anti-TNF drugs was $17,000 - $29,000 per patient. 20] These price quotes were from 2014; who wants to bet whether pharmaceutical prices have increased or decreased since this data was collected? Drug prices also reflect the cost of research done on Medicare patients. In a way, every American is bearing the cost of these drugs. Other researchers show the cost per infusion is between $2,000 and $9,000. This cost does not include the labor of nurses, doctors, and hospital staff to administer the drug, just the cost of the drug itself. 21]

For autoimmune conditions, it's important to note that these costs are continuing because the patient must stay on the drug to prevent a flare-up of the disease. This means a lifetime of dependence on expensive medications with nasty side effects. This pattern may be good for drug companies, but it isn't good for people. Money aside, the worst part is that these treatments only trade one problem for another. Let's move forward. Any time I hear about someone having an allergic/atopic condition such as eczema, asthma, or other autoimmune cluster symptoms, my immediate medical treatment involves eliminating sources of allergy and inflammation. Restoring gut health and improving the performance of detoxification organs such as the liver, pancreas, and kidneys comes next. Numerous research studies show promising results from non-invasive therapies that help support the body in restoring balance during atopic conditions. Multiple studies showcase the benefits of acupuncture in the treatment of asthma. One study showed marked improvement in quality-of-life scores when using acupuncture and conventional treatment methods. 22] In another study, participants were given acupuncture points to support breathing. Participants were also given an herbal combination that was applied to the skin. After 30 weeks, the participants who received the herbal support and acupuncture treatments showed a down-regulation of the allergic immune response and a decrease in the incidence of allergic-based asthmatic episodes. 23] Adding adjunct care to conventional treatment plans seems highly beneficial. We need less steroids and more natural solutions. Modulating the immune response naturally reduces the number of prescribed pharmaceutical drugs. The best way to mitigate side effects is to prescribe fewer drugs.

My Standard of Care

At Terrain Wellness, drugs are not our first reaction when patients come in with skin ailments like acne, eczema, psoriasis, or allergic rashes. The first thing to look at in these cases is the elimination of inflammatory foods while also improving digestive health. Unhealthy small intestines that are inflamed from poor diet and food allergies can lead to improperly digested food particles escaping the digestive tract and contaminating the blood and interstitial fluid of the body. This process of internal contamination from the intestines is called a leaky gut. These leaking food particles then antagonize our body's immune system, leading to autoimmune symptoms that *appear out of nowhere*. In my clinical experience, autoimmune conditions that happen "for no reason" are rare. There's always something deeper at play. For this reason, we reserve medications like antibiotics and steroids for temporary use in only the most serious circumstances. Our standard of care isn't just opinion; the research supports it. A study found that a combination of acupuncture and a gluten-free diet reversed urticaria and eczema associated with dermatitis herpetiformis, which had not responded to steroid treatments. Notably, the women in the case study showed no signs of celiac disease in both endoscopy and colonoscopy, yet blood tests were positive for the human leukocyte antigen DQ-8. 24] This is further evidence that gluten sensitivities are difficult to find and often go misdiagnosed with conventional testing. Herbal evaporative concentrates are the plant equivalent of a topical corticosteroid cream. These natural remedies are slow-cooked herbs simmered over low heat for multiple days. When finished, the herb reduction is black and has the consistency of a thick cream.

The herbal cream is applied directly to skin rashes, varicose veins, and other inflammatory skin conditions. You can find these herbal decoctions and more information on creating specific herbal remedies in various herbal texts. One of my favorites is *Herbal Antibiotics* by renowned herbalist Stephen Harrod Buhner, as well as *Medicine from the Heart of the Earth* by Dr. Sheryl Tilgner, an excellent herbalist and naturopathic physician. By utilizing herbal medicines, regenerative injection therapy, and acupuncture before resorting to steroids, we can significantly improve our quality of life. Inflammatory conditions like joint pain and autoimmune disorders also respond well to improvements in digestive health through naturopathic care.

We can even reduce inflammation and the need for steroids by addressing our psychological health and how we deal with emotions and stress. I understand the value of corticosteroids and have prescribed more than I ever wanted. However, for long-term sustainable health, a much better approach is to use the wisdom of herbal medicine and the modern knowledge of the biochemistry we cover in this book to optimize our health so that medications become unnecessary.

TLDR: Too Long Didn't Read

According to the research, steroids, as well as NSAIDs (Non-Steroidal Anti-Inflammatory Drugs) like ibuprofen, interfere with joints' ability to repair. This means that over time, NSAIDs and cortisone shots make joint conditions worse, not better. Much like steroids, anti-TNF agents reduce inflammation, but suppress the immune system. Before the COVID-19 pandemic, I never expected to work so extensively with corticosteroids. But, when patients arrived with shortness of breath and low oxygen levels, steroid-based asthma medications became a simple, effective way to help them through the worst phase of the illness. Corticosteroids can also be valuable for managing acute conditions related to allergy and inflammation.

However, long-term steroid use comes with significant health risks—many of which are overlooked in conventional medicine. One of the most concerning uses is "cortisone injections for joint pain." Research shows that both corticosteroids and NSAIDs (non-steroidal anti-inflammatory drugs) like ibuprofen interfere with the body's ability to repair joint tissue. Over time, this means these drugs may actually worsen joint damage rather than improve it.

Chapter 5
Microbiome 101

1 of 37,200,000,000,000?

We commonly think of ourselves as one person. I am one individual human with my thoughts, feelings, hopes, and fears. But what is one human made of? 78 organs (depending on who's counting), 206 bones, and about 3 times that many muscles. Okay, where did I get 37.2 trillion from? No, I'm not talking about the national debt either. Estimates vary, but researchers estimate that each adult comprises about 37.2 trillion human cells. 1] Yes, you're one person, but you're also a mega-structure of about 37.2 trillion cells. Each cell has a job, and within each cell are tiny organelles that have jobs, too. But these 37.2 trillion cells are only about half the story of what makes up the human body.

Each human body—made up of roughly 30 to 37.2 trillion cells—also hosts about 39 trillion microorganisms. Truth really is stranger than fiction: by cell count, you're more microbe than human. Yet when we think about health, we rarely consider the vast community of bacteria and fungi living inside us. When I bring this up with patients, I often hear, "But doctor, it's okay—I take probiotics!" We only think of microbes when they make us sick; we call them germs. You are one person trying to make peace with the 39 trillion microbes living in and on you. Most Americans have taken antibiotics in their lifetime and eat at least some processed foods. How many trillion microbes did the antibiotic kill off?

Does eating yogurt from a supermarket atone for our careless germ genocide? 39 trillion microbes. This is where my clinic, Terrain Wellness, got its name. Our bodies are more than bodies. Our bodies are the terrain within which trillions of tiny critters live out their entire lives for generations. In biology, animals influence the terrain, and the terrain influences what animals can live there. We can only solve complex health problems once we respect the terrain and its living creatures. What are these microbes doing inside of us? Modern medicine spends billions of dollars trying to make our 37.2 trillion human cells healthy and then tells us to eat yogurt.

> *Disclaimer: Yes! We're talking about germs and poop here, people. I get it; poop and germs might gross you out. But you cannot be healthy unless you make peace with all these poop germs. So, it would be best to learn who these microbes are and what they want. Laugh if you need to, squirm because you're uncomfortable if you must. Just stay with me and learn this vitally important material. Okay, good talk.*

Healthcare understands that the 39 trillion microbes living inside us are vaguely important for digestive health, but they rarely go deeper. This over-simplification of our human microbiome is grievously disrespectful to the complex ecosystem inside us all. In my clinical practice of medicine and according to the latest research, making peace with the bugs inside us is a big part of what most doctors miss. Microbes live on our skin, in our airways, and—most abundantly—in our gut. Many of medicine's mysteries may lie in this often-overlooked half of the human body. It's time we give the microbiome the respect it deserves.

> **"All disease begins in the gut."** 3] – *Hippocrates.*

Before discussing what can go wrong in our gut microbiome, let's discuss what a healthy gut looks like. Imagine a world where you have regular bowel movements at least once or twice a day. There is no straining to poop, no gas, no bloated belly after eating. There's no undigested food, blood, or mucus in the toilet when you poop. Your poop comes out like a long, easily passed snake that often sinks to the bottom. Not too hard and not too soft. You easily wipe clean, with no stickiness and no pain. You flush the toilet, you wash your hands, and your bowel movement is so uneventful that you forget about it. Mission complete. Sounds nice, right? Unfortunately, this isn't the case for many of the patients who come to see us. Yes, we want to know all the details of your bathroom adventures. It's weird, but it makes us better at helping you. We must hear about your digestion because every small detail is a clue. Strangely, your microbiome is communicating to you through symptoms.

Your Microbiome

Bacteria and other microorganisms make up a significant portion of your body. These microbes aren't just along for the ride; they aid in properly functioning multiple organ systems. "The human body contains trillions of microorganisms... Because of their small size, however, microorganisms make up only about 1 to 3 percent of the body's mass (in a 200-pound adult, that's 2 to 6 pounds of bacteria)." 4] The microbiome is all the microbes, their waste products, and their genetic material (bacteria, viruses, fungi, bacteriophages, and protozoa) that inhabit the human body. Most people think of the bacteria and fungi that aid in proper digestion and healthy bowel movements. However, the microbiome changes everything from our genetic expression to how the brain functions. The microbiome living inside each of us can influence human gene expression, the immune system, brain chemistry, nutrient absorption, and hormonal signaling, to name a few. What's your gut got to do with it? Simply put, everything. With new research just starting to take the microbiome seriously, the current healthcare model of the germ theory may be outdated. At the risk of over-simplifying, germ theory is the idea that you catch a bad germ, and the germ infects you and makes you sick. You get better by killing off the bad germ and eating some yogurt to return the good microbes. However, new research shows that we all have pathogens all the time. Pathogens are microorganisms known to cause illnesses that people casually call germs.

The interesting thing is that in healthy people, these pathogens are just there and don't make you sick. What we consider harmful germs frequently coexist inside us all the time. Labeling some microbes as good and others as bad might be an oversimplification. Researchers must investigate why these same germs cause disease in some but seem harmless in others. The simplistic idea that germs are "bad" so we should kill them does not align with this more complex understanding that healthy and unhealthy people often have the same germs. 4]

"I'm sorry, Dr. Dani, are you telling me that COVID affects some people differently than others?"

On the exhale of a weary sigh, "Yes."

Nerd alert! This next part gets a little technical, but I'll make it as simple as possible and summarize it as I go. Researchers took samples of intestinal tissues of people diagnosed with irritable bowel syndrome (IBS). Since areas of inflamed intestinal tissue coexist with those not inflamed, scientists took the same person's inflamed and non-inflamed tissues. They were looking for clues about why some areas were inflamed but not all areas. The inflamed intestinal tissue had a different genetic expression than areas with non-inflamed tissue. The genes in the inflamed tissue were altered. These altered genes had interesting differences in function; the inflamed tissue was able to repress bile, citric acid, fatty acid, and specific protein(s), whereas the non-inflamed tissue did not have these attributes. 5] What we experience as irritable bowel syndrome is related to altering the intestines' genetics. Where modern medicine explains away things like IBS and other ailments as autoimmune conditions, I ask why. Why did someone's intestinal genes change? And, not just random changes either. The changes were related to food. Our personal health decisions related to food, physical activity, and medications are part of very complex systems. Let's explore some more research. The standard American diet (SAD, pun intended) is high in industrially processed fats, processed carbohydrates, sugar, and artificial ingredients.

We all know that SAD leads to weight gain and maybe heart disease when we're old. But the mechanics of how these foods hurt us are much more complex than we realize. Research shows that the Standard American Diet (SAD) alters our gut microbiome, which in turn reprograms the genetic activity of our cells. In essence, what we eat reshapes our gut microbes—and those microbes send signals that influence how our genes are expressed. The cascade of changes triggered by the SAD leads to shifts in the microbiome that can promote obesity and, over time, increased risk of cancer.

"The obesogenic diet shapes the microbiome before the development of obesity, leading to altered bacterial metabolite production that predisposes the host to obesity" 6]

Are germs making us fat? Sort of. More precisely, imbalanced dietary choices caused an overgrowth of gut microbes that altered our gene expression, leading to obesity, inflammation, and autoimmune conditions. With what we've already learned about antibiotics, I'm sure you know by now that it's not so simple as killing off the supposedly "bad" germs. To be clear, I don't even think of these gene-modifying gut microbes as bad germs. They're just microbes doing the best with what they've been given. If we give them processed foods, sugar, artificial ingredients, and alcohol binges, then our poor little germs can only do so much. We must learn to make peace with our microbes, or they'll destroy us. If that felt too technical, here's the simple version: what we eat shapes our microbiome, and that, in turn, influences our health—even at the genetic level.

Your Mouth and Your Gut

The mouth is the gateway to the body. The colon is the exit. The mouth is where the outside world meets our inside world; it is the gatekeeper. Here, I like to use some terrain analogies to make it more interesting. Inside the mouth is like a swampy forest at the edge of your kingdom. After the swampland of the mouth, we travel through the fiery acid of the stomach. As we discussed elsewhere, the acid in your stomach is not a dragon to be defeated; it's a powerful guardian. Stomach acid kills off many unwelcome invaders that wander in while you're munching and chewing. Aside from barbecuing would-be knights who get too uppity, what do dragons do? They guard treasure. Don't get trapped in the lie of neutering the dragon in your stomach by taking antacids. He's there for a reason.

The dragon in your stomach kills off invaders, and his fire melts down the food you eat so that the pure gold can be refined. Stomach acid is your friend, and if he's angry, then there's something you need to learn. Of course, they make girl dragons, too, so make this fun allegory your own in whatever way suits you. No matter what though, you need to learn your terrain. Before becoming a doctor, I was a dental hygienist with plans to continue into dentistry, but that's a tale for another time. What's important now is that I've closely observed (and cleaned) more mouths than you can imagine. My work in dental hygiene allowed me to see some patterns. It's surprising how much you can tell about a person's health simply by observing their mouth. The gums of a person with diabetes, someone with an autoimmune disease, or chronic digestive disorders all have tales to tell that don't involve speaking. Of course, these clues led me to interesting conversations as I cleaned patients' teeth. The most interesting thing revealed in these conversations with dental hygiene patients was that they had never discussed these issues in detail with their primary care doctors. Diabetic patients get their diabetes treated. People with thyroid issues were prescribed thyroid medications. Those with autoimmune skin conditions got steroids. Patients with multiple issues saw a specialist for each of their issues. The specialists stayed in their lanes while the primary care doctor only spent a few minutes with each patient. Mouth after mouth, patient after patient. I met countless interesting people with interesting health conditions.

As time went by, patterns emerged. Certain medications would wreak havoc on a patient's oral health, not to mention deplete a person of vital nutrients needed to repair teeth and gums. My uncle is an equine veterinarian. One day, I asked him how they treated horses with infected teeth and periodontal disease. He uttered a huff of exasperation and replied tersely, "If we can't clean the horse's teeth, then we have to shoot them." Seeing my shocked expression, he explained that bad teeth in horses are a sign of past or present serious health problems in the horse. And if they can't get the horse's mouth healthy, the animal will slowly die of malnourishment. 7] I do not suggest we "put you out to pasture" if your mouth is a mess. But I want you to learn that if your mouth is a mess, it can affect your entire body. More people are becoming aware of the link between oral hygiene and immune system health, but there's more to it than that. The bacteria that make up a healthy mouth microbiome live in a balance called homeostasis. It's not so much about good and bad bacteria; it's more about how they are balanced. Even bacteria generally regarded as harmful germs don't cause an issue if their numbers are kept at a dull roar. Even bad germs can help protect our teeth from cavities and periodontal disease. Every 24 hours, these bacterial populations, called dental plaque, must be broken up from the surfaces of the oral cavity. Otherwise, they build up and become hardened bacterial colonies called tartar or calculus (8). No, not the math kind of calculus. The kind that builds up on teeth is a hard deposit of calcium and grime. As calculus builds up on your teeth, it provides a matrix for more bacteria to grow and over-populate your mouth. Infections develop, and the immune system spends valuable resources fighting germs trapped in your teeth.

This calculus matrix of calcium and bacteria will continually spread if not removed. Eventually, the calculus spreads under your gum line, attaching to the root surface of each tooth. When this happens, the gums begin to bleed and swell, a process called gingivitis. If gingivitis continues, the bacterial infection driven on by calculus deposits will spread so deep on the root surface that the gums no longer bleed and swell as much, but the worst is yet to come.

Sometimes, in as little as a few weeks, gingivitis can progress such that the jawbone itself begins to erode, a process called periodontal disease. The jawbone and the connective tissue that supports your teeth is called the periodontium. Periodontal disease eats away at the bone and soft tissues surrounding your teeth as the gums and tissue retract away from the infected calculus deposits. The bacteria that grow on the root surface form biofilms. Biofilms are the sticky matrices formed by bacterial colonies. Biofilms make it difficult for our immune system to find and kill pathogenic bacteria and infections. Why are we talking about this? So many reasons. Proper oral hygiene frees up your immune system to handle more important issues. Next, your teeth need to last for your entire life. Dentures are not an ideal solution. Losing teeth in your 40s, 50s, or 60s could mean living multiple decades with reduced quality of life. More than that, a diseased and infected mouth opens a highway for bacteria and other pathogens to enter the bloodstream. If gingivitis progresses with continued bone and gum loss, periodontal disease becomes a severe condition marked by rancid breath, ulcerations, bleeding, tooth loss, and bacteria entering the bloodstream.

FYI, bacteria in the bloodstream are then distributed throughout your organs. Trust me, you don't want germs in your heart. Gum disease affects the whole body. Blood tests on people with periodontal disease show elevated white blood cells and markers of inflammation, such as elevated c-reactive protein. Bacteria related to periodontal infection have also been found in the blood clots of some victims of heart attack. 9] Until gingivitis becomes severe, it's often painless and remains hidden under the surface of the gums. This means people don't realize how bad their infected mouths are. As it turns out, oral health also has something to do with our gut microbiome.

As studies emerge on the human microbiome, we're beginning to understand the connection between the mouth and the gut. The research shows that various diseases are being caused indirectly by mouth bacteria. Oral bacterial overgrowth disrupts gut flora, leading to systemic disease. For example, P. *gingivalis* is a bacteria commonly found in periodontal infection, has acid resistance. If allowed to increase, this type of bacteria can survive the stomach's acid and take over the digestive tract. Once there, it has been shown to colonize and may be connected to cancer development.

> *"P. gingivalis can be implicated in precancerous gastric and colon lesions, esophageal squamous cell carcinoma, head and neck (larynx, throat, lip, mouth and salivary glands) carcinoma, and pancreatic cancer."* 10]

Do you want to make a bad situation even worse? Combine gum disease with taking antacids. As mentioned elsewhere in this book, reduced stomach acid allows the wrong kind of bacteria to enter the gut. Antacids and small intestinal bacterial overgrowth (SIBO) both increase the risk of cancer and other serious health conditions. Periodontal disease and gut imbalance (dysbiosis) are associated with numerous health conditions. 11]

- Obesity
- Diabetes
- Atherosclerosis
- Rheumatoid Arthritis
- Non-alcoholic fatty liver disease

- Hormone imbalances
- Cancer

But wait, there's more. An imbalanced microbiome in the mouth causes problems everywhere in the body. The microbiome plays a crucial role in hormonal imbalances, so looking at a person's gut is a key piece to helping men and women who want to have their "hormones balanced." Digestion and the microbiome begin in the mouth, but they don't end there.

Gut Health & Hormones

Emerging research shows a connection between gut health and your ability to process hormones. During glucuronidation, the liver makes high levels of glucuronic acid. Glucuronic acid aids in detoxifying hormones, neurotransmitters, drugs, mold toxins, and cancer-causing agents from the body. This acid bonds to substances that need to be removed, forming a complex that is then moved into the small intestine and excreted from the body. Unless these substances are bound into a complex, they stay in the body and can't be eliminated. This binding and excretion process traps dangerous substances and releases them into the wild, where it cannot harm. The binding property of glucuronic acid is essential in eliminating toxins.

Old hormones can build up in the body to the point that if more hormones are released, the message won't be noticed because so much of the hormone has already built up. Do you remember the old television show *I Love Lucy*? In one episode, Lucy and her best friend, Ethel, are sent to work at the local chocolate factory. They find themselves overwhelmed as the chocolate comes down the conveyor belt at a speed they can no longer keep up with. Suddenly, they cannot package the chocolates quickly enough, and the delicate chocolate truffles pile up. The two characters in the TV show try hiding the unpackaged chocolates so their boss won't be mad at them.

Desperate to avoid getting in trouble, the two begin stuffing the sweets into their hats, shirts, and mouths. They are busting at the seams full of chocolate as they try to compensate for their inability to package chocolates fast enough. If you have yet to watch this episode, it's worth looking it up online and having a good laugh. This comical scene is more than just entertainment; it also (unintentionally) is a powerful illustration of what the body does when it's given too much to detoxify. Glucuronic acid plays a vital role in removing old hormones so the body can properly respond to newly released hormones. Much like Lucy and Ethel packaging the chocolate, when there are too many hormones in the gut from a congested liver and gut, the body cannot keep up, and the old hormones get stuck. When bacteria in the gut become imbalanced, the bound acid-hormone complex comes apart, and the old hormone is released back into the body at an inappropriate time, thus making our liver even more overburdened. This is where something called estrobolome comes in. Estrobolome is when certain gut bacteria keep you from eliminating estrogen. Excessive estrogen, known as estrogen dominance, can be a serious problem for both men and women. Too much estrogen can lead to issues like:

- Breast, uterine, & ovarian cancers in women
- Erectile dysfunction & breast development in men
- Endometriosis pain in women
- Thyroid issues
- Weight gain
- Insulin resistance (a precursor to diabetes)

The biochemistry involved here gets a bit complicated. But don't worry, I've come with receipts. Essentially, the bacteria and fungi in your gut, influenced by your oral hygiene and the foods you eat, will make or break you. Poor gut health wreaks havoc on your hormone balance. Let's dig a little deeper. Let's learn about beta-glucuronidase, a byproduct of certain intestinal bacteria you don't want to overgrow. Beta-glucuronidase is a substance that aids in the digestion of carbohydrates, an important energy source for the body. But this compound can also break the bonds between glucuronic acid and the hormone it's attached to. A small amount of beta-glucuronidase in the gut is beneficial as it acts as a digestive aid. If beta-glucuronidase levels are too low, the body may struggle to digest certain foods properly. At times, low beta-glucuronidase levels may indicate that the body has a high toxic load and is depleting available beta-glucuronidase. However, our focus here is on elevated levels. When beta-glucuronidase levels are too high, the compound breaks the bonds between glucuronic acid and the hormone it is bound to, effectively releasing the hormone or toxin. This unbinding allows estrogen and toxins to be re-absorbed back into the bloodstream from the intestinal tract. 12] This way, previously processed toxins and hormones can be pushed back into the blood multiple times.

The bacterial condition where processed estrogen is sent back into the bloodstream is an *estrobolome*. This imbalance forces the liver to reprocess old "bad" estrogen and toxins constantly. Over time, an unneeded toxic burden is put on the liver and creates a state of estrogen dominance. Sadly, this recycled estrogen is harmful to the body and not useful. Keeping these old hormones bound up with glucuronic acid and heading out the exit is important. In people with high levels of beta-glucuronidase this becomes difficult and intervention may be necessary.

Luckily, herbs and minerals, especially calcium-d-glucarate, keep waste estrogen in the gut from becoming unbound and unruly. But herbs and supplements won't make up for bad dietary fundamentals. With its excessive carbs and sugar, the SAD (standard American diet) encourages the bacteria that make beta-glucuronidase to become overpopulated. One of the reasons why our society has too much estrogen is this estrobolome condition. The simple answer is we eat too much sugar and junk food. Our comprehensive GI panels test patients' beta-glucuronidase levels to help us understand a patient's hormones and detoxification. We always look into gut health when a patient has hormone regulation issues. Estrobolome doesn't just stop there; the hormone imbalance creates a cascade of negative health consequences. High levels of beta-glucuronidase and the estrobolome it creates have been connected to the development of the following:

- PCOS
- Metabolic syndrome (Pre-Diabetes)
- Mood disorders
- Endometriosis
- Breast cancer
- Uterine cancer
- Worsening menopausal symptoms
- Colon cancer

- Prostate cancer

While I can only give medical advice to patients I treat, here are some guidelines to explore with your healthcare team.

When your beta-glucuronidase levels are too low 13]

- Replenish healthy gut bacteria using specific probiotics
- Investigate and eliminate environmental and toxic exposures

When your beta-glucuronidase levels are too high 13]

- Investigate and eliminate environmental and toxic exposures
- Eliminate all hydrogenated and processed fats from the diet
- Lower sugar consumption
- Stop smoking
- Eliminate alcohol
- Remove inflammatory and allergenic foods
- Hydrate
- Avoid antibiotics unless necessary
- Repair your gut and re-seed it with the correct probiotics

Remember, glucuronic acid is the one that binds to old hormones and toxins and carries them out of the body. If you have an estrobolome, increasing your glucuronic acid while decreasing beta-glucuronidase is a good place to start.

Natural Substances to increase glucuronic acid

- Calcium-d-glucarate
- Apple pectin
- Cumin
- Fenugreek seed
- Milk thistle
- Restoring proper calcium, magnesium & iron levels
- Cruciferous vegetables like brussels sprouts, cabbage, broccoli, cauliflower
- Oranges, especially orange peels

Gut Health & Mood

The gut contains its own nervous system, called the enteric nervous system (ENS). The enteric nervous system is a network of nerve bundles that communicate directly with your central nervous system via your spinal cord and into the brain. The enteric system is unique because it can also act independently of the central nervous system. In anatomy and physiology, professors sometimes call the ENS the brain of the gut. You didn't know you had a second brain, did you?

This brain of the gut uses hormones to send the messages necessary for its work. The chemical messengers used by the ENS are also part of why food, eating, and digestion is so emotional for humans. The hormonal actions of the ENS are crucial for you to understand. Poor gut health throws the brain and the gut into turmoil. Mood imbalances like depression, anxiety, bipolar disorders, and schizophrenia are connected to the health of the gut. Michael Gershon, a neurogastroenterology researcher and author of *The Second Brain*, explains how the gut uses around 30 neurotransmitters to do its job. These neurotransmitters also indirectly affect your actual brain. While serotonin is most known as the happy hormone, Gershon explains that about 95% of all the serotonin in the body is made and used in the gut. 14]

For this reason, digestive side effects are common in depression medications, especially selective serotonin reuptake inhibitors (SSRIs). There are so many serotonin receptors in the gut that when an SSRI medication is taken, it causes changes in bowel movements, stomach pain, and other gastrointestinal issues. Have you ever had a *gut feeling*? Have you ever felt an emotion that left you *sick to your stomach*? Have you ever been so excited you had *butterflies in your tummy*? Your brain and gut-brain use many of the same hormones. Now, the story gets even more interesting. The bombshell that some of you already guessed is that your gut bacteria influence neurotransmitters like serotonin. A 2018 research study found the following,

"Gut bacteria both produce and respond to the same neurochemicals." 15]

This includes GABA, serotonin, norepinephrine, dopamine, acetylcholine, and melatonin. These neurotransmitter chemicals are directly related to controlling mood and learning. Several studies have shown that people with IBS (irritable bowel syndrome) have an increased rate of depression or anxiety, as well as a decreased amount of cognitive flexibility in those with co-morbid gut conditions. 16] Poor gut health will make you hormonally depressed; the reverse has also been observed. Chronic emotional stress is harmful to digestive function over time. In this way, psychological problems can change your gut microbiome such that imbalanced bacterial colonies lead the body to all the harmful conditions we're discussing: Inflammation, weight gain, hormonal imbalance, and worsened mood disorders. Mood, depression, and poor gut health create a vicious circle.

Ironically, the comfort foods we eat when we're feeling emotional actually fuel this fire by feeding the bacteria that make beta-glucuronidase. The relationship between the brain and gut gets even more complicated, though. *Holobiome* is a private research company in Cambridge, Massachusetts. The company is isolating drugs made by the natural flora of the human microbiome. Yes, gut microbes are making drugs inside of you. We'd better be careful what microbes we encourage because those microbes can either poison us or help us. Holobiome researchers found that certain gut bacteria could not be grown without certain neurotransmitters—particularly gamma-aminobutyric acid (GABA), an inhibitory neurotransmitter known for its emotionally calming effects on the body. This means that our mental and hormonal health influences what bacteria grow inside us. Now it gets weirder: the research also uncovered that certain bacteria in healthy guts produce GABA. Healthy gut bacteria naturally produce innate anti-anxiety medication for you, the host. This microbiome-produced GABA relieves the patient while providing a substrate to grow the first bacteria. Yep, that's right; birds of a feather do flock together. It all begins with the gut. Everything from depression and anxiety to diabetes and estrogen-dominance patterns are greatly influenced by the tiny critters living inside of us. *Holobiome* researchers weren't finished, though. The species of bacteria called the Bacteroides group grabbed researchers' attention for its ability to make GABA. Predictably, these "GABA-producing bacteria" were packaged into medications and patented.

Once patented, *Holobiome* then teamed up with other researchers studying brain scans in depressed individuals. The researchers found brain scans showing hyperactivity in the prefrontal cortex, a pattern that has been associated with severe depression. They tested these individuals and found low levels of bacteroides bacterial species in the gut. 17] Resolving depression is directly tied to gut bacteria. An unhealthy gut microbiome is more than weight gain and vanity pounds. There's an undeniable link between an unhealthy gut and mood disorders like depression and anxiety. Certain gut bacteria can release unwanted estrogens and toxins back into the bloodstream. Other gut bacteria manufacture hormones that lower anxiety. And finally, the comfort foods that make us feel good at the moment contribute to gut health imbalances that cause a host of physical and emotional issues.

Case Study: Jack

Meet Jack. Jack is a 50-year-old man with long-standing gut issues and mood imbalances. Jack also has a son named Ben. We meet Ben elsewhere in this book, but we mention him here because the apple does not fall far from the tree. Ben has learning challenges related to

ADHD. With what we've learned above, who wants to guess whether gut health might influence attention? Good guess. Jack came to see us because he had unshakeable exhaustion. When I sat down with Jack for the first visit, he confided in me, telling me that he took ADD drugs (amphetamine-based stimulant meds). These stimulant meds are commonly used to treat ADD and narcolepsy.

> *Dr. Dani's thoughts... Doctors have prescribed amphetamine-based ADHD medications to millions of children due to school performance concerns. Ritalin is **methy**lphenidate, and Adderall is dextro**amphetamine**. 18], 19] Have you ever seen the TV show Breaking Bad where they make methamphetamine? While Ritalin and Adderall can be used somewhat responsibly in certain circumstances, their relation to illegal amphetamines like meth is unavoidable. There are significant costs—physically, mentally, and socially. As parents, we've allowed Big Pharma and doctors to put kids on these stimulant drugs, and now we wonder why methamphetamine abuse is an epidemic.*
>
> *We need to recognize our collective ignorance. Even those who didn't prescribe these meds were complicit—we didn't speak up, organize, or educate others. We act like school boards suddenly overstepped during COVID, but they've been recommending amphetamines as a first-line solution for decades. We all share responsibility. Now, an entire generation faces the fallout—drug-related homelessness, crime, and tragedy. Maybe it's not our kids who need fixing but the institutions who educate them. Good talk.*

Okay, back to Jack. In addition to ADD meds, Jack was also on two different types of acid blockers to keep his "life-long" stomach issues under control. He described his digestive problems as unrelenting, and the antacids were his constant companion. As a child, Jack had been hospitalized for a severe asthma attack. He was 30 pounds overweight and could not seem to lose weight easily. His mood would vacillate between anxious and depressed. Over the years, he'd been on various antidepressants to pull him "out of the hole." Jack was first interested in acupuncture but was willing to find out if I could help him with anything else. Jack was an artist by trade and was the primary parent at home. Between trying to pursue his work and keeping up with the kids, lack of energy was his main complaint. His goal for treatment was the stamina to keep up with his kids while having enough of himself left for his business and household.

When I met Jack, he was pleasant and gentle, but his face looked tired. He was tall and had good posture but dark circles under his eyes. It looked like he hadn't slept well in months. He explained that he was sleeping, but not enough. He explained that without a stimulant medication and lots of caffeine during the day, he wanted to sleep all of the time. Although the stimulants barely got him through the day, he'd have a rebound of energy at night, making it difficult to fall asleep. When he finally slept, he'd never wake feeling rested. Instead, he was stiff and tired, washing stimulant ADD medications down with coffee to prop himself up for the day. We discussed his eating habits and what triggered the acid reflux.

He was reactive to so many foods that I immediately started him on a special anti-inflammatory diet. I ran extensive blood and nutrient panels, looking for clues everywhere. Concurrently, I used the neuro-emotional technique (NET) to clear out somaticized stress patterns in his nervous system. Within a week of being on the anti-inflammatory diet, Jack cut his acid-blocking medication down by over half! Based on Jack's questionnaire responses, I also suspected that Jack had a genetic marker related to DAO (D-Amino Acid Oxidase). The DAO gene produces a specific enzyme that helps break down excess histamine in the body. Histamines are a type of hormone released by the body during allergic reactions and injuries. Histamine is important for immune response and cell repair, but consistently high levels throughout the body can be harmful. Jack was sensitive to histamine-rich foods. Some of these histamine foods are normally considered healthy; fermented foods like sauerkraut and miso may have some benefits but can also raise histamine in certain people. As it turned out for Jack, these common and often healthy foods were a big problem. Chronically high histamine levels are linked to conditions like asthma, eczema, excessive stomach acid production, and mood disorders such as depression and anxiety. As the mystery unraveled, Jack's story started to make sense. He shared more about his lifelong struggle with asthma, recalling childhood attacks so severe that they landed him in the hospital several times.

We continued to refine his diet to reflect his unique situation. We greatly reduced his consumption of histamine foods like pickled, fermented cheese, cured meats, and alcoholic beverages. We moved away from antacids and took steps to raise his stomach acid by supplementing with betaine HCL; please see the chapter on antacids if this part doesn't make sense. Within 3 weeks of making these nutrition shifts and raising his stomach acid levels, he started to feel "human again." He began weaning himself off of the stimulant medications. Around this time, I recommended that he start a series of IV therapy sessions to help replete his B vitamins (antacid meds harm B vitamin absorption). On his IV treatment days, he'd want to sleep for about 24 hours. But after 24 hours, he woke up with high alertness and energy for the next week. This IV therapy strategy worked well to get him out of the hole. Once we got him more stabilized, we modified the IV therapy dosages because the b vitamins became overwhelming. After reevaluating updated lab reports reflecting our changes, we switched him to lower doses of specific vitamins to modulate a biological process called methylation. After a few months of treatment at Terrain Wellness, his lifelong digestive issue was about "60% better." But something was still a bit off. The patient was ecstatic about his improved health but reported that he was still having issues with slow bowel movements and constipation. Hearing his symptoms and knowing his history of chronic antacid use, I tested him for SIBO (small intestinal bacterial overgrowth).

SIBO is an unpleasant condition that can develop in individuals who take acid blockers or have low stomach acid production. Symptoms include nausea, bloating, diarrhea, constipation, abdominal pain, feeling overly full after eating, and malnutrition. Jack tested positive for SIBO, so I prescribed a combination of herbs and the antibiotic Rifaximin. While antibiotics can disrupt gut health, Jack's intestines were already overrun with harmful microbes, making it necessary to start fresh. The treatment stabilized his digestion, but his mood began to fluctuate.

As we know, many neurotransmitters are produced in the gut. A healthy microbiome breaks down proteins into amino acids, which are precursors for neurotransmitters like serotonin, dopamine, and norepinephrine. Long-term gut dysfunction and methylation issues can impair this process, leading to mood instability. After a year of gut restoration and replenishing his nutrition, Jack felt amazing. His energy soared, and he began a daily meditation and fitness routine. With his newfound vitality, he stopped taking stimulant ADD medications.

Although we still fine-tune his treatment based on seasonal needs, Jack now lives medication-free and can do everything he enjoys. He even sent us a photo of his flat stomach—something he's never had before—thanks to his 30-pound fat loss. At 50, his digestion is normal as long as he sticks to foods that work for his body.

Gut Health and Cancer

As we've hinted a few times in this chapter, there's a direct connection between the gut microbiome and cancer. The gut microbiome plays a crucial role in our immune system. A 2017 study found the following,

> *"Although the microbiome influences carcinogenesis through mechanisms independent of inflammation and the immune system, the most recognizable link is between the microbiome and cancer via the immune system, as the resident microbiota plays an essential role in activating, training, and modulating the host immune response."* 20]

The gut is the training ground of your immune system. One of the best ways to increase immune function while decreasing autoimmune conditions is by restoring a proper gut microbiome. While certain genetics and lifestyle habits affect cancer rates, one of the most influential factors in cancer is immune system health. A healthy immune system finds and eliminates would-be cancers before they grow enough to be detectable. A person who lives to a ripe old age and has never had cancer could well have killed off a potential cancer before anyone noticed. Here's a paradox we must understand:

Everyone gets cancer, but not everyone gets cancer.

Healthy people are internally equipped with immune cells called Killer T Cells that fight and destroy developing cancers. For cancer to be a detectable disease, a few things must occur.

Steps in cancerous tumor formation:
1. A cell must mutate and become cancerous.
2. The body's killer (cytotoxic) T- cells fail to kill off the cancer right when it appears.

Cancerous tumors grow because killer T-cells fail to act in time. Human bodies cure cancer every day on their own, without anybody even noticing. Your body already knows what cancer is and why it's bad, this is why your body makes substances like TNF to rid itself of tumors. To understand cancer, we must respect that multiple failures have occurred. Modern medicine focuses on step 1 stuff like genetics and tobacco. Yes, these factors do make cancerous cells more likely to appear. But medicine needs to get more curious about the second part of cancer formation: why didn't the T-cells do their job and zap the cancer when it was a tiny single cell? Part of this may be a perspective and motivation problem. We humans are often only motivated to solve big problems. But in many cases, big problems are just small problems that we ignored. Researchers and pharma companies are driven in a certain direction because people will spend big bucks on big problems. Scientists are trying to slay the cancer monster and reap the hero's reward that comes with it. Less energy is spent on the small, boring stuff that would have stopped the monster from forming. Cancer is a disease that happens when the immune system fails to eliminate abnormal cells, but what causes this? One answer is toxic exposure. Over time, a body depleted of resources cannot support immune function and cell repair. Most people leading fairly normal lives may wonder where these toxins come from. The toxins come from environmental exposures that influence how and what type of bacteria are grown in your body. Imbalanced gut bacteria, like an overgrowth of H. *pylori*, which is connected to SIBO, have been tied to cancer. But we can't just say that H. *pylori* is bad. It's not that simple because H. *pylori*, at a healthy level, is part of the normal flora and prevents asthma, allergies, and possibly multiple sclerosis. 20]

As we learned elsewhere, a small amount of bacteria can be helpful; too much can cause harm or even cancer, and antibiotics damage microbiomes. Studies on mice have shown that antibiotics negatively affect the response of enzymes that control macrophages (the cells that eat invaders) in immune cells and increase markers for heart diseases. 21] Various studies have raised questions about the repeated use of antibiotics with the development of fatal types of breast cancer. 22] Antibiotics might kill off an offending germ, but artificially killing off a germ may change how our immune system responds. While the connection between the development of tumors and cancer has been established, numerous studies have shown that learning to modulate the microbiome could also offer hope in treating cancer. A 2019 study stated,

> *"While research is still at an early stage, there is potential to exploit the microbiome, as modulation may increase the efficacy of treatments, reduce toxicities, and prevent carcinogenesis"* 23]

The above quote is a little complicated, but you must pay attention to the microbiome and prevent carcinogenesis (how cancer starts in the body). Having a healthy gut not only prevents some cancers from developing, but it may also be vital to having medical cancer treatments work properly. For this reason, any chronic disease diagnosis, including cancer, should also guide patients toward whole-food nutrition and gut microbiome repair. Research is ongoing, but a proposed mechanism of how colorectal cancer (CRC) develops involves gut microbiome imbalance. The overgrowth of pathogenic bacteria in the intestines creates decreased oxygen and blood flow. As you recall, specific beneficial bacteria are needed to give proper signaling to the immune system, creating a synergistic "checks and balances" system that eliminates any tumor growth that may occur.

Low blood flow, lack of oxygen in the tissues, and a down-regulation of immune response may partly cause CRC to develop. Overpopulation of certain bacteria shutting off parts of our immune system sets the stage for cancer and other diseases. Cancerous tumors seem to develop where specific bacteria also thrive. Tumor growth creates a vicious circle where the area of the body is even more devoid of proper blood flow and oxygen. This environment encourages biofilms made of bacterial colonies that may mask the cancer from the immune system. A biofilm is a slimy layer of germs that sticks to a surface.

Bacterial biofilms create a camouflage where the immune system is so distracted by all the bacteria that it misses something worse: cancer.

In this toxic bacterial environment, cancer continues to develop. Bacteria like *Bacteroides fragilis*, a gram-negative anaerobic bacterium, are thought to play a significant role in the development of colorectal cancer (CRC) 24]. Research has shown a close link between *Bacteroides fragilis* and cancer. Some may be tempted to think of simple solutions, like taking drugs to eliminate the harmful bacteria. But is it really that easy?

Take H. *pylori*, for example. While antibiotics can eradicate it, we must consider the protective qualities of H. *pylori* and the collateral damage caused by such aggressive treatments. Antibiotics don't just eliminate H. *pylori*—they also wipe out beneficial, lesser-known species of bacteria vital for healthy bodily function.

It's time to end the war on germs. These microorganisms live inside us, and we must learn to coexist with them. By shifting our approach toward peaceful coexistence with microbes, we can unlock ways for our bodies to benefit from the protection that bacteria, viruses, and fungi provide. The gut microbiome is a vast topic, so we'll continue this discussion in the following chapters.

TLDR: Too Long Didn't Read

The types, ratios, and quantities of microorganisms living inside you greatly impact your health. Although a healthy adult human has trillions of microbes, most doctors only tell you to eat yogurt and take a probiotic. But, probiotics and yogurt can't fully change the fact that antibiotics and eating the standard American diet wreaks havoc on our gut microbiome. Gut health affects everything from your mood and hormone levels to the development of cancer and autoimmune conditions. We can't be healthy until we learn to live at peace with the trillions of germs inside each of us.

Chapter 6
Microbiome 201

"He had swept it out of existence, as it seemed, without any provocation, as a boy might crush an ant hill, in the mere wantonness of power." – H.G. Wells (The War of the Worlds) 1]

In the last chapter, we began to explore a few of the complexities that tie our fates together with microbes. We need them. There are trillions of microbes living inside us. Can we kill off a few billion here and there without consequence? Until the modern era, we didn't even know what germs were. Then, we woke up to the shock of our lives. Tiny, invisible invaders were responsible for deadly infections killing people. The solution was simple; strike first and strike hard. Kill the germs before they kill us. Industrial capability kicked in with disinfectants and antibiotics, and a kind of *War of The Worlds* ensued where germs were mass exterminated with no questions asked. To be sure, previously fatal infections were solved, and the miracle of modern medicine, germ theory, was born.

What's Wrong with Germ Theory?

Germ Theory proposes that microorganisms, known as pathogens, are a direct cause of disease. While this is true for many, but not all, diseases, it doesn't offer a complete explanation. For example, both sick and healthy people are exposed to the same germs—so why does one person get sick and the other doesn't? Germ Theory is factually correct, but it's incomplete.

We need more than just Germ Theory to explain this. Moreover, the theory's focus on fighting germs can be questioned. Is it better to eliminate all germs from our environment, or is it more beneficial to focus on building a body that is healthy enough to resist the harm germs cause? Germ Theory emphasizes waging war on microbes, but what are the consequences of this approach? In a conventional war, the battlefield becomes a wasteland—if our bodies are the battlefield, we risk damaging ourselves in the process. If we think objectively, there might be times when *killing the bad guy* causes more harm than benefit.

Microbes are essential for various digestive, hormonal, and immune processes in the body. While it's true that some microbes can make us sick, it's equally true that we need them to survive. This complexity shows that Germ Theory is an overly simplistic view, treating microbes as generally harmful while ignoring the vital role of beneficial microbes.

The adoption of Germ Theory has evolved into a philosophy with its own goals and values. While it's based on observable facts—germs are involved in many disease processes—it overlooks the larger picture. Having an infection does mean harmful microbes are replicating in the body, but what other factors contribute to the illness? Germ Theory's conclusion that killing germs is always the best way to fight disease is debatable, and many observable facts challenge this notion.

Conditions necessary for infection:

1. Microbial exposure
2. Susceptible host

Germ theory wants to solve sickness by getting rid of condition 1, microbial exposure. Attacking condition 1 works in emergencies, but germs are everywhere, and we need microbes to live. In our day-to-day lives, it's probably a better plan to focus on condition 2: not being susceptible hosts. After decades of industrialized warfare against germs, medicine realized that some so-called germs help us digest food. To be clear, the war on germs didn't stop. But big medicine did start telling patients to eat some yogurt to replenish the good microbes. To this day, the war on germs continues. Antimicrobial soaps fly off the shelves and we're still making new antibiotics despite evidence that our war against the germs is a losing battle. We're fighting the germs even though the smartest people in the room know that our efforts will result in creating more super-bugs for tomorrow. This futile process would be comical if it wasn't also terrifying.

The process of learning about microbes is interesting.
1. Germs exist, and they can kill us!
2. But— not if we kill the germs first.
3. Germs evolve and fight back when we kill them.
4. Wait, some "germs" are on our side!?!?
5. Germs and people have been cohabitating for centuries, and we must learn to live at peace with them.

The idea that germs exist and can cause illness, was revolutionary for its time. Germ Theory is not wrong per se, but the conclusions drawn from it are not always wise. The idea began with factually correct scientific observations, but the decisions made based on the observations are still up for debate. Here are some key scientific observations about illness:
1. Bacterial overgrowth is directly tied to many illnesses.
2. Medical treatments that kill off bacterial overgrowth can resolve these illnesses.

However, we often build debatable opinions around these facts. In modern culture, we unconsciously blend fact with opinion. Here's where we begin forming opinions based on the facts mentioned above:

Germ Theory says:
>*Bacteria cause disease*

My response:
>*Sort of. But supposedly bad bacteria also live inside healthy people too.*

Germ Theory says:
>*I can avoid illness by killing off all germs and vigilantly avoiding exposure.*

My response:
>*Yes and no. While some microbes are genuinely harmful, avoiding all germs can actually weaken the immune system by preventing it from strengthening over time.*

The common US practice is to protect children from household germs by regularly disinfecting the home, while artificially exposing our kids to quasi-pathogens (vaccines). While many doctors take this approach, it could give childrens' immune systems an unrealistic view of environmental threats. We're teaching young immune systems that deadly viruses (vaccines) are everywhere, but germs on the kitchen floor are rare. We don't yet know the potential long-term effects of this skewed immunological perspective.

Germ theory says:
> *Antibacterial soaps, disinfectants, and medications are the primary defense against germs*

My response:
> *Mostly not true. Sure, it's smart to be extra cautious in places like hospitals, homeless camps, open sewers, or around used needles and garbage dumps— these places carry some really dangerous pathogens. But it's actually normal and healthy for our bodies to be exposed to germs every day. Regular exposure helps train our immune system. On the flip side, if we go overboard with cleaning, we can end up leaving our immune systems unprepared when we do come across something harmful.*

Since germs are everywhere, the best defense is to live a healthy lifestyle encouraging a robust and balanced microbiome. Returning to our two conditions for infection, microbial exposure, and susceptible host, the better long-term solution is to make oneself more resilient. In this way, you're not a susceptible host. Sure, take extra precautions when you're in a high-risk environment. But remember that a balanced microbiome will naturally repel infection. Yesterday's cultures had rituals and spiritual explanations for disease. Today, science claims to have left religion behind; many people today believe that spiritual explanations are useless or even harmful traditions that we cling to for comfort. And yet, germ theory's followers believe in rituals, too. Using antibacterial soap everywhere in the home is a ritual to make us feel good. For most households, antibacterial soap does not lower your chances of getting sick. What about society's lingering obsession with wearing face masks in public?

I'd bet that anyone still wearing a mask years later probably also got multiple doses of the vaccine that was supposed to stop the spread, prevent infection, and keep people from getting seriously ill. During COVID, a lot of the medical practices started to look pretty ridiculous. If the vaccines really worked as promised, why are people still masking? The whole mask and vaccine thing doesn't really make sense anymore. But, the medical establishment will never admit they were wrong because it would mean that they got fooled while also leading others astray.

"The authors find that infection with SARS-CoV-2 occurred in 1.8% of the participants in the treated group (recommended masks for three hours per day) versus 2.1% of the participants in the control group. A difference of about 17% over 60 days appears statistically insignificant." 4]

In the citation above, the authors found a 17% improvement in outcomes from wearing masks. On the surface, this sounds like a significant difference. But what they're really talking about is a reduction from 2.1% to 1.8%. If doctors were upfront about the real data—telling people that wearing an uncomfortable mask in public only reduced their chances of getting COVID from 2.1% to 1.8%, would entire regions have enforced strict mask mandates? As the quote points out, the difference is statistically insignificant. The harsh truth is that both COVID vaccines and masks failed to stop the spread. Sure, we can argue that COVID could have been worse without the vaccines, but such "what if" arguments aren't scientific. The vaccine didn't stop the spread. Mask mandates didn't stop it either. Even those who supported the masks and vaccines could see through the so-called science if they were paying attention. Rachel Gutman-Wei put it this way in her article in *The Atlantic*, published in February 2022:

"As of March 1, District residents will need to cover up in order to attend school, go to a library, or ride in a taxi. But gyms, sports arenas, concert venues, and houses of worship—you know, all the places where people like to breathe hard or sing and shout in close proximity—will be facial free-for-alls... Good luck complying in a restaurant, bar, or airport food court. Pointing out the logical flaws in mask mandates is easy." 5]

We had to mask up in a library, but not at a sports arena. The illogical COVID pandemic response proves that medicine is quickly abandoning reason in favor of rituals that are logically flawed to their core. Other rituals within modern healthcare are harder to spot, though. We're commonly told that eating probiotic pills or yogurt will forgive our use of antibiotics and processed foods. Germ theory was a step forward in our understanding, but it's not the final step in wisdom.

Making germ theory the highest authority leads us to kill off good bugs if it means taking out bad bugs, too. The basic facts that germ theory recognized were revolutionary for the time, but our understanding has moved past it in fundamental ways. Please don't misunderstand me, Germ Theory has helped us cure and understand many diseases. However, taking the idea too far has led us to many other problems. There is a growing link between autoimmune conditions and the types and quantity of gut microbes present. Germ theory's focus on killing microbes leads us to gut microbe imbalances that can have real-world health consequences that we'll explore now.

Bacterially damaged gut linings let components of poop into your bloodstream.

- Dr. Danielle Lockwood

Gut Health & Autoimmune Conditions

In my clinical practice of primary care medicine, I repeatedly bang my head against an undeniable truth. You can't reverse an autoimmune process until you have a healthy gut. A healthy gut is one where the human body works in harmony with the bacteria and fungi living inside of us. One study found that certain mice get autoimmune diseases when exposed to certain bacteria. Point blank: scientists injected the bacteria E. *gallinarum* into mice and an autoimmune process was triggered. How did the bacteria create an autoimmune condition? This specific bacteria breaks down gut lining, allowing partially digested food waste into the animal's bloodstream.

Bacterially-damaged gut linings let components of poop into the bloodstream. From there, these waste products hit detoxification organs like the liver, and your body spontaneously becomes allergic to itself. These same researchers then looked at liver biopsies of humans who had known autoimmune diseases such as lupus erythematosus and found that some of them did indeed have *E. gallinarum* in the samples. 6] A 2018 study in the *Expert Review on Gastrointestinal Hepatology* wrote,

"Many studies have shown the relationship between autoimmune diseases and the gut microbiome in humans: those with autoimmune conditions display gut microbiome dysbiosis." 7]

Dysbiosis occurs when there's an overgrowth of harmful bacteria or a shortage of beneficial bacteria in the gut, leading to an imbalance that's closely linked to autoimmune conditions. In the previous chapter, we saw how antibiotics and junk food can damage the gut microbiome. Now, we're learning that this damage is a major contributor to autoimmune disease. Although modern medicine is aware of this, the current standard of care doesn't fully reflect this reality. If you visit a doctor for an autoimmune condition, you'll likely hear a brief explanation that the immune system is simply overactive and attacking itself because of bad luck or genetic factors. The typical solution? Medications to suppress the immune system. But will suppressing the immune system restore a healthy gut microbiome? Will it prevent food waste from passing through a damaged intestinal lining?

Immunosuppressive drugs are proverbial band-aids that do nothing to solve gaping wounds. Medicine's surface-level thinking fails to repair the underlying cause of the autoimmune disease. In my practice, I started getting results for patients when I helped them restore overall balance in their whole body. With balance restored, autoimmune disease often simply resolves itself. Even with my background in acupuncture and natural medicine, I had a hard time believing that autoimmune disease was reversible until I saw it myself. Don't get me wrong—resolving these issues requires a team approach, several months of effort, and properly identifying what's causing the immune system to react this way.

Even still, it's very possible to see all signs of autoimmune diseases go into remission. Some autoimmune diseases are more insidious than others. Sometimes, the damage from autoimmune conditions and the drugs used to treat them may not fully disappear. Some patients already have irreversible side effects from the immunosuppressive drugs they've been prescribed. For other patients, full recovery is achieved with little to no long-term effects. The question remains: are the treatment strategies in conventional medicine resolving autoimmune disease, or do they just get people on yet another drug that they must keep taking? Would Big Pharma rather have people not need medicine, or have a population ridden with autoimmune diseases that's dependent on expensive pharmaceuticals? Of course, sickness is good for business. But this doesn't mean a conspiracy theory per se. It just means that more money and research are directed toward expensive drugs and less toward prevention.

A 2012 publication from the *Indian Journal of Pharmacology Society* corroborates this reality. 8] The publication highlighted that, despite advancements in pharmaceutical drugs "treating" autoimmune disease, no drug on the market has been able to put autoimmune disease into remission. Pharma makes more money on people who continually need a drug rather than a one-time cure. At the time of the study, autoimmune was the 10th most common cause of death in developing countries. This study categorizes the two current philosophies on treating autoimmune diseases.

Conventional Treatment of systemic autoimmune diseases (SAIDs):
1. Symptomatic or replacement therapy
2. Immunosuppressive or immunomodulatory therapy 8]

An example of the first strategy is how most doctors treat thyroid diseases. The doctor sees that the thyroid is not working so they simply up the dose of thyroid drugs. Or, the thyroid is over-producing, so they suppress the thyroid using different drugs. Don't get me wrong; there's a time and place to prescribe thyroid medications. But I don't use thyroid drugs for every thyroid problem. These medications are there to prevent thyroid collapse. Importantly, I'm also guiding my patients to resolve the underlying issues of autoimmune disease.

The second conventional strategy is how most doctors treat Crohn's' disease, ulcerative colitis, psoriasis, multiple sclerosis, asthma, and eczema. These doctors suppress the immune system so it stops attacking the body. Autoimmune diseases are related to infection and exposure to toxins. Immunosuppressive drugs are symptom management and don't address anything about why a person is sick. Managing symptoms isn't good enough. Yes, the short-term use of steroid drugs is warranted in severe reactions and temporary situations. This is especially true in life-threatening inflammatory attacks such as anaphylaxis. But using immunosuppression as a long-term treatment is lazy. It takes patience, deep investigation, and a rich understanding of the nature of autoimmune diseases that most conventional doctors don't have time for.

Pressured by insurance companies, supervisors, and the structure of the hospital system, most doctors lean on predefined protocols that make up a generic standard of care. Patients given the generic 'standard of care' feel somewhat better for a while but are left dependent on a drug to keep masking their continued problem. Immunosuppression doesn't really work that well, though. It's time for doctors to do better. Ironically, patients on immunosuppressive therapy have a higher risk of developing another autoimmune disease. In general, a person with one autoimmune disease is 30% more likely to have multiple autoimmune diseases.

At best, immunosuppressive agents temporarily allow us to ignore the problem; at worst, we may even be adding fuel to the already raging autoimmune fire. 9] Like germ theory, autoimmune treatment seeks to fight an adversary. Let's change the focus. We must create an internal body state that no longer encourages autoimmune patterns. Modern lifestyles are full of pesticides, fungicides, artificial dyes, chemicals from plastics, antibiotics, antacids, and pain medications. These modern inventions are harmful to the gut. Even if you don't directly use pesticides and other chemicals, they're being used all around you. Most people living modern lifestyles are in cities and suburbs, and those who eat processed foods and have taken medications are at high risk of poor gut health. This poor gut health leads to inflamed intestinal linings that allow waste products and even pathogenic bacteria from the gut into the bloodstream. This mechanism of action is called a leaky gut. As internal organs are exposed to contamination from the intestines, the results are an autoimmune reaction.

Certain food debris leaking from the digestive tract into the bloodstream can interfere with receptors in the body, causing the body to interpret its own cells as harmful. This process leads to inflammatory autoimmune reactions. So, what types of foods are associated with this reaction? We don't always know exactly what's doing it, but genetically modified foods and heavily treated crops like corn, wheat, soy, seed oils, and processed packaged foods are harmful to gut health. What we don't know fully is how much these foods are inherently inflammatory. Or, is the harm more related to how Big Ag and Big Food process these substances? The answer may be some of both. In any event, the link between food ingredients and autoimmune conditions is strong.

Celiac disease is a common autoimmune condition where people react to a wheat protein called gluten. Exposure to gluten causes people with celiac disease to have an impaired intestinal lining. This compromised intestinal wall is believed to allow other allergens into the bloodstream. Not surprisingly, a study found that people with celiac disease had a higher incidence of developing diabetes and thyroid diseases. This link suggests that celiac disease shares a common developmental pathway with other autoimmune diseases. 10] Research has shown that the presence of certain gut bacteria can induce an TH17, an inflammatory cytokine. TH17 modulates inflammation in our mucosal linings throughout our digestive tract. Increased TH17 has been associated with autoimmune disease. 10] Gut health is directly related to autoimmune conditions.

Hunter-gatherers and the Digital Age

For thousands of years, humans lived in small tribes of hunter-gatherer groups. When we think of hunter-gatherers, we picture foraging for nuts and seeds, gathering small grass seeds, and hunting animals. But it's important to also realize that primitive human societies lived in every climate. Their cultures and practices were each well-adapted to their unique environments. From what scientists can piece together, these pre-modern societies did not get autoimmune disease. One study conducted on the hunter-gatherer Hadza tribe of Tanzania showed a diverse microbiome makeup different from what is seen in modern diets. 11] Their lifestyles also lack time indoors, smog, antibiotics, chemical soaps, pesticides, other medications, and electromagnetic radiation from electrical devices.

We may not know all the factors at play, but we do know this tribe thrives on unrefined, seasonal foods and daily movement. For a deeper dive into the impact of modern technology on our health, I highly recommend *A Hunter-Gatherer's Guide to the 21st Century* by Dr. Bret Weinstein and Dr. Heather Heying. The book explores how our modern lifestyle conflicts with our natural biology, leading to chronic diseases and mental health issues, and offers practical advice on aligning our lives with our innate needs. It's an eye-opening read that challenges our assumptions about progress. 12]

Collectively, we naively assume that we can take humans and alter everything about their food, lifestyle, and surroundings without unintended consequences. Let's examine some consequences now. In the research studies mentioned above, bacteria from the groups Firmicutes and Bacteroidetes dominated the stool samples from the Hadza tribe, in contrast to those from the city-dwelling cohort they were compared with.

Researchers also measured Short Chain Fatty Acid (SCFA) levels. SCFAs are beneficial substances made by "good bacteria" inside the body. SCFAs are important in regulating the immune system and help with protection against germs. That's not all. SCFAs also improve nutrient absorption. The research found higher levels of SCFAs in the Hadza tribal members compared to city dwellers. 11] Higher SCFA means increases nutrient absorption and boosts the immune system. Emerging research found spore probiotics in the stools of hunter-gatherer tribes. These spore-based probiotics come from native soils that haven't been treated with industrial pesticides and fertilizers.

Since these spore probiotics live out in natural soil, they've been consumed by humans and animals for ages. These spores act as seeds that may replant healthy gut bacteria. A 2017 randomized and placebo-controlled study published in the *World Journal of Gastrointestinal Pathophysiology* found that spore probiotics helped people resist endotoxins produced by harmful bacteria. The research also showed that spore probiotics were associated with gut lining repair. These probiotics can get past the acid of the stomach into the intestines. Once there, they help regulate gut PH and promote the production of SCFAs. 13]

Furthermore, spore probiotics lower triglycerides within 90 days of use. 14] Some spore probiotics influence the immune system in other ways. It turns out that many probiotics, and especially spore-based probiotics such as Bacillus subtilis activate an area of the immune system called Gut Associated Lymphoid Tissue (GALT). GALT is made up of clusters of immune cells called Peyer's patches that are arranged in a network. The GALT makes up over 70% of total immune function. Most of the immune system is in the gut. The gut microbiome is a primary influencer of immune system health. Our modern lifestyles negatively affect gut health, which in turn negatively affects our immune systems. Yet again, we see a vicious circle emerge surrounding gut health, diet, and pharmaceuticals. But we're not done yet; the body of evidence tying gut microbes to immune health is deep and compelling. Research published in 2008 found that specific spore probiotics could activate toll-like receptors and antigen-presenting cells in the body. These specific signaling molecules train our immune system to fight infection and eliminate foreign growth and tumors in the body. Spore probiotics also increase T-cell and B-cell response and increase long-term adaptive immunity (14). Restoring proper gut health is an important and overlooked step in treating disease. Do scientists need to make new and better drugs? Or, do we need to simply reclaim the good practices that we've since left behind?

The Western Diet is pornography for your tastebuds – Richard Lockwood

Gut Health and The Western Diet

While hunter-gatherer diets varied, things like vegetables, nuts, seeds, meat, low sugar, and low carbohydrate eating methods were nonetheless common. Also common was time outdoors in nature. People (and the microbes living inside those people) had generations to acclimate to their unique flora and fauna. Now, all of a sudden, we're all eating the Western Diet with its processed foods. What's the Western Diet? It's anything at McDonalds. It's also anything found in the snack aisle of your grocery store: macaroni and cheese, crackers and chips, pasta, most commercial breads and pastries, breakfast cereals, soda pop, juice boxes. Even the supposedly healthy options of the foods above are still processed foods. What's always surprised me is just how accepted and habitual these junk foods have become in our society. When we eat, we're not just feeding ourselves. We're also feeding the trillions of gut microbes living inside of us. Bad food means the bad germs inside of us get stronger. Listen, I like chocolate here and there. But even though I eat it sparingly, there's an emotional component to it. I think it's okay to have some cake on your birthday and have some pie on Thanksgiving. But we can't make these sweet treats part of our daily routines and expect to be healthy.

You need to eat a lot less processed food. Period. Start by eliminating the low-quality, habitual ones like soda pop and low-quality snacks. If you really need to, make your treats rare and of high quality so it feels special. Above all, avoid using food to numb your feelings or pass the time. Bored, mindless eating, and eating to manage emotion are both bad ideas. Be mindful, savor each bite with gratitude, and set it aside before you're full. Work on your intimate relationships, read the book called *Attached* by Dr. Amir Levine, and learn how you emotionally connect with others. 15]

We are emotional creatures, and healing around food will also touch on relationships, love, desire, fear, and need. Get right with God. It seems cliché or like we've moved beyond ideas about God, but our deteriorating physical health is a sign that we've forgotten some basic truths. Sure, many of us are spiritual, but we've left behind the difficult spiritual work of repentance and forgiving others. Repentance is simply admitting that you were wrong and asking God to help you do better. Forgiving others means you make a conscious decision to rip up and throw away all of the mental *I-Owe-You's* from all the times you've been cheated, lied to, wronged, abused, or mistreated. No matter what you believe about God, even if you think God isn't real, if you submit to the process with an open heart, truly repent, ask for help, and forgive others, you'll see your health and well-being improve over time. Living in unforgiveness or bitterness, or refusing to repent, causes things like food, sex, drugs, social media, and other comforts to become false gods that slowly harm us. Healing our relationship with food may be the single most important thing we can do for our gut health. We must get right with food. For me, there's no getting right with food without getting right with God. While a number of my readers find Christian morality very uncomfortable, now it's time for all of the Christians to get uncomfortable.

Here's an analogy that may hurt, but go with me for a minute. If you let it become habitual, junk food can become pornography for your taste buds. This isn't just my idea; medical research shows numerous patterns in the parts of our brains that desire food, sex, and emotional intimacy. 16] We even have entire TV channels, websites, magazines, and social media influencers devoted to watching other people make and eat food! I've even heard people use the phrase *food porn* to describe the common practice of sharing pictures of decadent meals with their friends.

Food and sexual reproduction are our two strongest human needs. We must get this right, or we'll have very deep-seated issues. Junk food and pornography are both cheap, easy, and feel good at the moment. For both food and sex, there's big money in exploiting these human needs in unhealthy ways. Out in the world, we see throngs of people leading sexually-unfulfilled lives who have turned to food to cope with loneliness. Think about it: fast food chains and big food companies make billions exploiting people's needs in a harmful way. How many lives have McDonalds and Coca-Cola ruined? Illegal drugs, alcohol abuse, and illicit sex are generally frowned upon in Christian churches across America. But, food addiction is alive and well in the church despite the fact that the Bible warns that making the stomach into a god leads to spiritual and physical destruction. 17]

Illegal drugs also tap into these deep human needs, but drugs are expensive and illegal, while sweet treats are cheap and acceptable in polite society. Food, drugs, and porn all leave us feeling lonely, empty, unhealthy, and perhaps shameful. Pornography exploits our deep desires and fills them in a way that leaves us unhealthy, unfulfilled, and lonely.

Worst of all, pornography scratches the itch without fulfilling our deep purpose for building intimacy, trust, and a loving family that will be meaningful and supportive.

In the same way, the Western Diet feels good in the moment, but over time, our bodies become poisoned and incapable of reaching their true potential. We don't usually think of it this way, but things like obesity, diabetes, heart disease, and autoimmune conditions rob us of decades of joy. Worse still, the preventable diseases associated with the Western Diet mean that we'll never reach our true life potential. Sounds a bit like porn or illegal drugs, doesn't it? Have a slice of cake on your birthday, but beware: processed foods can become porn for your taste buds. These foods are habit-forming, addictive, and harmful.

A quick stroll down the snack food aisle might temporarily satisfy a craving, but it won't truly fulfill you. Every day, I meet people who would never allow something like pornography in their homes, yet they feed their kids a standard Western Diet. Of course, occasional treats and celebratory foods can be fun and uplifting—I'm not saying, "Don't enjoy life." But, these foods should be enjoyed in the right context as treats, not as a lifestyle. Just like with sex, celebratory foods can become addictive and harmful if used out of context. On the other hand, healthy, nourishing foods are more like finding a meaningful relationship—they take effort, and they don't offer instant gratification. Healthy foods require more time to prepare and aren't as easy to come by in our fast-paced, convenience-driven world. Eating well demands self-discipline and planning ahead. Vegetables and naturally raised meats might not satisfy our cravings right away, but taking the harder path leads to long-term fulfillment in both food and life. In times of plenty, spiritually minded people have temporarily abstained from food as a way to restore spiritual sensitivity to God. Fasting—abstaining from food—has been a tradition for thousands of years. True fasting involves a deeper sacrifice, not just giving up habits like temporarily smoking or alcohol for Lent. It's about denying something essential to create space for reflection and lasting change.

Food is Emotional

As in relationships, our food choices are also deeply tied to our emotional and spiritual maturity. Sure, just eat healthy foods in proper proportions to your needs. Simple, right? Not so much. Like resolving a pattern of broken or non-existent relationships, healing our relationship with food will take dedication, perhaps professional therapy, and a willingness to question lifelong ideas and behavior patterns. In the Bible, Jesus says that we need to spiritually die or cut off certain parts of ourselves in order to be blessed. 18] According to Jesus, hanging onto our negative or harmful patterns leads us to death. He told people an analogy, saying it was better to cut your own arm off and be saved rather than die with our arms attached.

Don't actually cut your arm off. But be willing to periodically cut off something in your life that has become harmful. Similarly, eastern mystical traditions of meditation also involve a surrender where we set aside or "die to" our need for constant inner chatter and desire for outside stimulation. Life experience and what I've seen in my medical practice both prove that we can't transform our food choices (or our relationships) using surface-level tactics.

There's also a symbolic death in facing uncomfortable feelings and having hard conversations. The person we were yesterday was wrong about some things. Admitting that fact and symbolically dying to it guides us toward a better future. Many times, we're not even aware of our deeply held beliefs, but these secret beliefs end up controlling us. An example might be, "Everyone leaves me, but chocolate is always there." My husband even once saw a meme that said, "Pizza is my boyfriend." All jokes aside, food is deeply tied to our intimate desires.

Most addiction recovery programs involve admitting when we're wrong, forgiving others even if they don't deserve it, and asking God to help us. These programs work because they recognize that repentance, forgiveness, and asking God for help are fundamental laws of the universe. I know I'm talking a lot about emotional health and spirituality here when the topic is gut health. There is a connection though, our emotional and spiritual state is a primary driver in the food choices we make. In turn, food choices are the primary factor in our gut microbiome. Sure, there are also medications and environmental factors, but food is still the biggest thing we can control every day.

Here's the pattern:
- Emotional/Spiritual Health → Food Choices
- Food choices → Gut Microbiome
- Gut Microbiome → Whole Body Health

We'll explore the emotional and spiritual aspects of food later, but for now, let's focus on the research about the gut microbiome. Studies show that when humans shift from traditional diets to the processed foods of the Western Diet, there's a noticeable decline in beneficial spore-type bacteria in the gut. In mice fed a Western Diet high in processed ingredients—like sugars, refined carbs, hydrogenated oils, processed meats, and dairy—researchers found an increase in Bacilli (bad bacteria) and a decrease in Bacteroides (good bacteria). These mice also gained significant fat. Later in this book, we'll learn that the body stores excess fat to help trap and isolate toxins, reducing the load on the liver.

Gout & Your Gut

Let's talk about gout for a bit. Uric acid is one toxic byproduct that gets stored inside body fat. Having too much uric acid would make weight gain advantageous to the body trying to bind up this toxin. For this reason, obesity may be a last-ditch defense mechanism that the body uses against gout because it provides a way to safely store uric acid that it can't get rid of. Excessive uric acid in the body primarily results in Gout, a disease where painful uric acid crystals form in the joints. [20] Uric acid may also be involved in other serious health conditions. Multiple Sclerosis (MS) is a degenerative neurological disorder. One study showed that patients with MS often have gout, too. Uric acid is a byproduct from the breakdown of corn syrup, hydrogenated oils/trans fats, processed meats, refined sugar, and alcohol. Colloquially, gout is sometimes referred to as the *Disease of Kings* because only wealthy nobles could afford the opulence associated with heavy alcohol use and junk food.

Today, processed foods and alcohol are cheap and widely available. High levels of uric acid in the blood can signal that the kidneys are struggling to filter properly, which can lead to gout, kidney disease, cancer, heart disease, and high blood pressure. Interestingly, higher uric acid levels and increased incidents of gout have been observed in patients with rheumatoid arthritis three months after starting treatment with TNF inhibitor drugs. 21] Paradoxically, however, uric acid is also an antioxidant. This means that, like everything else, balance is key.

In my clinical practice, when I see high levels of uric acid in the body, it's a biological cry for help. Excess uric acid is the body sounding an urgent alarm to lower inflammation and increase detoxification immediately. In this analogy, gout is an urgent warning that the hypothetical building (your body) will soon be engulfed in flames. Uric acid plays a role in mediating proper immune response. The presence of uric acid crystals in the body triggers an inflammatory immune response similar to when a bacteria invades a cell. 20] Gout can contribute to inflammatory and autoimmune conditions, particularly ones affecting joints. One major way to quickly break this inflammatory autoimmune chain reaction is to improve gut health. The research is clear: allowing certain healthy probiotics to increase in the gut reduces autoimmune symptoms. 22]

Scientists have linked gut imbalances to the following autoimmune diseases 23]:

- Rheumatoid arthritis
- Type 1 diabetes
- Lupus erythematosus
- Multiple sclerosis
- Hashimoto's thyroiditis
- Crohn's disease
- Ulcerative colitis

The trajectory of the research is clear: the causal link between poor gut health and autoimmune conditions has been established. I would go one step further and argue that improving gut health will make a difference for you no matter what autoimmune or inflammatory condition(s) you already have or have risk factors for. We've gone deep on gut health in these last two chapters, but there's still more left to uncover. Join me in the next chapter, where we'll peel off one more layer of this fascinating onion. If your care provider never told you how complex gut health is, it may be time to fire your doctor.

TLDR: Too Long Didn't Read

Germ theory: This school of thought says that germs are everywhere, and we need to kill the germs before they kill us. I counter that germ theory may be taking the above conclusion too far. Indeed, germs are everywhere, and they can and will make you sick. A simpler alternative is that since germs are a fact of life, we need to learn how to live in a world of germs. Killing all germs all the time doesn't work. Both sick and non-sick people are exposed to germs every day. The better way is to avoid the worst germs while strengthening yourself so normal germs won't hurt you.

Western Diet: The Western Diet is the default way that most Americans eat: processed foods, fried foods, lots of carbohydrates, fast foods, sugar, corn syrup, artificial sweeteners, preservatives, etc. The standard Western Diet is killing us because these ingredients cause us to have more bad gut bacteria. Heart disease, diabetes, autoimmune conditions and so much more are all tied to processed foods and the gut bacteria that come with that diet.

Emotional eating: Why can't we quit the basic Western Diet? We all know fast food and sugar are bad for us, but most of the country is still eating it regularly. The answer is that food is deeply tied to our emotions and motivation. Making the right choices is hard because what feels good now feels bad in the long run. Many of us are susceptible to getting stuck in addictive spirals involving food. The way out is to be deeply honest about our emotional pain and take ownership of our negative patterns.

If these emotional eating patterns become food addictions, then physical changes will not be enough. Spiritual healing from addiction comes through repenting of our mistakes and confessing things we may regret, forgiving others so we let go of bitterness, and asking God to help us be transformed to live better. Most addiction recovery programs involve admitting when we're wrong, forgiving others even if they don't deserve it, and asking God to help us. These programs work because they recognize that repentance, forgiveness, and asking God for help are fundamental laws of the universe.

Autoimmune and inflammatory conditions: Poor diet is more than unwanted weight gain. Our food choices change our gut bacteria, creating a pattern of inflammation, hormone imbalance, mood disorders like depression, and autoimmune conditions. We need to break this vicious circle by improving our gut health and transforming our food choices.

Chapter 7
Microbiome 301

"All disease begins in the gut." -Hippocrates

We're spending a lot of time on the gut for a reason. Digestive health is the foundation upon which we build everything. If we get gut health wrong, nothing will be right. In this chapter, we've got some serious work ahead of us. First, we need to do some mental exercises to get us ready to face some hard truths. Then, we'll review real-world examples of how gut health influenced COVID-19 outcomes. Lastly, I'll show you how to fix our broken health from the ground up. Or should I say: from the gut up? No matter what future "pandemics" come your way, you'll be harder to kill if you go with your gut.

In the first days of the COVID-19 pandemic, a few brave doctors and nurses blew the whistle that physical health greatly improved outcomes. The best defense against any disease is to be healthy. This has always been true. Medications and hospitals are not the foundation of physical health; living a healthy lifestyle is the foundation. Even if everything goes right (which it never does), drugs, vaccines, and lockdowns can never replace an active lifestyle supported by nourishing foods. Period. Unfortunately, whistleblowers were banned from social media, and the government largely ignored the relationship between personal health and your risk of dying from COVID. The news focused on ventilators, not weight loss. Healthcare officials should have stressed the importance of basic health and wellness fundamentals. Ventilators, vaccines, and Remdesivir lead to billions in pharma and hospital revenue; broccoli and taking a walk outside are almost free. Is it surprising what treatments they wanted to focus on? Hospitals and Public health leaders should have been shouting on the hilltops for the population to get healthy immediately. What's this book called again? Oh, that's right, "Fire Your Doctor."

Health officials deemed COVID serious enough to shut down businesses and restrict freedoms, yet highlighting the link between diabetes, obesity, and COVID risk was avoided for fear of "fat-shaming." While mocking others is wrong and hurtful, in a free society, people have the right to express their views—even if we don't always agree. As adults, we must take responsibility for our health and actions. Sometimes the truth is uncomfortable, but it's necessary for growth. If we're too unwilling to hear the truth, we're tacitly demanding that everyone lie to us.

Like most women, I'm sensitive about my body. God just made me this way, and I accept it. But I'm also strong enough to hear hard truths. Sure, it might hurt my feelings, but being a strong leader means I care more about the truth and doing what's right. You can't be a leader and be self-focused. My purpose in life is more important than my feelings. I'd rather feel embarrassed than leave my husband without a wife, my children without a mother, and my patients without the healthcare they need. Standing in the fire of hard truths forces me to be strong in my faith in God, and it solidifies my commitment to my purpose. Open up the closet and take out your big-kid pants (or, if you're my husband, the pants are in a pile in the corner); one leg, two legs, now look in the mirror and repeat after me:

"I am responsible for my own health. Nobody cares as much about my health as I do. If I won't fight for my health, nobody else will. Even if it's not my fault, I take responsibility anyway."

Okay, good talk.

Our society is mad at the government for not being honest. But millions of Americans are also saying, don't you dare hurt my feelings! The authorities decided that we were all too fragile to have the truth on the front page, even though they knew the truth: obesity worsens outcomes from COVID-19. Sure, you could find this basic fact if you dug for it, but all of the public messaging on the news and from politicians omitted the importance of basic nutrition, physical fitness, and vitamins. Let's take a moment and grow more mentally resilient by considering some harsh realities. Maybe you don't believe some of the below, but do your own research and at least consider it. Okay, let's face some uncomfortable truths (don't worry, we already know them):

- Government social security is not enough to retire on.
- Government cheese is an inferior product.
- Government housing projects created a humanitarian nightmare.
- Trump promised to drain the swamp, but government corruption is worse than ever.
- Both sides of the political aisle have been corrupted.
- The self-styled *anti-racist* Left chose Biden, an aging white man who supported racial segregation. 2]
- If companies like Chase Bank and Pepsi support an uprising, then it's a marketing campaign, not a revolution.
- Bush, a so-called Conservative, passed the *Patriot Act*. This single law may be the most anti-freedom document in American history. 3]

I'm deliberately picking on both parties here to illustrate a point. The establishment routinely does the opposite of what they say they stand for. Why are we talking politics in *Fire Your Doctor*? Because, no matter which way you lean politically, don't entrust your family's health to the government and a corrupted two-party political system. Now that we've practiced wrestling with difficult facts, it's time to look at two hard truths the news wants to avoid. Vaccinated or not, non-elderly people in robust physical health were never at high risk from COVID-19.

Here's the harder part:

Most Americans are not in robust physical health. In fact, the majority of Americans have terrible personal health. I'm not saying this to be mean, but here are some facts we need to face.

- Over 70% of Americans are either overweight or obese. 4]
- One in three Americans has diabetes or prediabetes. 5]
- Half of American adults have high blood pressure. 6]

On the rare occasions that I've spoken publicly about the Pandemic, most people told me how angry they were at the government's pandemic policy. Sure, we can have a conversation about government corruption and failed leadership. Yes, the government lied to us and failed us. But, the bitter reality is that half of the country has high blood pressure, and 70% of us are overweight. What's worse, that the government failed us or that we as a country have failed ourselves? The biggest factor when it came to COVID has always been personal health. Our failing personal health is our problem, and blaming the government won't fix it. Okay, I get it. These truths hurt, but the truth will also set us free. Now that we've faced the truths about our health and that our leaders can't/won't fix it, let's learn how to fix ourselves.

Gut Health & COVID-19

The positive correlation between diabetes, obesity, and severe reactions to COVID-19 was known early on in the Pandemic. But, correlation is not the same as cause and effect. The actual causal link between these comorbidities and COVID is more complicated. Recent studies outline the connection between those who have more deleterious symptoms of COVID-SARS-2 virus with alterations in gut bacteria. In plain English, the research shows that bad gut bacteria makes COVID worse. As we've learned in previous chapters, diabetes and weight gain are also related to bad gut bacteria. The researchers found that:

> *"Associations between gut microbiota composition, levels of cytokines, and inflammatory markers in patients with COVID-19 suggest that the gut microbiome is involved in the magnitude of COVID-19 severity, possibly via modulating host immune responses. Furthermore, the gut microbiota dysbiosis after disease resolution could contribute to persistent symptoms, highlighting a need to understand how gut microorganisms are involved in inflammation and COVID-19."* 7]

There's a lot to unpack here. The gut microbes associated with severe reactions to COVID are linked to inflammation markers in the body. In some individuals, life-threatening "cytokine storms" occurred in the late stages of the virus. Higher levels of bacteria that raise inflammation and cytokines appear to be how obesity and (pre)diabetes tie into COVID. Additionally, the research indicates that so-called "long-haulers" or "post-COVID syndrome" could be perpetuated by these inflammatory gut bacteria. Lastly, the gut microbiome modulates the immune response. Immune response and low inflammation are crucial in fighting off any disease, especially with C19. As a side note, long-hauler symptoms, called post-viral syndrome, are not new. Many established viruses are associated with lingering effects, especially in people with a weakened immune system or at risk for diabetes. For those who may not know, metabolic disorder means diabetes or pre-diabetes. In 1988, researchers made the following observations:

> *"...post-viral fatigue syndrome is a common disorder... patients complaining of exhaustion, fatigue, muscle aches and pains, and invariable psychiatric symptoms such as emotional lability, poor memory/concentration, and depression. Present-day research points to the cause as a metabolic disorder secondary to persistent viral infection."* 8]

So, let me get this straight: the post-viral symptoms that are being linked to diabetes have been known for at least thirty years. There's really nothing new in that, is there? In my clinic, many patients tell me they've "never been right" after recovering from an illness. This is another area where public healthcare messaging really failed the American people. We needed to hear the hard truth: blood sugar fluctuations from eating too many carbs, sugar, and artificial sweeteners harm our immune systems and reduces our ability to recover after disease. With the Pandemic dragging on for multiple years, people had time to get healthy.

Instead, we were told that the beach was closed, truckloads of sand were dumped onto skateparks, schools were closed, and loss of socialization harmed millions of American kids. Then, we were told to get the vaccine, or you're a bad person. Get the vaccine, or your grandma's going to die. Get the vaccine, or you're fired. Those who declined the vaccine were threatened with a *winter of sickness and death* by the President of the United States, Joe Biden. On every news network, on billboards, on every social media app and website, we were told the same message: the vaccine is the only thing that will save you. The authorities and the news didn't want to focus on crucial truths like:

- COVID kills by causing runaway inflammation
- 70% of the country could significantly reduce their COVID risk through simple diet and lifestyle changes.

(Pre)diabetes, obesity, food choices, and unhealthy gut microbiome create an inflammation process in the body; this combination increases all disease risk and significantly shortens life expectancy. 9] The medical community has known this for years. Is it any surprise that these preventable risk factors also decrease your body's ability to fight off COVID? The government's pandemic response cherry-picked data and pretended that masks, injections, and social distancing were the primary factors in surviving. The real truth is that being healthy has always been more important than any medical intervention.

The public was never told why obesity and diabetes are so bad for COVID either: these lifestyle health conditions accompany bad gut bacteria that raise inflammation and lower immune response. Regardless of what choices anyone made about accepting or declining a medical intervention, can we really consent if we aren't given all of the choices?

We were told that the Pandemic was life and death, and the vaccine was the only way out. Local restaurants serving whole foods were closed, and McDonalds and other fast-food giants stayed open. While governors became dictators that demanded businesses be closed, fast food chains selling food that leads to diabetes were left as the only places to eat. To be clear, I don't support any lockdowns at all, but I find it conspicuous that unhealthy restaurants were open, but local places were forced to close. Two weeks to flatten the curve turned into years of ridiculous restrictions; these extended lockdowns would have been enough time for people to lose weight and improve their gut and metabolic health. Why didn't more authorities try to improve COVID recovery through diet and lifestyle? I'm not sure, but it's interesting that healthy people living healthy lifestyles means less money for hospitals, drug companies, and junk food makers.

Fever, Immune Response & Gut Health

I'm sure nobody paying attention is surprised that our leaders made laws and policies that help pharma and fast-food giants while hurting the public. I could write a whole book about how the government and media manipulated people into taking a medical treatment while ignoring healthy-living fundamentals. This was a crime against humanity. But this sad reality also comes with a silver lining: we are not sitting ducks. Regardless of our current health condition and despite our past mistakes, if we're alive, we can make different choices. We need to get healthy now. We need to improve our gut health now. We need to stop taking medical advice from entities that are bought and paid for by fast food and drug makers. As a country, we need to make sure that these corrupt entities are never allowed to coerce the public by lockdowns and mandates again.

But our main focus must still be improving our personal wellness. You can't change the system if you're dependent on the system. **You can't be independent of the broken healthcare system if you're unhealthy.** There's something even more fundamental than political change that must occur. The fastest way to break free of the broken system is to build strong immune systems by getting healthy. This is done in several ways. Part of building immunity is exposing our immune system to pathogens. Humans are social creatures, and we build immunity by interacting with people and their germs.

We don't need lockdowns; we need to be around other people. Also, we need to stop the insanity of masking and trying to disinfect everything. We have survived as a species by getting sick.

In the grand scheme of things, we only just discovered things like soap very recently. Germs and even viruses have been with us since the beginning. Nearly 8% of our DNA is from viruses, and 40% is encoded with some portion of genetic remnants of viruses. 10] Bacteria, viruses, and other pathogens have been humanity's fellow travelers throughout the ages. There's something even more fundamental than political change that must occur. The fastest way to break free of the broken system is to build strong immune systems by getting healthy. This is done in several ways. Part of doing this is exposing our immune system to pathogens.

Bacteria, viruses and other pathogens have been humanity's fellow travelers throughout the ages. When modern people get sick, we tend to view fevers (abnormally-raised body temperature) as bad because we feel bad. But it's not so simple as that. Fever is a natural part of the body's immune response. Why are we taking a bunch of pain relievers and anti-fever medications when fever is part of the immune response? Yes, there's a point where an extremely high fever above 104°F (40°C) can be very harmful. But, when a person is getting sick, I usually recommend guiding the fever with herbs and hydrotherapy to keep it under 104. Fevers under 104°F are the mark of a healthy immune response.

Stop suppressing your immune response by suppressing every fever. Every rule has exceptions. Fevers in newborn babies require physician oversight. Also, seek medical care if you have a fever of unknown origin or fevers associated with red, swollen joints. Use the above information as guardrails, but other than that, let the body burn if that's what the immune system needs to do. Some people even use saunas or soak in hot baths as a treatment when they get sick; just keep your temperature under 104°F. When exposed to heat, the body releases something called "heat-shock" proteins in response to elevated temperature.

These proteins protect cells from damage and reduce physical stress in the short term. Heat-shock proteins are released as the body's temperature goes up during a fever or when exposed to a hot bath or sauna. Heat-shock proteins have also been shown to have a modest protection effect to heart cells after a heart attack. 11] Moderate fever when you're sick is a sign that your immune system is working. So why are we talking about fever in a chapter about gut health?

Because **weakened immune systems that can't mount a proper fever response are related to poor gut health.** Making it even worse is that weakened immune systems push people to use antibiotic drugs that do even more damage to gut health. This cycle of impaired immunity, weak fevers when sick, and bad gut microbes is self-reinforcing. Eventually, this process increases the risk of autoimmune disease and other health problems.

Vaccines, Gut Health & Adverse Events

From the time we're little we're told that vaccines are *safe and effective*. If that's a scientific fact, there must be a scientific reason why. Otherwise, it's religion and not science; I believe in God, so I'm okay with faith. But, I'm very careful who/what I put religious faith in. I won't try to prove God to you, but that is one place I don't have a problem putting faith in. However, I don't have faith in science because faith is anti-scientific. Science is supposed to be the opposite of faith. Faith trusts and believes. On the other hand, science is about questioning, testing, looking for bias, retesting, and verifying previous tests. We're told that vaccines are science, and then we're told that we must *trust the science*. Science is the unbiased and systematic study of how and why. Faith trusts. Science wants to know why and how. Therefore, *trust the science* is a religious statement of faith that is very unscientific. Science asks how, why, prove it, and prove it again.

Over time, science changes its mind. Past science has proved certain things to be true only to have later science question and disprove yesterday's "facts." This process of proving and disproving is supposed to lead to better knowledge over time. Science only progresses so long as we continually question what we think we know. Here is a question. Are vaccines safe and effective? Is every vaccine safe in every case and for every unique person? Or, are vaccines safe and effective because they're rigorously tested, retested, and monitored for problems after release?

Here's a little-known fact: not every vaccine makes it through testing. Research shows that 54% of vaccines fail at some point during clinical development, and 17% of those failures are due to patient safety concerns. 12] Some supposedly good vaccines make it through short-term testing and then later fail in the third or fourth round of human trials. Even worse, there have even been vaccines that passed all human trials and were released to the public only to be banned over safety issues later on. Most recently in the spring of 2024, the AstraZeneca COVID-19 vaccine was pulled from the market due to risk of heart complications. Even more concerning, at least some health officials were aware of the possible cardiac risk to patients long before the injections were removed. 13] What does this tell us? It tells us that vaccines are not inherently safe; they're only safe in proportion to how good the testing protocol is. Any hope of vaccine safety requires excellent testing protocol combined with an unbiased reporting of side effects.

Vaccines Are Not Automatically Safe

Vaccines are only as safe as their testing and time out in the public proves them to be, but they are not inherently safe. Yes, I know, vaccines have become a political flashpoint in recent years. But, even the staunchest supporters of vaccines must understand that every medical intervention has pros and cons. This chapter is far from a complete look at the benefits and weaknesses of vaccines, but we need to look at how vaccines interact with gut health. With regard to vaccines, the unquestionable religious statement is that vaccines are safe and effective.

Half the audience is rolling their eyes and telling me to take my tinfoil hat off, but hear me out. Did you know the FDA has banned certain vaccines because of safety problems? Yes—some were pulled from the market due to harmful, even fatal, side effects. So, let's make a distinction here. The truth is that no medical treatment is automatically safe. Treatments (including vaccines) are only as safe as our testing procedures verify them to be. We're told that vaccines are safe and effective because they merely train the immune system to do its job better. Easy-peasy, case closed: vaccines simply train the immune system using a harmless stand-in instead of the dangerous virus. Right? Sort of, but it's complicated.

Unscientific assumptions surrounding *safe & effective*:
- "Training the immune system" to do its job better assumes that the immune system is strong enough to receive training.
- It assumes that all vaccines will undergo long-term testing over a decade or more. 13]

- "Training the immune system" assumes that it will learn the right lesson from our training.
- It assumes that our immune system will properly apply what it learned at the right time and in the right way.
- It assumes that we know what to train the immune system to focus on.
- It assumes that our training won't make our immune systems specialists at the expense of general capacity.
- It assumes that having an immune system specially trained to respond to hundreds of viruses will still remain balanced and able to respond to unique circumstances.

The talking heads tell us that vaccines are **always safe** and **always effective**. Really? But, what about the vaccines that have been deemed unsafe by the FDA? Are those safe, too? Were they safe when approved and magically became unsafe? Or, did the testing procedure let a bad vaccine through the cracks? Don't get me wrong, I'm not saying that a particular class of medical interventions is good or bad. Vaccines are a category of medical treatment that can be good or bad: but most are somewhere in the middle.

Science declaring that vaccines are safe and effective is making an unscientific generalization. Which vaccines? Given to which type of patient? At what dosage and booster schedule? So, what does the real science say? It says that vaccines have benefits but there are also very complex interactions occurring that science doesn't fully understand. Multiple research articles have connected vaccinations such as Tetanus and the flu shot with various autoimmune conditions, such as reactive and rheumatoid arthritis and Guillain-Barre syndrome. 13] Why is this? We don't know. But it's possible that while we're training the immune system to fight a virus, the immune system might also learn the wrong lesson and begin attacking itself too. Giving toddlers dozens of shots in a short period of time could be compared to exposing them to the world's most dangerous threats all at once. Yes, deadly viruses do exist—but is it always wise to expose young children to so many, especially all at once? In this analogy, while their immune systems might learn to defend themselves, they could also end up overwhelmed—like developing a kind of biological PTSD that affects both their mental and physical health.

Following this analogy, it's possible that immune systems could become hyper-vigilant, imbalanced, or self-destructive if over-exposed to what they think are killer viruses via immunizations. Hyper-vigilance may cause the immune system to overreact because it believes killer viruses are constantly being injected. Could this hyper-vigilance cause the immune system to eventually just start attacking everything, even its own body? The research is ongoing, but there is scientific evidence linking autoimmune conditions with over-vaccination. Adverse events following immunizations (AEFIs) do occur and are often underreported or overlooked

> *"The scientific knowledge about AEFIs is limited because their notification is frequently overlooked by physicians (under-notification) and because the available adverse event data frequently show only temporal relationships between vaccination and the onset of an AEFI."* 14]

Sharing on Facebook® that you experienced a vaccine adverse event can feel like modern-day witch-burning. Still, these reactions are real—and they're not new. Scientifically, adverse events related to vaccines were documented well before COVID. The following reactions have been reported in individuals who received vaccines and experienced side effects as a result of their body's response:

- Hypotonic Hyporesponsive Episode (HHE);
- Multiple Sclerosis (MS);
- Apnea in the preterm newborn (APTN);
- Guillain-Barré Syndrome (GBS);
- Arthritis/Arthralgia (AA);
- Immune Thrombocytopenic Purpura (ITP).

In previous chapters, we learned how gut health and good/bad gut bacteria tremendously affect our immune system, autoimmune diseases, diabetes, inflammation, and cancer. Now, we also have to layer upon the immune-modifying effects of widespread vaccinations for an ever-growing list of viruses. The health considerations, adverse events and side effects associated with vaccines don't act in a vacuum. They intermingle with the effects of processed foods, antibiotics, industrial chemical exposure, and our modern sedentary lifestyle. Research has linked vaccines like Tetanus and the Flu vaccine to rheumatoid arthritis and Guillain-Barre syndrome in some instances. 12]

Other researchers have connected the pathogenic overgrowth of a common gut bacteria, *Prevotella copri*, with early-onset rheumatoid arthritis. 15] This is just one example of how seemingly safe and effective treatments could have serious health consequences that may not be readily apparent. We're told that arthritis is just autoimmune and happens because of bad genes or for no reason. But while genetics and luck play a role, modern science also plays God with drastic changes in our diets, medicine, vaccines, and lifestyles. Is it wise to assume that playing God has no unintended consequences? This leads me to a few points I want to clarify when it comes to vaccines.

First: you never know how any drug will work in your body. Safe for someone else doesn't mean safe for you. Some people can safely drink alcohol in moderation, while others become fatally addicted. Human biology is unique.

Second: if you have a personal or family history of autoimmune disease, it may be wise to use all medications with caution, including vaccines.

Third: Poor gut health makes vaccines less safe and less effective. Vaccines won't work right unless the immune system is healthy. Poor gut health and autoimmune disease go together, and this can lead to complicated, negative vaccination outcomes.

Finally: vaccines are like any other medical intervention. They have risks, benefits and side effects.

No medical intervention is right for everyone. Medicine is not a one-size-fits-all for everyone all of the time. The problem with our modern culture around vaccines is that it's suppressing and censoring debate and open discussion. Most people are not being told the whole truth about vaccines. Patients can't really consent to a treatment that they don't understand. Our culture has abandoned informed consent with regard to vaccines. As decision makers of our health and our families' health, it is important that we have the choice to delay or decline any treatment the government recommends. Vaccine mandates and penalties for those who don't get vaccinated are a form of manipulative coercion that strips away our fundamental human right to say *no*.

Restoring Your Guts to Glory:
Ways to Build or Rebuild a Healthy Gut

Choose vaginal birth when possible. Your microbiome starts at birth and usually comes from your mom. You know all that gooey stuff that covers the baby when it gets pushed out of the mom? Yep, that slime is full of bacteria that should be implanted in your gut. Babies born via cesarean section had gut flora that was made of bad hospital germs including Klebsiella and Pseudomonas. These hospital-based microbes made up almost 30 percent of a newborn's gut bacteria when tested up to a year after birth. Numerous studies have linked a correlation between babies born via natural birth and those born via cesarean. 16] Babies born vaginally tend to have greater microbiome diversity, which supports the development of a healthy gut. Emerging research also suggests that maternal nutrition can influence a baby's gut health even before birth. Scientists have studied fetal waste—known as meconium—and amniotic fluid to estimate the state of the newborn's gut. However, the findings remain inconclusive, as researchers couldn't fully isolate the samples from external bacterial contamination.

Post-birth, however, factors such as maternal age, antibiotic use, feeding regimen, and genetics influence the baby's gut health. Babies born naturally from healthy moms are exposed to healthy vaginal flora, Bifidobacterium, Bacteroides, Clostridia, and Parabacteriodes. These healthy microbes are just a few of the anaerobic bacteria isolated from naturally-born infants. In babies born via cesarean, the gut flora is dominated by the Firmicutes group of bacteria, a phyla of bacteria usually seen only after the first year of life and in the GI tracts of many adults. To boil all of the above down and make it simple: Natural vaginal birth from a healthy mother gives the newborn baby a good start toward the healthy gut microbes they need. On the opposite side, C-section births give the baby hospital germs in their gut and set the baby up for poor gut health from day one.

Choose Breastfeeding when possible. Further colonization of healthy gut bacteria comes from human breast milk. Breastfeeding also gives the baby healthy bacteria that lives on the mother's skin. The milk also contains complex sugar molecules that feed the gut and help build a healthy gut lining. Finally, breast milk has an immune defense built in. Human breast milk contains protective immune system enhancers such as secretory IgA, calprotectin and lactoferrin. These natural immune enhancers educate the immune system. These, in combination with the healthy gut flora from vaginal birth, also reduce allergies and asthma. 17] The topic of breastfeeding is a difficult one for me. I had a difficult time breastfeeding and did not produce enough milk for either of my kids. I had trouble with my son who had a tongue tie, and I didn't produce enough milk to sustain him. I gave him colostrum and supplemented it with breast milk until he was six months old, after that I made him a homemade goat's milk-based formula that contained probiotics and goat colostrum.

The fact is I knew all of the research on the benefits of breast milk for the gut, the immune system, and the proper development of babies, and yet I had to compromise. Even still, the nutrition from breast milk is absolutely the best. With my second child, my husband researched the macro and micronutrients found in human breast milk and developed a goat milk formula that had our new baby thriving in no time. Her formula also included probiotics to support gut flora production. We tried to find ways to build their gut health because I did not make enough breast milk. I mention this here because I know other mothers struggle with breastfeeding. I am here to say there are options that can help with gut microbiome for those who don't make enough milk.

Introduce whole, nutrient-dense foods first. Give babies lots of prebiotic foods such as root vegetables. Foods like yams, jicama, potatoes, green bananas, squash, and apples. These break down to create a substrate that helps promote healthy gut bacteria. For babies, say *no* to rice and wheat cereals. Rice, wheat, and corn fillers cause bloating in babies. Breast milk contains an enzyme called pancreatic amylase, which helps break down starches. Without those breast milk enzymes, wheat and rice are even worse for a baby's gut health. We also limit processed carbohydrate foods (bread, crackers, candy, french fries, etc.), Especially before nine months old, it's best to avoid feeding babies processed foods. Instead, offer gut-healing options like bone broth, stewed meats, and vegetables. These provide the healthy fats and proteins essential for brain development and support the growth of beneficial gut bacteria. After my kids turned one, we began introducing some grains—but only after they'd eaten their meat and veggies. This approach prevents their stomachs from filling up on simple carbs and ensures their bodies are getting the nourishment needed for healthy growth and a strong gut.

"Lick the dog." Germs are a natural part of life—we've coexisted with them for all of human history. Instead of trying to eliminate them completely, we should focus on living and adapting alongside them. I generally advise against the regular use of hand sanitizers, antibacterial soaps, and constant disinfection. Daily exposure to everyday household germs helps build a stronger immune system. When it comes to kids, I often joke that they should "lick the dog"—and honestly, a little germ-sharing between kids and pets isn't a bad thing. The goal is to diversify the immune system and microbiome through regular, natural exposure. My kids crawl on the floor and sometimes even eat off of it—and I'm okay with that.

Bring on the bugs. Both of our kids have also grown up with dogs and cats in the house and farm animals like chickens free-ranging in the yard. Multiple studies have shown a reduction in allergic conditions to infants exposed to a household pet. 18] Germ theory emerged after scientists such as Louis Pasteur and Robert Koch discovered microbes. Koch was a physician and microbiologist who published Koch's four postulates on disease in 1890. These postulates were used to establish the basis for microbes or germs causing disease. They were the mainstay up until 1965 when the Bradford Hill Criteria for disease took over. Germ theory and Bradford Hill did advance medicine, but it's not the whole story. We have seen a decrease in many infectious diseases, but a stark increase in autoimmune disease. Evidence shows that childhood diseases can protect kids from allergies later on. 19] Genetic sequencing of bacteria, viruses, and fungi that inhabit our body shows that microbes play a complex role in our overall health. Put simply, disease prevention is more than killing germs. We need regular exposure to household germs. There are also countless helpful microbes that we need to be fully healthy.

Avoid antibiotics when possible. The overuse of antibiotics is covered elsewhere in this book, but it's worth repeating: antibiotics wipe out your healthy gut microbiome. Sometimes they're necessary, and when I do use them, I always follow up with gut repair. The damage from a single round may not show up for weeks or months. When people ask why they get sicker with age, it's not just aging—it's a weakened immune system. The best way to rebuild that system is to clean up your gut. Overusing antibiotics also fuels the rise of drug-resistant superbugs. The more we rely on them, the stronger and deadlier the germs become.

> *"In 2015, antibiotic-resistant pathogens were estimated to cause over 50,000 deaths a year in Europe and the USA. The toll is projected to rise to 10 million deaths per year worldwide by 2050. These figures suggest we are reaching the end of the antibiotic era."* 20]

Antibiotics don't just kill harmful bacteria—they also wipe out beneficial microbes. This can lead to dysbiosis, an imbalance that allows bad bacteria to take over. Dysbiosis weakens nutrient absorption and vitamin production (like B, D, and K), all of which are vital for immune function. As a result, your body becomes more vulnerable to infections. It's also linked to chronic issues like diabetes, heart disease, obesity, depression, anxiety, autoimmune disorders, and more—even after just one round of antibiotics. One simple way to protect your gut is to avoid unnecessary antibiotics and limit disinfectant use.

Choose food free of pesticides & herbicides. Glyphosates, commercially known as Roundup®, are sprayed heavily on US commercial crops as a weed killer for genetically modified food crops. Roundup® was developed by Monsanto company, a large U.S. based agrochemical company. Roundup® is known for its ability to kill a wide variety of plants, except for crops that are genetically modified to resist the weed killer. Sounds *safe and effective*, right?

Let's back up for a moment and examine Monsanto's past products: PCBs, DDT, and Agent Orange. 21] In case you don't know, these previous Monsanto products have all been banned because they're very harmful to humans and animals. Monsanto's reputation was so tarnished that when Bayer (yes, the makers of aspirin) acquired it in 2016, they quickly dropped the Monsanto name. Soon after, Bayer was hit with a $10 billion fine because people developed cancer due to glyphosate exposure. Research has also shown that exposure to Roundup® increases levels of a protein called zonulin, which was discovered by Dr. Alessio Fassano and his team at the University of Maryland. Zonulin combines with proteins in wheat and gut bacterial overgrowth, triggering autoimmune diseases such as celiac disease and type 1 diabetes in genetically susceptible individuals. 28] This means that Roundup®-treated wheat can create a wheat allergy where there would never have been one before. Furthermore, excess zonulin from Roundup® exposure harms the tight junctions that seal our gut lining. Roundup®-treated wheat leads to intestinal tight junctions that are swollen and open. Damaged tight junctions create a condition called leaky gut, making a person more susceptible to autoimmune diseases. Exposure to glyphosate (Roundup®) has been shown to increase the destruction of beneficial gut bacteria, allowing disease-causing bacteria to thrive. Then, a vicious circle ensues.

The overgrowth of harmful bacteria causes the body to make even more zonulin as a way to regulate the immune system. Exposure to Roundup® has been linked to obesity, Alzheimer's, Parkinson's, autism, depression, infertility, and cancer. 26] Glyphosate has also been linked to chronic joint pain, particularly in athletes like golfers and soccer players who spend time on freshly sprayed, pesticide-laden lawns and fields. These chemicals contribute to widespread inflammation and joint tissue breakdown. Once the body is detoxified from these harmful substances, pain often subsides, allowing for joint function to improve and rehabilitation to take place.

These diseases may take decades to show up, which makes it harder to legally prove that Roundup® caused the damage, which is the only reason that glyphosate is still around. In time, though, Roundup® will likely be banned, and then they'll promise that a new chemical is safe. Any good gut repair plan must include the elimination of commercial pesticides in food sources whenever possible.

Commercially- produced GMO food crops are habitually sprayed with Roundup®. Avoiding processed foods and foods made with GMO wheat, corn, and soy is a good place to start.

While zonulin is an important discovery related to the microbiome, health, and disease, it's not my primary marker for assessing impaired intestinal barrier function. It's just one of several markers that may indicate gut barrier damage. Additionally, zonulin can appear in other parts of the body as a signal to trigger an immune response, so it's not specific to the gut. Its presence could also point to other underlying health issues that have yet to be fully understood.27] The body is inherently complex, so it's important to view immune and gut function as part of a bigger picture, rather than focusing on just one marker.

Almost everyone has gut microbiome issues. Almost everyone in the modern world has been exposed to antibiotics and pesticides. As a child and teen, I was given several rounds of antibiotics, which led to a lifetime of gut issues—today, my gut health remains one of my weakest links, aside from my muscles. If anything goes wrong in my body, it's usually my gut.

The good news is I've made significant progress in improving my gut health. This journey has given me valuable context and experience to help others heal their guts at our clinic. Today, we have viable alternatives to antibiotics for treating many conditions. While antibiotics are sometimes necessary, most of the time, they're not. Combinations of herbs, nutrition, and probiotics can address bacterial overgrowths while also supporting a healthy gut microbiome.

Your gut health is at the core of your internal terrain. Protect it, and it will keep your immune system strong, ensuring pathogens stay at bay.

Age gracefully. Aging has a significant impact on gut microbiota. We're told that this just happens when we get old, but I counter that it's a lifetime of choices finally catching up.

Why is Poor Gut Health Linked to Aging?

Decades of eating the Western Diet has finally caught up.

Years of using antacids has repeatedly harmed normal digestion and allowed bad bacteria to flourish. Low stomach acid allows the overgrowth of certain bacteria like *Helicobacter pylori*, further inhibiting natural digestive secretions.

- Using antibiotics has killed off good gut microbes, allowing bad bacteria to flourish.
- Taking NSAIDs, pain medications, antidepressants, heart medications, and other drugs has been shown to break down healthy gut barriers and slow the motility of the gut.
- Combined effects of all these factors have been amplified over decades of neglected gut health.

All of these factors contribute to a gut that lacks biodiversity and has an increase in pathogens. Healthy probiotic levels are essential for nutrient absorption and the production of short-chain fatty acids. The presence of a Western Diet significantly reduces beneficial bacterial species, especially in elderly populations living in nursing. The poor-quality commercial food served in these facilities, combined with widespread antibiotic use, is likely the cause of the gut health issues observed in these settings.

A decline in healthy gut flora leads to reduced bioavailability of B vitamins and essential amino acids. Research shows that elderly patients who consumed a diverse, whole food diet maintained gut microbiota similar to that of healthy young adults. These healthy centenarians lived more than a decade longer than those who did not follow a whole-food diet.23]

Kill & repopulate. There comes a point when a patient's gut health is so overwhelmed by parasites, harmful fungi, and pathogenic bacteria that a complete reset is necessary. At our clinic, we may run comprehensive gut panels to identify exactly what's growing inside you—the good, the bad, and the necessary. Symptoms are not always a clear indicator that your gut needs attention. Often, gut health issues are masked by prescriptions or high inflammatory markers in the body. That's why, regardless of whether obvious gut symptoms are present, we encourage nearly all patients with chronic conditions like autoimmune disease, pain, or mood disorders to evaluate their gut health.

Once we know what's going on, we eliminate the pathogens and repopulate the gut with healthy flora. Think of gut health like a garden: we need to remove the weeds while replanting the crops we want to grow. When your garden is healthy, the good plants crowd out the weeds, making it harder for them to take over. After we've restored healthy gut microbes, we focus on repairing the tissue damage caused by harmful bacteria and continue nurturing the microbial populations that make up a thriving gut environment.

Fecal transplants. No talk about gut health would be complete if we failed to mention poop. It's pretty amazing what we can find by looking at poop. I remember going to an outdoor science camp when I was in 4th grade. I sold wrapping paper and candy bars for months to raise enough money to go. When we got there, it was a glorious wonderland for a nerdy science girl like me. We mapped constellations and used our night senses by taking hikes in the dark. However, the most interesting thing we did at camp was dissecting excrement. You can learn a lot about an animal by looking at their poop. I took that lesson to heart, poop dissection led to my interest in digestion, the mouth's microbiome, and eventually dentistry. I learned that certain bacteria ran in certain family lines. Later, while in college, I even participated in a research study on spit for $16. Hey, a college kid's got to eat. My point is, we can learn a lot from waste and fluids. When I heard about using a healthy person's poop to fight against intestinal infections like *Clostridium difficile*, I wasn't surprised. 25] A healthy microbiome with beneficial bacteria has something called bacteriocins. Bacteriocins are powerful anti-microbial agents that are even stronger than potent antibiotics like vancomycin or metronidazole. A healthy microbiome will actually kill off bad germs, but without the side effects of antibiotics. Fecal transplants also affect the production and expression of genes. One study found,

> "*a fecal transplant, however, drastically increases global DNA methylation in previously germ-free mice.*" 25]

Let's break this down: germ-free mice are free of any known pathogens. Healthy poop was given to the mice, then the mice started making genes used to fight infection. Poop is powerful. Fecal transplants restore microbiomes ravaged by surgery, medications, or severe infection. This gentle approach helps heal previously damaged guts without the need for continued drug use, promoting lasting gut health.

Use the right kind of probiotics. In years past, doctors were ostracized and even jailed for suggesting that their patients take bacteria in order to heal their bodies. Doctors were mocked, called "quacks," and had their medical licenses revoked for saying that certain bacteria could be used to support a healthy gut. While traveling, I once met a doctor who was trained in Brazil. We talked for over an hour about how doctors in other countries are trained. Where he was trained, all doctors prescribed a probiotic any time they prescribed an antibiotic. My jaw nearly dropped. When I seemed surprised, he asked me, "Aren't doctors trained that way in the US?" Sadly, not most doctors. To illustrate the power of probiotics, researchers tested kids for severe diarrhea caused by the rotavirus. The researchers found that kids infected with rotavirus had low gut bacterial diversity when compared to uninfected kids. 23] Microbial diversity in the gut protects against infection. Conversely, a lack of different types of bacteria in the gut increases risk of infection. Diverse, healthy gut microbes discourage bacteria from forming colonies. In the rotavirus study, the infected kids given probiotics were able to clear the diarrhea within three days. Proper probiotics not only protect against infection, but they also help you recover faster. Interestingly, other viral infections, such as HIV and Hepatitis C, are also correlated with low gut microbial diversity. 23]

Keep in mind that quality matters; not any probiotic will do. Also, there are certain conditions where a probiotic will make the problem worse. If you suffer from SIBO (Small Intestine Bacterial Overgrowth), probiotics can worsen the gut imbalance. If your gut symptoms increase when taking probiotics, it's a sign that you may not have the right probiotic or you have an infection like SIBO. In such cases, it's important to seek out a naturopathic doctor who has a deep understanding of the gut microbiome and its impact on overall health.

Consume the whole food and nothing but the food. Dr. Weston Price, a Cleveland dentist, traveled the world to explore the causes of tooth decay and crooked teeth. He studied isolated tribes with traditional diets—rich in meats, fats, plants, nuts, seeds, and unpasteurized milk. These tribes had straight, healthy teeth and little disease. Their diets included nutrient-dense foods like butter, fish, eggs, shellfish, and organ meats. Many tribes also followed customs around reproduction: both parents consumed healthy nutrition before conceiving, and mothers spaced pregnancies to fully recover their nutrition between births, promoting better health for both mother and child.

Years later, when Dr. Price returned to these tribes after they adopted modern diets, he saw a dramatic decline in oral health. Children had narrowed faces, crooked teeth, and weaker immune systems, highlighting the negative impact of modern diets and lifestyles.29] Traditional eating benefits the whole body, positively influences our genes, and is key to maintaining beneficial gut microbes.

TLDR: Too Long Didn't Read

The Western Diet disrupts the gut microbiome and contributes to a range of preventable health issues. These comorbidities significantly increase the risk of severe and fatal cases of COVID-19. While the government's response to COVID was a mix of incompetence and corruption, we the people also bear responsibility for our poor health and fitness.

Vaccines are often labeled as safe and effective, but the research shows they're not universally safe for everyone. Both vaccine efficacy and immune system function are heavily influenced by gut health. Poor gut health can increase the likelihood of vaccine side effects. While vaccines do have benefits, the over-vaccination of our population may be a mistake. Ultimately, the safety of medical treatments, including vaccines, depends on robust testing protocols and transparent side effect reporting systems.

There's a lot you can do to improve gut health:

- Avoid the Western Diet

- Eat a natural whole foods diet
- Have a natural, vaginal birth
- Avoid antibiotics whenever possible
- Avoid GMO foods and anything treated with Roundup®
- Consider fecal transplant in severe cases of gut imbalance
- Not all probiotics are the same
- Probiotics can make certain conditions like SIBO worse

Chapter 8
Overfed, But Hungry

"Actual happiness always looks pretty squalid in comparison with the overcompensations for misery." -Aldous Huxley, Brave New World

Now that we've gone deep into the guts of gut health, it's time to look closer at what we're putting into our guts: commercially-processed foods. Industrial food production is one of the defining features of modernity. Supermarkets being full of processed foods has changed more than our waistlines though; it's also changed our moral values and how we view the world. Even people who believe in God have experienced this slow perspective shift. For too many people, instant messaging, instant food, and instant gratification have become habitual. Once we relied on belief in God, personal struggle and delayed gratification. Now, our culture trusts in money, technology, science and government to meet our needs.

In a way, science and technology have become the new gods of our culture. These new gods promise us a paradise of plenty and a life centered around convenience. In the developed world, we're free to sip zero-calorie drinks while we recline on memory foam in climate-controlled comfort. The niceties of modern living, even for lower-income people, would seem like a literal heaven on earth for our ancestors. Yesteryear's hunter-gatherers, farmers, fishermen, warriors, blacksmiths, cobblers, bakers, and even kings could have never imagined a modern grocery store, let alone Amazon Prime®. Every appetite and desire has been commoditized by technology: fast food, drive-throughs, and delivery orders from phone apps. Our human addiction to instant gratification goes well beyond food. Our culture is awash with cheap distractions like reality TV, credit cards, scrolling on social media, dating apps, and even online pornography. The gods of technology and instant gratification have invaded every aspect of our lives. But there is some hope. Becoming intentional about the food we eat (and don't eat) is one of the fundamental battlefields where we can push back against this powerful force. Many religious traditions emphasize the practice of fasting (abstaining from food for a determined period of time) as a discipline for spiritual growth. According to thousands of years of religious tradition, we can reclaim part of our lost humanity by limiting or eliminating certain foods. This spiritual principle rings especially true in our world where instant access to low-cost food-as-entertainment is available 24 hours per day.

Note: When I mention the spiritual and physical benefits of fasting, I am in no way condoning eating disorders. A proper fast has a clear beginning and end. Likewise, fasting cannot be used as a crutch to compensate for over-indulgence periods. The goal here is to be well-nourished and well-balanced in our health and body weight.

Beyond just physical health, fasting and maintaining healthy boundaries with food may also impart an emotional and spiritual benefit as well. We are at a very unique time in history where we're spiritually starved but physically spoiled. Eons of physical hardship and torment failed to kill the human spirit; in fact, those physical hardships may have made us spiritually stronger. But now, the luxury and comfort we always wanted may be leading to our physical, spiritual, and emotional deaths. The Devil is not without irony: famine, war and hardship have failed to kill the human race, so now he's giving us the most difficult temptation of all: abundance and excess.

Modern culture gives us exactly what we want. When do we want it? Now, of course. There's only one problem. Getting everything we want is killing us.

Everything You Want, Nothing You Need

Over 60 percent of all calories being consumed by Americans come from a category of food called Ultra Processed Food (UPF). These recreational foods are often eaten for entertainment or pleasure. UPFs encompass foods such as candy, soda, chips, cookies, cakes, and other highly refined and shelf-stable foods. A June 2020 study published in The American Journal of Clinical Nutrition found that eating Ultra Processed Food leads to shortening of telomeres, indicating premature aging. 1] Now you're asking me, what's a telomere and why do they matter? Telomeres are a part of DNA involved in cell replication. Telomeres are how your DNA gets copied and preserved inside your body's cells. Shortened telomeres are a marker for aging that leads to errors in your body's DNA. These errors harm your body's DNA. This damage is directly linked to illnesses like cancer and diabetes.

The research shows that processed foods harm your DNA (and a lot of other things) over time. Junk food is more than unwanted weight gain, it harms your body all the way down to your DNA. The September 2020 *European Association for the Study of Obesity* found that as little as three servings of UPF per day doubled the odds of premature DNA telomere shortening. 2] Internal medicine researchers with the *Journal of the American Medical Association* (JAMA) found that ultra processed foods were not only lacking in nutrition, but they also led to diseases such as diabetes, obesity, heart disease and cancer. JAMA describes ultra processed foods as "energy dense, rich in refined carbohydrates, saturated (hydrogenated) fats, salt, and contain low dietary fiber." 3] Beyond the high calorie, low nutritional profile, the research also shows how UPFs are produced harmfully. These foods expose people who consume them to chemical additives and known carcinogens such as acrylamide. 4] Let's take a moment and think about our great-great-grandparents. Maybe you've seen a picture of them. What is one thing you may have noticed? You may have noticed how slim and vital they were. That's because they ate completely differently than we do now. Our ancestors ate very different food, and they also spent a lot more time being active. Today, millions of Americans spend 8 to 15 hours sitting every day!

> *"One in four American adults sit for more than eight hours a day, according to new federal research from investigators at the Centers for Disease Control and Prevention."* 5]

Sitting and lack of physical activity has led to an onslaught of serious health conditions including increased rates of cancer, cardiovascular disease, diabetes and chronic pain. One study from 2010 noted that males who sat for more than 6 hours a day had a 40% increased rate of premature death compared to their active counterparts. 6] Just getting up and doing something, anything seems to be better than sitting or lying around all day.

Our ancestors ate much less than we do today, especially in large families where food was scarce. Back then, having 7-10 children was common, so there simply wasn't as much to go around. Before the rise of industrially processed food and mass agriculture, food wasn't cheap or abundant. Portion control was built-in, as families had to share what little food they had. Also, the food they ate was real and nutrient-dense, so people ate less but felt fuller longer. Today's mass-produced foods are engineered for two main purposes:

1. Be so good it's addictive
2. Be cheap to make

Recreational food and beverage is about maximizing taste and cheapness is how we end up with people addicted to foods that taste good in the moment but produce harm over time. Certainly, our ancestors faced hardships like famine and disease in ways that we don't understand in the modern world, yet. Let's be honest: most of us don't want to give up our WiFi and indoor plumbing. But, the mass migration away from naturally raised meats and fresh fruits and vegetables has certainly had an impact. In his piece, *"Six Rules for Eating Wisely"* published in *TIME* magazine, Michael Pollan instructs us to avoid any food that our great-great-grandparents wouldn't recognize: "Imagine

how baffled your ancestors would be in a modern supermarket… (most items) aren't foods—quite—they're food products." 7] The modern world brings many unspoken assumptions.
We assume that…

. . . we can replace pasture-raised livestock with meat raised on colossal factory farms and not notice a difference.

. . . we can replace naturally grown crops with genetically modified crops sprayed with pesticides and fertilizers without side effects.

. . . we can replace hours spent outside being active with hours of screen time indoors.

. . . We can regularly eat processed foods like chips, soda, and crackers without immediate health consequences.

. . . we can use pharmaceuticals to avoid the consequences of our bad habits.

. . . we can consume artificial sweeteners and get the reward of sugar while avoiding the harm.

As you may have guessed, none of the above assumptions are automatically true. Factory farms and genetically modified crops are less nourishing than traditionally raised meats and vegetables. Can we really genetically engineer wheat and corn that grows faster than normal while being planted in depleted soil without giving something up? Screen time can't replace outdoor activity and real-life human interaction. Processed foods are not good for you. Genetically modified crops are not a free lunch. Diet foods are a lie.

The Diet Food Deception

The one thing that's worse than a lie is a deception. A lie is a fact that is knowingly false. A deception is a process of coercing someone to follow a completely false reality. Unfortunately, the most effective deceptions are built on factually true statements, or at least contain some truth in them. Let's explore one of the greatest deceptions perpetrated against the American people. Above, I stated that diet foods are a lie. In a way though, these processed foods are actually a deception that's worse than a plain old lie. Diet food makers imply that their products will help us lose weight. That's the lie.

The deeper deception within diet food is the myth that we can proverbially have our cake and eat it too. Here's a 'brilliant' idea from the multibillion-dollar food industry: What if we made cookies and soda, but instead of sugar, we used artificial sweeteners? That way, customers get all the pleasure of sweets but none of the sugar and added calories. It's perfect, guilt-free fun! Right? Wrong. Diet sugar-free foods are indeed lower in calories. But the deception is that diet foods are good for you; actually, the opposite is true. Diet foods are more harmful than actual sugar. It seems crazy at first, but if diet foods actually worked, then why is obesity worse than ever? That's because even though diet foods are lower in calories, they won't help you lose weight. The research shows that even though zero-calorie sweeteners are not sugar, they fool the body into thinking it's sugar, making the body respond hormonally with a huge insulin spike.

Diet foods can actually make insulin resistance worse. Insulin resistance is the mechanism behind type II diabetes. When the body is constantly exposed to sweet foods, it responds by releasing more insulin. Artificial sweeteners like Splenda® and NutraSweet® also trigger an insulin response, much like real sugar. Over time, if your body is always releasing insulin, it builds a tolerance to it, and eventually, your natural insulin stops working effectively—leading to diabetes. As insulin resistance progresses, losing weight becomes increasingly difficult. Consuming more diet foods with artificial sweeteners further damages your insulin response and even lowers your metabolism. This diet food deception can easily spiral into weight gain and diabetes.

In simple terms, diet foods with artificial sweeteners can actually contribute to diabetes and make it harder to lose weight, going against their intended purpose. A large French study published in the *British Medical Journal* found that regularly consuming aspartame (NutraSweet®) and sucralose (Splenda®) significantly increased the risk of stroke and heart disease. 9] Sure, you're cutting calories. But cutting calories with artificial sweeteners is a dangerous shortcut, not a solution. Insulin resistance and the biochemistry of artificial sweeteners is complicated. Here's what you need to know; diet foods are bad and if you eat them, you'll feel bad. Predictably, the food industry is fighting this inconvenient fact with the usual propaganda. If you Google® artificial sweeteners you'll find what used to be trusted news sites telling everyone that these chemicals are safe, and you can eat diet foods without fear. Despite this, the research is clear about fake sugar and insulin resistance. People are attracted to the enticing deception of guilt-free sweets. Sadly, diet foods are the new cigarettes. Popular news sites get advertising money from diet food makers (and drug companies) and are biased.

In the past, Big Tobacco lobbied and bribed their way into decades of denying that smoking was bad. Tobacco companies sponsored studies and doctors to tell everyone that smoking was fine or that "the research was inconclusive." Nonetheless, the truth came out slowly and the research was always undeniable. Decades later, we all know smoking is bad. To be completely honest, in the back of our minds, we knew it was bad back then, too. We just didn't want to believe it. Diet foods are marketed on the deception that ingredients don't matter, and you can taste sweets without paying the price. In the diet food deception, being healthy is equated with simply limiting calories. But, the quality of food matters a lot. If the whole story was just calories in calories out, the diet food movement would have solved our weight issues through the power of science. But, decades into diet soda, diet cookies and low-fat: our nation is more obese and unhealthier than ever.

Nothing got solved because the solution was really a deception. The food industry has tricked us into believing that convenience and cheapness should come before our health. We've been conditioned to accept processed, nutrient-poor foods as normal, when in reality, they're not food at all—they're a concoction of chemicals, preservatives, and artificial ingredients designed to keep us hooked. Eating healthy isn't just about the calories we consume; it's about the quality and diversity of those calories. The body requires whole, nutrient-dense foods in the right amounts to function at its best. It's not just about cutting calories or eating less—it's about eating better.

Processed foods, while often convenient and addictively tasty, are a far cry from what our bodies were designed to thrive on. People who consume these foods are more likely to face chronic health problems, from heart disease and diabetes to autoimmune diseases, skin issues, and even cancer. It's shocking that many of these products are still widely accepted as food. They're not much different from drugs in that they can be addictive, dangerous, and, in many cases, life-threatening.

What's even more disturbing is the way these foods increase calorie intake without offering real nourishment. Like drugs, they entrap us in a cycle of over-consumption and dissatisfaction. We eat more and more, but our bodies remain malnourished, starving for essential nutrients. In a world where we're consuming more calories than ever, the real tragedy is that we're still nutritionally deprived. What should be a balanced, fulfilling diet has turned into a dangerous game of excess without any true benefit for our health.

This is a wake-up call for us all—food is supposed to be fuel, not a trap. It's time to prioritize real, whole foods that nourish us from the inside out.10] A 2017 article published in *Critical Review of Food Science and Nutrition* stated the following:

> *"We verified that most vitamins are deficient in obese individuals, especially the fat-soluble vitamins, folic acid, vitamin B12, and vitamin C."* 11]

This translates to more calories and less nutrients available to think, move, repair, and breathe.

Modern Medicine & "Diabesity"

Diabesity is a modern medical term that joins diabetes and obesity. This makes sense because there's a strong correlation between diabetes and obesity. Most metabolic issues like diabetes and slowed metabolism are connected to a dysfunction in blood sugar. Diabetes doesn't start suddenly. Metabolic issues develop insidiously over many years of eating processed foods, diet foods and living a sedentary lifestyle. If modern medicine took the time to actually look, we'd see the early signs of diabetes much sooner than an actual diagnosis of diabetes becomes apparent. That is, if we bothered to conduct detailed hormone testing and preemptive screening with patients. Clinically, the development of insulin resistance, hypoglycemia and hyperglycemia leads to a cluster of symptoms called metabolic syndrome long before full-blown type II diabetes shows up. Metabolic syndrome is a group of symptoms that increase your risk for heart disease, stroke, and diabetes. There are five major categories, and one would qualify as having *Metabolic Syndrome X* if one has at least three out of five symptoms.

Symptoms of Metabolic Syndrome X:

- High blood pressure
- Raised blood sugar
- Abdominal fat
- Increased cholesterol
- Elevated triglycerides

At Terrain Wellness, we prioritize the criteria of Metabolic Syndrome X because it is far more clinically relevant than overall weight or Body Mass Index (BMI). While BMI can be a useful tool in some cases, it doesn't always reflect a person's true health, especially for those with higher muscle mass. For example, my husband's BMI is near the "overweight" category due to muscle and bone density, but he is actually very lean. While a BMI chart can alert you when things are significantly off, it's not the most accurate or effective measure of metabolic health.

Most people don't need a BMI chart to know when there's a health issue. While weight gain is often accepted as part of aging, it's not inevitable. The real danger is Metabolic Syndrome, which is more harmful than carrying extra pounds and makes weight loss much harder. That's why our clinical approach focuses on reversing Metabolic Syndrome first—improving metabolic health makes weight loss easier.

Achieving metabolic health starts with eating natural, nourishing foods—no cheese puffs, chips, or artificially sweetened yogurt. Most Americans need to drastically reduce their intake of sugar and processed carbohydrates. At our clinic, we build on this foundation by restoring gut health through herbs, supplements, and individualized functional nutrition. Additionally, we incorporate mind-body medicine, acupuncture, and focused movement to rebalance and reverse the harmful lifestyle and emotional patterns that contribute to poor metabolic health.

In most first-world countries, we're in a pattern of consuming more calories from empty foods and too few nutrient-dense foods. This diet of processed foods makes us sick, which of course means we need drugs to combat the effects of poor nutrition and lifestyle choices. The food industry makes billions selling us processed and fast foods that lead to illness, while hospitals and drug makers make even more billions selling us the cure. Medications such as acid-blockers, antibiotics, cholesterol-lowering drugs, blood pressure medications, and blood sugar medications are all linked to poor lifestyle choices.

Taking a drug doesn't address the root cause of poor diet and a sedentary lifestyle—it only masks the symptoms of unhealthy choices. In a way, these drugs are deceptive because they enable bad habits while concealing their consequences. Statins, among the most prescribed medications in America, are a prime example. Common statins like Lipitor®, Zocor®, and Altoprev® are prescribed to lower cholesterol, which is often cited as a major contributor to heart disease. But are they really effective? Despite widespread statin use, heart disease continues to soar. Data from the *National Health and Nutrition Examination Survey* shows that statin use among Americans over 40 increased from 20% to 28% between 2003 and 2012, yet the rate of heart disease remains alarmingly high.12] With 28% of the population over 40 prescribed a statin, a vast fortune is being made on these drugs. Nearly 35 million Americans take statins, resulting in almost 13 billion pills sold each year by Big Pharma. For those without insurance, a bottle of 30 Lipitor pills can cost over $400, according to SingleCare.com. 13] This means Big Pharma has between 100 and 200 billion dollars up for grabs so long as doctors keep prescribing statins.

Statins are highly profitable, with millions of people taking them, which creates a potential for bias. However, that doesn't automatically mean Big Pharma is wrong. It was proposed that if everyone took statins, heart disease would decrease, but sadly, that's not the case. Dr. Aseem Malhotra, an award-winning cardiologist, highlights several issues with statins. Many doctors claim that statins are safe and that side effects are rare, but Malhotra reveals that research supporting statins has been influenced by corporate interests. He questions whether cholesterol should even be the primary factor in heart disease risk. If it's not, then lowering cholesterol may not help prevent heart disease. Malhorta's position is backed by the data, because millions of statin prescriptions haven't reduced heart disease.

Research from the *British Medical Journal* shows that taking statins only increased life expectancy by 3 to 4 days. Given such a small impact, it might be within the margin of error. In my medical opinion, prescribing statins to 28% of adults over 40 is unwise when the benefits are so questionable. While statins may make sense in certain cases, for mass use across millions, the benefits should be much more significant.

The research indicates that, even if statins lower cholesterol, they don't actually help us live longer. So, what about safety? According to Malhotra's clinical data, up to one in five people taking statins experience side effects. Rather than turning to statins, Malhotra and an increasing number of healthcare professionals advocate for a Mediterranean diet and moderate exercise. It's no surprise: pharmaceuticals aren't the solution. We need to return to the basics of healthy living—eating real food and leading active, fulfilling lives.

By now, it's clear that you might need to consider firing your doctor, especially if you were prescribed a statin. Statins are widely recognized as a poor choice for many, but there are still a few important things you should understand about these drugs.

Statins cause significant deficiencies in CoQ10, a naturally produced compound in the body. CoQ10 is a powerful antioxidant that helps produce energy in your cells' mitochondria. As we age, our natural levels of CoQ10 naturally decline, and certain conditions like heart disease, Parkinson's, chronic migraines, or illness recovery can further deplete it. Unfortunately, cholesterol-lowering drugs also reduce CoQ10 levels.

The common side effects associated with statins, such as fatigue and muscle pain, are likely tied to this CoQ10 depletion. In severe cases, the shortage can lead to rhabdomyolysis, a potentially fatal condition. Rhabdo occurs when muscle fibers break down and release debris into the bloodstream, which is then filtered by the kidneys, turning urine dark reddish or brown. This condition can result in kidney failure, cardiac arrhythmias, and in extreme cases, even death.

"...statins are commonly associated with muscle complaints, termed statin-associated muscle symptoms (SAMS). Symptoms range from minor muscle aches to more severe muscle pains, severe cramps, muscle weakness, and, in rare instances, rhabdomyolysis." 22]

The mainstream view on statins is that rhabdomyolysis is rare, but the frequent and painful muscle side effects suggest tissue damage is happening. Statins are just one example of how medications can deplete nutrients and harm our health. You can't use prescriptions to offset poor diet and lifestyle choices without causing more damage. This issue extends beyond statins—diabetes meds and antacids can lead to serious vitamin B12 deficiencies.

Vitamins, derived from the Latin words for life (vita) and amino acid (amine), are essential for our bodies to function. Yet, we often overlook their importance. In reality, vitamins are critical life substances. Most major medications contribute to nutrient deficiencies, which is why we routinely supplement vitamins for anyone on medication long-term. Lab tests confirm what we already know: many Americans are overfed but severely lacking in basic nutrients.

Diabesity and the Gut

Diabesity, a term combining diabetes and obesity, emerged alongside the rise of corn syrup, processed foods, sedentary lifestyles, and increased reliance on prescription medications. It didn't exist 100 years ago, indicating that modern factors are to blame. As discussed earlier in this book, food affects gut microbes, which in turn influence metabolic health. The science is clear: an overgrowth of certain gut bacteria contributes to higher obesity rates. A 2005 study in *Obesity Alters Gut Microbial Ecology*, states that:

"Differences in gut microbial ecology between humans may be an important factor affecting energy homeostasis; i.e., individuals predisposed to obesity may have gut microbial communities that promote more efficient extraction

and/or storage of energy from a given diet, compared with these communities in lean individuals." 16]

In clinical practice, my team has experienced this idea first-hand with patients having trouble losing weight. Just so we're clear, weight loss is multifactorial. Calories, exercise, hormones, and food choices all matter regarding weight. But, in clinical practice we find that when we rebalance patients' digestive systems and restore healthy gut microflora, we observe that weight loss becomes much easier to do. When it comes to weight loss, everyone wants to focus on genetics. While it's true that some people will genetically gain or lose weight more easily, things are a lot more complicated than the DNA we've inherited. Our health is much deeper than factors outside of our control. Sustainable weight loss is directly tied to digestive health. Factors like blood sugar, hormones, immunity and inflammation are important factors in weight loss that are all influenced by our gut health. Going a level deeper, many common prescription drugs have also been shown to negatively influence our gut health. Prescriptions solve one problem while creating new problems that in turn call for more prescriptions. Again, we're caught in the vicious circle of bad food leading to bad medicine as our health spirals downward. While our goal may be focused on one thing, like weight loss, the reality is that we may need to solve numerous smaller issues before we can effectively lose weight and keep it off. Genetics are a factor, but the factors in our control will make the biggest difference. A 2016 Article in *Genome Medicine* found,

> *"Although genetic variants have been associated with susceptibility to developing obesity and type 2 diabetes, the heritability of these variants is fairly modest. The gut microbiota has recently been recognized as a key environmental factor driving metabolic diseases. In fact, the gut microbiota is even seen as a separate endocrine organ, which is involved, through a molecular crosstalk with the host, in the maintenance of host energy homeostasis and in the stimulation of host immunity." 17]*

The quote above highlights how crucial our gut microbiome is, almost functioning like an additional organ. Everything starts with the gut. Another shift in recent generations is the widespread use of oral contraceptives. A 2016 study found a measurable link between *the pill*, micronutrient deficiencies, and obesity in premenopausal women.18] The pill disrupts healthy gut bacteria, impairing digestion and reducing nutrient absorption. These factors must all be considered when evaluating health and weight loss. Prescription medications, in particular, can harm our digestive health. When assessing our diet, it's important to consider how well our bodies can digest the foods we eat. Effective weight management starts with gut health. A 2017 study compared various weight loss strategies, including bariatric surgery, diet restriction, and gut-health measures like prebiotics that nourish beneficial gut bacteria. The researchers aimed to determine whether weight loss surgery or gut health was more effective for weight loss. Here's what they found:

> *"These results show that restrictive diets and bariatric surgery reduce microbial abundance and promote changes in microbial composition that could have long-term detrimental effects on the colon. In contrast, prebiotics might restore a healthy microbiome and reduce body fat."* 19]

We don't need to starve ourselves. We don't need extreme weight loss surgery. We just need to get back to the fundamentals of real food and healthy gut microbiomes. In the study quoted, foods that help restore gut health produced positive results without risking the negative side effects of surgery. This study wasn't an anomaly, and the converse also holds true. Poor gut health leads to diabesity. Another systematic review found that bad gut bacteria led to a complex biological reaction that causes damaging inflammation and insulin resistance. 20] Remember that insulin resistance is the mechanism by which our metabolism is ruined, leading to diabetes. Food is fundamental to our health.

Conclusion

This chapter on food is barely scratching the surface of a complex topic. There's a lot more I could write about foods here: pesticides, farm-raised fish, industrially produced livestock, soy, and low-quality vegetable oils. While I briefly touch on some of these issues in other chapters, these topics are so big that they're probably best left for a future book. What you need to know now is that natural foods are the foundation of health. Refined sugars, soda, fast food, corn syrup, and prepared snacks are not real food and should be avoided. In order to restore the health of our society, we must use food and a naturally healthy lifestyle as the foundation for our health. Medications and the hospital system are not the foundation of health. Rather, these pharmaceutical interventions should be used cautiously and sparingly. As we've learned elsewhere in this book, the intricate balance of healthy gut microbiomes is foundational to restore health.

TLDR: Too Long Didn't Read

Even though the science is complicated, the answer's simple:
- Choose natural foods.
- Avoid processed foods.
- Find a doctor trained in functional medicine to help you get off prescriptions.
- Get outside and move.

Chapter 9
Your Thyroid: The Canary in The Coal Mine

"Wouldn't that be nice professor? The one simple elegant equation, to explain everything." -Stephen Hawking, *The Theory of Everything*

Holistic medicine being what it is, at times critics have derided it as a fanciful panacea, an unrealistic theory of everything. I would push back against these critics by asserting that when we solve a few fundamental health problems, hundreds of diseases (that are really symptoms) seem to resolve themselves. Our goal is to find out what's behind the problem that we see. The terms *holistic* and *root cause* have become vapid buzzwords that are losing their inherent value. For this reason, I try not to rely on buzzwords and instead focus on solving definable problems for patients. To this end, when my husband and I were developing the founding principles of Terrain Wellness, we came to a place where we had to pick one easily identifiable way that we could help people.

We asked ourselves:

- Who is my patient?
- What's my patients' problem?
- How can I solve it?
- How can I explain it in 30 seconds?

At first, this problem was tough because I can help almost any patient in the world using the principles defined in this book. We had to start with just one problem that was obviously underserved by mainstream medicine. The first problem we tackled was thyroid dysfunction. The tiny, butterfly-shaped gland in our necks can degrade into numerous health problems that conventional medicine isn't solving. Patients have suffered for years, sometimes decades under medical care that disregarded their symptoms and dehumanized them through lack of care. Conventional medicine seems to say to patients:

Your thyroid's broken.
We don't know why, and frankly, we don't care.
You'll need lifelong medication and treatment.
Call us when it gets unbearable, and we'll offer you another quick, useless prescription.
Sorry, not sorry.
—Your old doctor

While the above sentiment is not stated this way, this is how hundreds of my patients were treated by their old doctors. What's this book called again? Oh yeah, *Fire Your Doctor*! This lack of curiosity on the part of physicians is almost criminal. Why are most doctors just assuming that your thyroid is bad because "autoimmune" and just put you on artificial hormones? This is not what we're taught in medical school. What we're taught in medical school is that proper thyroid function is part of a much larger, finely balanced endocrine system. When any one part of the system has an issue, it causes the other hormones to become imbalanced, too. Our bodies are playing a hormonal symphony that must be tuned with the proper tones, rhythm and harmony. Otherwise, we all become a hormonal cacophony, a total mess where one instrument overrides the other. In my clinical experience, thyroid dysfunction is not a disease to be suppressed; it's a symptom of a much deeper hormonal imbalance.

"*Resistance to thyroid hormones are associated with obesity, metabolic syndrome, diabetes, and diabetes-related mortality.*" 1]

This was a quote from a 2019 research article in the research journal *Diabetes Care*; it speaks volumes about how important proper thyroid function is for metabolic health and the entire body. Many people know that the thyroid is a butterfly-shaped gland that sits in the middle of your throat. But most people tend to ignore this crucial gland until they begin to experience the painful symptoms of dysfunction. This gland regulates several vital body functions, including:

- temperature
- heart rate
- muscle strength
- cholesterol levels
- menstrual cycles
- breathing
- body weight
- nervous system signaling

To put it lightly, if your thyroid isn't happy, you aren't happy either. For both an increase in thyroid function, (hyper)thyroidism and a decrease in function (hypo)thyroidism, the symptoms can be very similar. Both create body temperature regulation issues, hair loss, depression and anxiety, muscle weakness and pain, and disruption in normal menstrual cycles. They are both connected to infertility, and they are both commonly caused by an underlying autoimmune process. For low thyroid function, this is often associated with something called Hashimoto's thyroiditis. For an overactive thyroid, the autoimmune process is called Grave's disease. If left improperly managed, Grave's disease will eventually turn into a low thyroid process, and the thyroid symptoms will look more like low thyroid function over high.

Symptoms of Thyroid Issues

Let's take a moment and review some common symptoms associated with the thyroid. Also, note that most people start to feel some or all of these negative symptoms before their condition is serious enough to show up on a conventional thyroid test panel. That's because thyroid blood test panels only indicate when your situation is bad enough to need prescription drugs. The problem didn't start overnight; it took years to develop. By paying attention to these symptoms before they get that bad, you'll be using the proverbial "ounce of prevention" instead of needing the "pound of cure" later on.

Hypothyroid Symptoms 2]
- Fatigue
- Sensitive to cold
- Weight gain
- Constipation
- Depression
- Lack of energy
- Muscle weakness
- Muscle cramps and aches

Hyperthyroidism Symptoms 3]
- Anxiety
- Difficulty Concentrating
- Frequent bowel movements
- Goiter or thyroid nodules
- Hair loss
- Hand tremors
- Feeling hot
- Heart fluttering/palpitations

While the above symptoms accompany thyroid issues, these lists are not complete. The main thing that you need to understand is that these problems go way beyond just the thyroid. This mysterious butterfly gland doesn't just "go bad" for no reason. There are bigger patterns at work here; modern medicine confuses our symptoms with the disease.

Thyroid issues are a symptom

> *You can have it fast,*
> *you can have it good,*
> *you can have it cheap.*
> *...pick two. -Unknown*

The so-called evidence-based medical approach is to treat the thyroid. The thyroid can't really be treated properly without addressing the much larger system of chemical messengers inside the body. You cannot effectively treat the thyroid unless you're also treating the big picture of the endocrine/hormonal system. Your thyroid is a key player in a hormonal signaling system called the hypothalamic-pituitary-adrenal axis, or HPA for short. 4] One common path to thyroid dysfunction is excessive cortisol. Cortisol is a stress hormone made by the adrenal gland. Maybe your old doctor put you on Synthroid, but what did they do to investigate and reduce your cortisol levels? Insurance-based medicine seeks to provide care as fast as possible and as cheap as possible; don't act surprised that normal healthcare lacks quality.

Cortisol is a stress hormone. We need cortisol to live, but thyroid problems occur when this hormone is too high for too long. Cortisol helps the body come down from adrenaline (our fight-or-flight hormone), but it has a number of other effects too. While the hormone adrenaline is commonly known, fewer people know cortisol and what it does in the body. We can't truly understand the thyroid gland until we learn a lot more about cortisol. I don't want to say that cortisol is bad, the truth is that it's complicated.

Cortisol levels rise every morning when we wake from sleep so we can handle the everyday stress that just being awake and conscious brings with it. Without proper cortisol levels, a condition called Addison's disease occurs. Addison's disease is typified by extreme fatigue, unhealthy weight loss, fainting, low blood pressure, diarrhea, vomiting, abdominal pain, joint and muscle pain, depression, and hair loss. 5] In extreme cases, low cortisol can lead to a life-threatening condition called acute adrenal failure. While too little cortisol is dangerous, it's much more rare than excess cortisol. When our lifestyle, emotional states, and the foods we consume create a constant state of stress on the body, cortisol levels can skyrocket out of control. Excess cortisol in the body over time brings on very specific physical presentations in the body. Patients in this state will present with belly fat that may often obscure the groin, fat on the back of the neck and red, rashy skin. They carry most of their fat in their torso, and the legs and arms lose muscle. This condition is called Cushing's Disease. 6]

Effects of excess cortisol (Cushing's Disease):

- Increased belly fat, especially the lower abdomen just above the groin
- Weight gain
- Loss of muscle size & strength in arms and legs
- Flushed, round face
- Mood swings (depression, anxiety, irritability)
- Muscle weakness
- High blood pressure
- Osteoporosis
- Blocking of insulin
- Increased risk/worsening diabetes
- Thyroid disruption

While we may not all have the above symptoms, we need to be aware that excess cortisol can be harmful well before Cushing's Disease occurs. Cortisol blocks insulin from acting on fat and muscle cells where it allows glucose/sugar to be utilized, leading to insulin resistance. 7]

Later on, insulin resistance leads to type II diabetes. The negative effects on insulin response force your liver to make more glucose, slowing your liver's function and driving your body to make even more insulin. Increasing insulin is an attempt by your body to correct the problem of not getting enough glucose into your cells. This creates a vicious circle of cells starved for glucose along with higher and higher levels of insulin. The body compensates by adding more insulin to counteract the effects of cortisol blocking glucose from getting into cells normally. Insulin resistance means your cells are starving while at the same time your blood sugar is getting dangerously high.

So, how do cortisol and insulin resistance harm the thyroid? When cortisol becomes too high for too long, it blocks the hypothalamus in the brain from telling your pituitary gland to produce TSH (thyroid stimulating hormone). Cortisol also signals the body to stop converting the inactive form of thyroid hormone T4 into the active usable form of thyroid hormone called T3. We cannot resolve thyroid issues without first getting control of cortisol and insulin. All of these factors are well understood in medical science, yet very little of this deep knowledge is actually put into practice in the normal thyroid treatment. 8]

At best, patients are given vague advice to lose weight, handed a pamphlet, and sent home with a thyroid prescription. But to make lasting changes, we must first address cortisol. Thyroid imbalance is often a symptom of broader endocrine disruption. So, how do we manage excess cortisol? Physically, we need regular exercise, a whole food diet with plenty of vegetables and quality protein, and a healthy gut microbiome. But one of the most important steps is managing emotional stress. It's easy to blame external factors for our stress: traffic, work, family, politics. At the end of the day though, these outside forces don't control our internal state. Our emotional and spiritual well-being plays a crucial role in our physical health.

This is a tough truth, but it's one we all need to hear: Life isn't stressing you out—your response to it is. If life feels overwhelming, it's important to take ownership of the stress we're creating ourselves. Once we do that, we need to avoid the bad and embrace the good. Avoid unhealthy coping mechanisms like emotional eating, drinking alcohol, withdrawing emotionally, or escaping into screens. Instead, focus on the good: seek counseling, exercise, connect emotionally with others, set emotional boundaries, practice prayer and meditation, and surrender what you can't control to God, resting in His peace. So now we've solved the thyroid mystery, right? Wrong. Cortisol, stress, and our spiritual state are all factors, but there are still some things to learn here.

My Doctor Ran My Labs

Even as an experienced physician, I remind myself that balanced hormones create a symphony of beautiful music. But when one section of the orchestra is off, the symphony turns into a chaotic mess—like cats fighting in a dark alley behind a dumpster. I examine numerous charts, diagrams, and drawings to understand how we can influence repair and fine-tune these hormonal instruments. The thyroid cannot be treated as a standalone gland; it must be viewed as part of a complex system that requires careful, strategic balancing. In the conventional medical model, thyroid treatment looks like this:

1. Run a "thyroid lab", check thyroid stimulating hormone or TSH.
2. Either the test "looks good" or "looks bad"
3. If it's bad, the doctor prescribes a thyroid drug
4. Repeat TSH testing, increase meds over the years
5. Your thyroid continually deteriorates over many years
6. When thyroid is completely destroyed, it is surgically removed
7. You end up on thyroid hormone replacement for the rest of your life

While there are many problems with the above standard of care, one of the most insidious problems is the definition of good and bad thyroid lab results. In these lab tests, "bad" is defined as "needs a thyroid prescription." Conventional doctors do nothing if it's not bad enough to need a prescription. But, there's a lot of nuance between *good* and *bad*. Patients usually start showing symptoms of thyroid dysfunction well before a basic TSH lab test puts them in the bad range. Why not treat thyroid issues before they get "bad" and need drug interventions?

As physicians, we can do much better than the current standard of care. At Terrain Wellness, we do. People come from all over the country for our help with thyroid issues. What we do isn't magic; we treat the thyroid as part of a much larger hormonal system. Over time, we've learned a thing or two.

The key to treating the thyroid is diagnosing the problem with far more precision than routine lab panels allow. Sometimes, thyroid issues stem from the brain, adrenal glands, or liver. Other times, long-standing digestive issues prevent proper absorption of essential micronutrients like zinc and selenium. Autoimmune conditions can also play a role. At some point though, calling everything autoimmune is just lazy. When we properly treat the thyroid, we focus on reducing inflammation by addressing pathogen and toxin exposure, as well as balancing gut health. Thyroid problems often involve multiple body systems that need support.

We do prescribe thyroid hormone, but we're specific about the type and tailored to the individual's needs. Throughout this process, we also look for other endocrine imbalances or issues with different body systems, as comprehensive thyroid care requires understanding the body as a whole. Simply put, we can't treat the thyroid in isolation if we want our patients to have healthy thyroids.

Better Testing, Better Doctors

As I mentioned above, conventional testing for thyroid function is abominable. I say this because we have had patients being managed by an endocrinologist for years (a conventional medicine specialist who treats only hormonal and metabolic conditions) with no relief. These supposed medical specialists are often underserving patients. After years, sometimes decades of neglect, these patients finally get angry enough to try something new. Patients are often referred by friends, co-workers or family members who we've helped. Even though nothing should surprise us anymore, we're still shocked by the lack of comprehensive testing within the medical establishment. Why aren't all doctors looking at the whole hormonal picture?

The path for most doctors is woefully simple: test thyroid levels, and increase the Levothyroxine. Levothyroxine is a synthetic form of thyroid hormone called T4. The body must convert this inactive thyroid hormone into the active T3 form. But, what if you're not healthy enough to convert inactive T4 into active T3? Many patients are nutritionally depleted of micronutrient co-factors such as zinc and selenium; making T4/T3 conversion is slow and inefficient. Even the prescribers are prescribing wrong. For this reason, we often find that patients do better on a combination dosage of T3 active and inactive T4 hormones. We also supplement with common minerals and herbs that are important to thyroid function.

Why We Won't Use Your Thyroid Panel

Sometimes, patients want to skip our lab testing protocol because they "already have labs" from their old doctor. Here's what you need to know: part of the reason your old doctor couldn't help you is because the tests they ran are garbage. Customary testing at a primary care, OBGYN and surprisingly at endocrinologist offices consists of TSH (thyroid stimulating hormone) and maybe (if you're lucky) Free T4.

What's the problem with that? TSH and T4 levels don't actually tell us if you have enough of the active hormone. The routine lab tests don't tell us if we're dealing with an acute thyroid condition or a long-term autoimmune process. Even in patients with all of the symptoms of thyroid dysfunction AND the customary garbage labs out of conventional range, people's old doctors have still told them "You're fine." The level of doctor incompetence around thyroid care is unimaginable, but painfully real. As I write this section, I'm furiously typing as I recall the years of pain that the medical establishment has caused my patients due to their abysmal standard of care. I get heated over this topic. While I'm upset on behalf of my patients, I'm furious on behalf of the millions of people in this country who have untreated and mismanaged thyroid issues. It's well past time to raise the standard. In our office, we've greatly enhanced the usual thyroid panel by testing for the following: TSH, Free T4, Free T3, Total T4, Reverse T3, thyroid antibodies and T3 uptake. We also compare your test results to optimal lab values. Depending on what our enhanced testing protocol uncovers, we may order comprehensive nutrient and digestive panels to make sure each patient has all the cofactors needed to process these hormones. In contrast to the medical establishment, which routinely ignores patients who say their thyroid "doesn't feel right," we run truly in-depth diagnostics to get to the bottom of things. If you're sick of being gaslit for wanting more from primary care, maybe it's time to fire your doctor.

Traditionally, conventional medicine's core competency has always been acute care and emergencies. But during COVID, even that core competency was eroded. When it comes to long-term hormone management, naturopathic, integrative and functional medicine are much more comprehensive and achieve far better results. Despite years of learning and tons of "research," the thyroid solution in conventional medicine almost always seems to be increasing your thyroid medication. There's very little individualization in conventional treatment plans and their optimal ranges are anything but.

Labs and Optimal Range

There's another, more insidious problem with routine medical lab testing. Any testing protocol has to compare something to a known precedent. That precedent is called the standard range. Standard range in lab testing is supposed to mean the ideal hormone levels that a person should have. What standard range really means is normal. Spoiler alert: **normal is not healthy!** Let me break this down in plain English. Standard thyroid panels compare the test results to the average person coming onto the lab for your area and demographic. This means that everyone's lab tests are graded on a curve. The problem with grading hormone panels on a curve is that the average 40+ American is overweight and has either pre-diabetes or is full-blown diabetic. Lab tests assume that the normal person they test is healthy and that their labs are compared to a healthy population. In reality, the labs just pull average and median test values from a sample of people who live within a certain radius of the lab.

Since most people aren't in optimal health, comparing yourself to the "normal" or "average" range won't help you get better.

Conventional lab ranges only tell you that you're not "dying" or about to die, but they don't offer much insight beyond that. When you rely on standard thyroid panels, they won't detect a problem until you've already lost at least 60% of thyroid function. The truth is, the conventional system is underserving patients, and many aren't receiving the thyroid care they need. The good news is, you don't have to continue suffering. Later in the book, we'll discuss how to find a better doctor who can provide the care you deserve.

Case Study: Natasha

Natasha is a 45-year-old overachiever in every area of her life—except one. She's a successful marketing director, a mother of three, and an all-around fantastic person. But despite her achievements, she was always tired and wanted to get to the bottom of it. Like many of our patients, Natasha found us through a referral. When she came in for her initial visit, she appeared well-groomed and happy but seemed to be struggling to keep her eyes open. She had been seeing her primary care doctor for years, who had been managing her low thyroid with Levothyroxine. Recently, she had also consulted an endocrinologist to get a more thorough work-up, but her symptoms persisted. Despite adjustments to her medication, she still wasn't feeling better.

Being meticulous, Natasha brought over ten years' worth of lab results, neatly sorted in a spreadsheet. At a glance, I noticed a pattern—despite her thyroid hormones being considered "in balance" by her doctors, her thyroid antibodies were extremely high.

Note: Natasha had actually begged her endocrinologist to run antibody tests after reading about thyroid conditions, and they agreed to test her. Most recently, her TSH was elevated and well beyond the conventional range, even with the standard, limited tests. It was clear that her thyroid was being mismanaged.

We began by running our enhanced thyroid tests, which her old doctor had never done before: reverse T3, free T3, free T4, total T4, and a baseline TSH. We also ran a basic wellness panel to check her immune system, liver, and kidneys, and added an iron panel and vitamin D check just to be thorough—things her endocrinologist had missed. The results were revealing. Natasha was not absorbing nutrients properly. Additionally, her immune system was working overtime due to an undiagnosed infection.

Our initial tests prompted further investigations, so we ordered additional tests to evaluate her adrenal glands, a viral panel, and her digestive health. This may seem like a lot of testing, but Natasha had been suffering for a decade, and even her endocrinologist wasn't providing answers. We had to do better.

Armed with a much more comprehensive understanding of her health, my team and I created a truly individualized care plan, or "Roadmap," tailored to Natasha's specific needs. We call it a roadmap because it's not just about making the best of where you're at—it's about leading you somewhere new. Our roadmaps are simple, clear, and goal-oriented. In Natasha's case, we outlined treatment goals for the first phase, which included a detailed meal plan. Food is often overlooked in conventional medicine, but it's essential for healing—no thyroid health roadmap is complete without it. All our patients attend a dedicated nutrition session where we develop a step-by-step plan using healing foods to restore thyroid function.

Now, back to Natasha's results. Her stress hormone profile showed a constant state of fight-or-flight, with a "flat line" curve indicating long-term chronic stress. This level of stress harms almost every aspect of your health, and in Natasha's case, it was particularly damaging. She lacked something called the Cortisol Awakening Response (CAR), a key factor for resiliency and coping with stress. When the CAR is absent, it negatively affects the thymus gland, an essential control mechanism for the immune system. Natasha's immune system wasn't able to protect her from tissue damage, pathogens, or tumors, which explained her immune issues and connection to autoimmune disease.

But we weren't finished. Natasha's comprehensive GI panel revealed improper fat breakdown, a lack of healthy gut bacteria, overgrowth of harmful bacteria, a protozoan infection, and Small Intestine Bacterial Overgrowth (SIBO). On top of that, her iron, zinc, and B vitamins were all low. Despite her outward appearance of being fine, Natasha had numerous underlying health issues that could have been very serious if left untreated. This wasn't just a thyroid problem; it was a systemic issue that conventional care couldn't address.

Her thyroid showed low active thyroid hormone (T3), very high TSH, and low free T4. She was also positive for a reactivated Epstein-Barr virus. It's safe to say Natasha had been badly mismanaged by both her endocrinologist and her primary care doctor. With everything going wrong in her health, no wonder Natasha felt exhausted. Finally, her symptoms made sense. She had been running on empty for years.

We immediately started Natasha on an adjusted thyroid medication, including a small amount of T3 hormone. We also gave her a micro-dosed hormone to help reduce inflammation related to autoimmune conditions. To address her nutrient deficiencies, we began repleting her vitamins and minerals with a series of IV infusions to bypass her gut dysfunction and deliver nutrients directly into her bloodstream.

Within two weeks, Natasha told our staff, "I feel like I woke up from a deep fog I've been in for years!" She realized she had been struggling through life on sheer willpower, not actual energy. After six weeks of treatment, we ran another lab panel and found that her thyroid hormones were within the optimal range, and her antibodies had started to lower. Over the next few months, Natasha's sleep improved, and she woke up feeling well-rested, no longer needing an afternoon nap. She had the energy to exercise consistently, and her complexion began to glow. The dark, puffy bags under her eyes were gone.

At the twelve-month mark, Natasha was a completely transformed person. We continue to support her evolving health, especially her gut health, which will take time to fully restore. But now, Natasha is living her life with hope for the future and the energy she needs to do amazing things.

Closing

Natasha's story may seem extreme, but her experience of being ignored and mistreated by conventional medicine is sadly common. Thyroid dysfunction isn't an isolated problem; it's a symptom of deeper, often complex, health issues. Insurance-based medicine tends to prioritize speed and cost, but healthcare can't be fast, cheap, and good all at once. Unfortunately, the short-cuts of conventional thyroid care often end up being slow, expensive, and ineffective.

In the race to be cheap for insurance companies and quick for appointments, the focus shifts to prescribing medication, lining the pockets of drug makers. This results in the worst possible combination: slow, expensive, subpar care.

Through investigative medicine, comprehensive lab testing, and the principles of naturopathic health, we're getting closer to a holistic approach to wellness. We'll never reach perfection in our earthly lives, but by using the full range of tools available to us, we can continually improve.

If your thyroid is being mismanaged, it might be time to *fire your doctor*.

Signs that you need naturopathic thyroid care:

- Muscle pain/weakness, swelling
- Feeling cold
- Hair loss
- Brain fog, fatigue
- Weight gain or rapid weight loss
- Constipation or loose stools
- Dry/rough skin & hair loss
- Irregular/heavy periods
- Depression/anxiety
- High cholesterol
- Infertility
- Temperature intolerances

- Trouble sleeping
- Swelling on the neck/ goiters
- Tremors or heart palpitations

Optimizing Weight & Metabolism with a Thyroid Condition

One simple way to improve your hormone health at home is to make some simple lifestyle changes before you need medical intervention. Talk to your physician and consider the following health tips.

Managing weight & metabolism with hypothyroid:
- Watch insulin levels, NOT calories
- Deploy patience
- Avoid inflammatory foods like gluten/wheat, dairy, corn, sugar & soy
- You MUST get good sleep
- Focus on weightlifting and building strength more than cardio
- You MUST reduce your emotional stress
- Correct all nutritional deficiencies
- Eat some fats to slow insulin response
- Eliminate stealth pathogens and support healthy immune function
- Reduce hidden sugars, even those marketed as healthy
- Make sure you have the right medication and are monitored regularly

General rules for optimal weight and metabolism with hyperthyroidism

- Treat the cause: remove stealth infections & pathogens
- Get on the proper medication
- BEWARE: once properly treated, you may become hypothyroid
- Fat is still your friend
- Increase calcium (hyperthyroidism leads to bone loss) eat foods like broccoli, kale, sesame seeds, dried figs, sweet potatoes, butternut squash, collard greens, chard
- Increase vitamin D3 intake – cod liver oil, or liquid/chewable supplementation

General rules for optimal weight & metabolism while having Euthyroid/sick/suboptimal thyroid

- Support immune system function
- Implement stress reduction techniques daily – complete the stress cycle
- Get better thyroid panels
- Have thyroid labs rechecked to make sure your thyroid remains in an optimal range
- Screen for toxins and mold
- Screen for stealth infections such as parasites and Lyme or Lyme co-infections

TLDR: Too Long Didn't Read

Thyroid issues are among the most common health concerns I encounter, affecting both women and men. The standard approach to thyroid treatment often involves waiting until dysfunction is severe, then masking the problem with prescriptions. Conventional care seems to treat thyroid imbalance as something normal, expected, and inevitable, leading to millions of patients with complex hormonal issues that remain untreated.

Factors like estrogen dominance, insulin resistance, chronic stress (excess cortisol), and certain medications can all negatively impact thyroid function. By addressing these underlying hormonal and lifestyle factors, we can achieve a more comprehensive thyroid recovery. My goal isn't just to manage symptoms but to help patients reclaim their hormone health so they no longer need prescription thyroid medications.

Chapter 10
Adrenals: Rest, Sex and Hormones

"I feel thin, sort of stretched, like butter scraped over too much bread"
J. R. R. Tolkien, The Fellowship of the Ring 1]

"Come to me, all you who are weary and burdened, and I will give you rest." -Jesus, Matthew 11:28 2]

One of the biggest complaints we get from patients is that they feel burnt out, exhausted, and tired. Some chalk it up to stress; for others, it's anxiety, fear, or just feeling spread too thin between work and family obligations. No matter the reason cited, a great number of our patients feel like they don't have enough energy to meet the demands of their lives. Fatigue can show up in many forms and have many causes. For some people fatigue looks like they can't run as fast or as long as they used to; their athletic performance is suffering.

Exhaustion can also invade the bedroom via lost libido; it's very common for patients to feel sexually frustrated, and many can't even remember the last time they had a good orgasm because it's been so long. Patients report compensating by habitually using excess caffeine just to stay awake. In a cruel irony, some fatigue patients feel exhausted all day and are tortured by insomnia during the night, feeling wired and unable to shut down. Fitful nights of interrupted, inadequate sleep, broken up by days punctuated by lack of energy and mental clarity.

When my team sees this clinical presentation, the first thing we think of is this:

What in the world is going on with their stress response system?

Which is always followed up with:

We need to check their adrenal and mitochondrial function.

The adrenal glands are small, mountain-peak-shaped organs located on top of the kidneys. While most people associate them with adrenaline, these glands play a much broader role. They produce and secrete vital stress hormones like cortisol, epinephrine (adrenaline), norepinephrine (noradrenaline), and aldosterone. What many don't realize is that the adrenal glands also produce small amounts of sex hormones. In post-menopausal women and middle-aged men, the adrenals become a key source of estrogen, progesterone, and testosterone. Yes, healthy women produce small amounts of testosterone, just as healthy men produce small amounts of estrogen.

Fatigue, exhaustion, insomnia, and issues with sexual performance or desire are common complaints I hear from patients. However, it's important to understand that the symptoms patients experience vary greatly because hormonal imbalances can affect numerous bodily functions. To better understand this, we need to revisit the tiny structures inside each of your body's trillions of cells—mitochondria. You may remember these from biology class as the powerhouse of the cell, but they do much more than just produce energy. Most cells contain about 1,000 to 2,500 mitochondria, with energy-demanding cells like muscles housing over 5,000. Mitochondria also play a role in immune function and detoxification by releasing substances that trigger the Cell Danger Response (CDR). The CDR is the body's defense mechanism against trauma or toxic exposure, helping to protect and heal the body.3] The CDR is supposed to be a temporary state that reverses independently. But, in cases where the CDR lingers on, it can produce numerous negative health effects.

Risks of Ongoing Cell Danger Response 4]
- Free Radicals inside cells
- Damage to DNA
- Metabolic disorder (diabetes and insulin resistance)

- Gut microbiome disorders

- Behavioral changes like ADHD, asthma, autism spectrum, Tourette's syndrome, bipolar disorder, epilepsy, suicidal ideation, etc.

- Autoimmune diseases such as lupus, rheumatoid arthritis, multiple sclerosis

- Cancer

- Heart disease

- Chronic inflammation

- Alzheimer's and Parkinson's disease

As you can see, staying in the Cell Danger Response (CDR) for too long leads to numerous debilitating and life-threatening health conditions. While ongoing CDR creates problems starting at the cellular level, hormonal processes also play a significant role in the body's overall function. One key hormone involved in this process is cortisol, which is produced by the adrenal glands. As we discussed in the thyroid chapter, cortisol is crucial for survival as it helps us recover from stressful events. Unlike adrenaline, which lasts only moments, cortisol can remain active in your system for days. While cortisol is necessary, too much of it over time causes harm.

By examining fatigue from both the cellular and hormonal levels, we can begin to address the chronic fatigue many of our patient's experience. In the past, cortisol would be released after the adrenaline-rush of life-threatening events, such as fighting off a tiger or defending a village from Vikings.

These stressors typically had clear, physical resolutions:
A) We killed the tiger.
B) The tiger killed us.

In either case, there was a definite, physical outcome that involved physical activity. Furthermore, surviving a tiger attack would likely make the warrior feel empowered, blessed, and capable. In contrast, modern stressors—such as rush-hour traffic, dealing with politics, or facing looming work deadlines—are often intangible, non-physical, and have no clear beginning or end. Unfortunately, sitting in traffic doesn't feel as heroic as defending your village against a predator. Traffic, political stress, and work demands can't be physically vanquished like a tiger or a Viking.

Imagine, for a moment, that you're a hunter-gatherer with zero contact with the modern world. You've just defended your village by killing a man-eating tiger. In the following evenings, you'd sit around the campfire, wearing your tiger-fur jacket, telling stories of bravery, overcoming adversity, and being grateful to the Creator. Now, compare that with modern stressors: constant, intangible, and poorly defined. Physical threats can be overcome, but abstract stressors like traffic cannot. Modern stress can feel unending and unbeatable.

Your hormones don't care whether you're fighting Vikings or constantly under work-related stress; cortisol is the go-to hormone in either case. In a sense, hormones act like drugs your body gives itself. And like any drug, the more you use it, the more tolerance you build. Constant stress leads to a never-ending cycle of adrenaline and cortisol. Since cortisol can stay in the body for days, your stress hormone levels can continue to rise.

Meanwhile, the cells in your body begin to downregulate their receptors in an attempt to protect themselves from internal damage. As a result, the body releases even more cortisol to produce the same effect. This creates a vicious cycle, similar to the process of insulin resistance that we discuss elsewhere in this book.

While we've talked about cortisol at length, let's take a quick dive into endocrinology to gain more insight. Healthy individuals need cortisol to function. Upon waking, a healthy person will experience a Cortisol Awakening Response (CAR), which involves a spike in cortisol during the first hour of being awake. The CAR indicates that waking up naturally increases stress levels compared to when you're asleep. In a healthy person, cortisol spikes upon waking and then gradually decreases throughout the day.

However, people dealing with chronic stress and fatigue often lack a healthy CAR. When this happens, cortisol is broken down into cortisone—the same cortisone that reduces inflammation but can damage joints over time. Because cortisol plays such an essential role in stress response, we conduct extensive lab tests on patients experiencing fatigue and stress. When we measure a fatigued patient's cortisol levels throughout the day, the results often show a flattened curve instead of the normal peak-and-taper pattern.

This healthy cortisol peak and taper process is essential for sustaining energy throughout the day. By evening, a healthy person will have very low cortisol levels, signaling the body to prepare for restful sleep. In contrast, stressed-out and fatigued patients often show either a flattened cortisol curve or a high peak that never drops to the optimal low level by bedtime.

The absence of a healthy CAR indicates severe adrenal dysfunction, a weakened immune system, and a reduced ability to recover from illness. Hormonally, this is why you may feel both tired and wired at the same time. A key sign of adrenal dysfunction is difficulty getting going in the morning. You might feel groggy and exhausted, often needing caffeine just to get started. By the afternoon, typically around 2-3 p.m., you may crave high-sugar foods like chocolate or salty snacks like chips to push through the last few hours of work.

Of course, relying on caffeine, sugar, and junk food is not a sustainable path to long-term health. Eventually, these crutches stop working, and that's when people are really in trouble.

The Adrenal, Thyroid & Blood Sugar Connection

You may notice elsewhere in this book that cortisol features heavily in many instances of thyroid dysfunction. While occasional excitement can make life fun and interesting, chronically experiencing stressful fight-or-flight responses leads to a number of harmful effects on the body, not the least of which is **adrenal and thyroid imbalance**. During times of stress, the adrenal glands release (nor)adrenaline into the bloodstream to prepare us for "fight-or-flight" in response to danger. But how does the body recover from being on high alert? The answer is that the fight-or-flight response also releases a stress hormone called cortisol. Cortisol puts the immune system into overdrive while also slowing digestion and inhibiting thyroid function (triiodothyronine (T3) and thyroxine (T4)). Here's where it gets a little bit complicated. In small amounts, cortisol is an anti-inflammatory hormone that prevents muscle, joint, and nerve tissue damage. For this reason, cortisone is used as a drug to treat painfully inflamed tissue. But, exposure to high levels of cortisol actually causes inflammation while inhibiting tissue repair over time. As an aside, new research shows that cortisone injections for arthritis pain actually do long-term damage to joint cartilage, making joint pain worse in the long run. 6]

So, if cortisol is anti-inflammatory, how does it cause inflammation? I'm so glad you asked. With continual high exposure to cortisol, the body develops a tolerance to the hormone's anti-inflammatory effects. Cortisol is the body's tool to fight inflammation; chronically high cortisol levels make that tool stop working. In this way, too much cortisol leaves the body without a natural process to reduce inflammation. 7] As a result, too much cortisol prevents the body from protecting its muscles, joints, and nerve tissues from damaging inflammation.

While cortisol in the proper amount can stimulate the immune system, excessive cortisol over time drains the immune system of the resources it needs to fight off infection. Because of this process, excess cortisol leads to increased inflammation and an ineffective immune system. The body just stops responding to cortisol. These harmful conditions open the door to a host of health conditions, from heart disease, obesity, thyroid problems, an increased risk of stroke, and numerous autoimmune processes. While cortisol is necessary for life at the right time and in the right amount, ongoing (chronic) stress brings out cortisol's negative aspects.

Excess Cortisol Over Time:

- Inflammation

- Slowed digestion

- Immune system dysfunction

- Autoimmune diseases

- Hypothyroidism

This cluster of symptoms is often referred to as adrenal fatigue. When adrenal fatigue is present, it causes a cascade of negative effects on the body's delicate hormone balance. From the hormone imbalance of adrenal fatigue comes weight gain, inflammation, autoimmune disorders and insulin-resistance (pre-diabetes). When people become stuck in this downward spiral, they report feeling "off." The symptoms can be unclear, but the patient will usually report having a slew of problems including weight gain, fatigue, trouble sleeping, waking up tired, sugar and salt cravings, energy at night but needing caffeine to keep them going during the day.

These patients may even notice that exercise feels more exhausting than energizing and that they get sick more easily and frequently catch Colds. These are all symptoms of chronic fatigue (adrenal fatigue) from the body being in fight-or-flight too often. This continuous fight-or-flight response will decrease vagal tone, which is the nervous system's ability to rebound from stress. Decreased vagal tone will lead to lethargy; these tired-out patients have activated the dorsal branch of the parasympathetic nervous system. The Dorsal branch is not the part of the parasympathetic system that helps with rest and digestion, but the aspect that keeps us feeling like we are walking through mud or constantly teetering on the edge of feeling like we are about to get sick. It's important to clarify that chronic fatigue is different from an adrenal insufficiency condition called Addison's Disease, which is an autoimmune disease that inhibits the ability to produce enough adrenal hormones. Addison's Disease is a serious endocrine disorder that can lead to a medical emergency. In contrast, adrenal dysfunction is not life-threatening per se but can lead to the development of various autoimmune conditions and eventually end in Addison's Disease. To help you better understand just how interconnected all of these hormones are to each other, please refer to the diagram, *Hormones in Balance*.

As you can see, achieving true hormonal balance requires addressing and evaluating all the body's systems. When men and women over the age of forty come into our office, they often request hormone replacement therapy. However, what they truly want isn't just hormones—they want to stop feeling tired and regain their energy. They want to be able to lose weight and feel as vibrant as they did when they were in their 30s. Despite what many might assume, this lack of energy and difficulty losing weight are not primarily due to a sex hormone deficiency, even as people age.

Issues with sex hormones are often a symptom of a larger, systemic hormonal imbalance, typically involving adrenal fatigue, thyroid imbalance, mitochondrial dysfunction, gut microbiome disruption, and metabolic health problems like blood sugar imbalances. Energy, weight management, healthy sleep, and sexual health are all deeply rooted in our hormonal balance, but they are also closely tied to how well our metabolism is functioning. To address these issues effectively, we must treat them at their foundational level.

In many cases, once we address imbalances like adrenal fatigue, mitochondrial dysfunction, and metabolic health (including blood sugar balance), issues related to sex drive and energy often resolve without the need for testosterone or estrogen replacement. The real underlying causes are frequently related to blood sugar issues, insulin resistance, cortisol dysfunction, thyroid imbalances, and mitochondrial health. By improving metabolic health, we can better regulate blood sugar and insulin levels, which in turn supports hormonal balance and overall energy levels.

That being said, we do believe that bioidentical hormones can play a vital role in helping individuals feel their best, and we use them often. However, we don't turn to them immediately. Bioidentical hormones should always be used with a clear understanding of the hormonal hierarchy and how the systems need to be balanced in the correct order. For example, treating adrenal fatigue, correcting thyroid dysfunction, and optimizing metabolic health—especially blood sugar regulation—before introducing hormone replacement therapies often yields much better results.

In some cases, where natural hormone balance cannot be achieved, bioidentical hormones remain an excellent option. But even in these cases, hormones are far more effective when the rest of the body's systems, including metabolic health, are functioning optimally. Using hormone replacement to merely mask underlying issues such as adrenal fatigue, thyroid dysfunction, or blood sugar imbalances doesn't address the root cause and doesn't truly solve the problem.

When it comes to hormone health, the old adage rings true: there's the fast way, and there's the right way. Trust me, choosing the right way will always serve you better in the long run, and you'll thank yourself later.

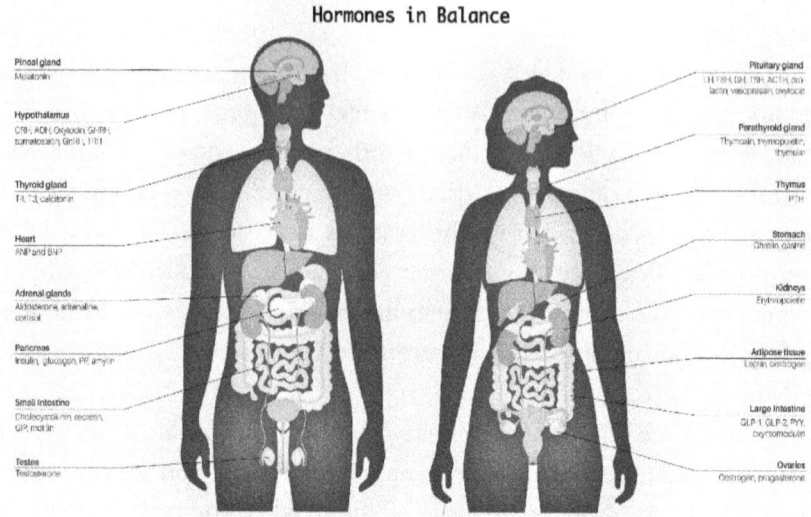
Hormones in Balance

The Mitochondria-Hormone System Connection

As we discussed at the beginning of the chapter, mitochondria are a type of organelle located within almost all of your body's cells. Mitochondria are directly responsible for creating energy within cells that your body can use to perform work. But mitochondria also play a less well-known role in hormone synthesis. Poor mitochondrial health results in poor steroid hormone production. This is part of why I don't start patients on hormone replacement without first addressing mitochondrial function. This isn't just my opinion, though. A 2013 study from the journal *Molecular and Cellular Endocrinology* found that the mitochondria contain enzymes that help the adrenal glands, gonads, placenta and brain convert cholesterol into compounds that the body then uses to make sex hormones.

The research also found two enzymes in kidney cell mitochondria that activate and breakdown vitamin D. Mitochondria directly influences the production of the mother hormone, called pregnenolone. Pregnenolone is an important precursor to all the major sex hormones such as estrogen and testosterone. Without pregnenolone, you will also not be able to make cortisol. Just as mitochondria can influence the production of hormones, hormones can also influence the health and function of the mitochondria. For this reason, we need to understand both in order to balance hormonal systems. 8]

Without proper function of the mitochondria, your adrenal glands and sex hormones can never be optimized. Going a step further, proper mitochondrial function is necessary for your entire endocrine system. So, how do we start repairing mitochondria? The first step is to shut down the excessive Cell Danger Response, or CDR for short. CDR is triggered when your body's cells are exposed to overwhelming stress. Stressors can be exposure to a pathogen, toxins, physical injury or emotional trauma. This leads to a cascade of events where the mitochondria switch from an energy powerhouse to a depleted battery. So, instead of mitochondria creating usable energy in the form of Adenosine Tri-Phosphate (ATP), it's forced to use its ATP to send signals to neighboring cells that danger is near. Once activated, the CDR must complete its full cycle for the condition to resolve. The CDR cycle starts with injury and ends with healing. As people age, their mitochondria become less efficient at completing and resolving a full cycle of CDR.

In cases of chronic fatigue and lack of energy, patients may well be stuck in the middle of the CDR cycle. Being stuck in an incomplete CDR means the cell's power-supply is being continually diverted into sounding a perpetual alarm, leaving greatly reduced energy available for daily life, exercise, and fun activities. Supporting healthy mitochondria helps slow the aging process while increasing energy levels. There's another layer to consider here. In situations where patients have been exposed to pathogens and toxins, they experience a two-part attack on their mitochondria. As we discussed, the first attack is that the CDR diverts mitochondria from providing enough energy to get through the day.

The second attack is oxidative stress inside of cells producing reactive oxygen species (ROS). These ROS complexes are used to neutralize toxins and pathogens. Oxidative stress can come from exposure to plastic residues in food and water, volatile chemicals, and processed foods. Higher oxidative stress in the body speeds up aging—

think gray hair and wrinkles. It also makes hormonal imbalances more common and severe. Plus, things like cancer, heart disease, and dementia are linked to oxidative stress. If you want to slow down aging and improve your quality of life in the long run, reducing oxidative stress is key. Bottom line: You won't get your energy back or balance your hormones without taking care of your mitochondria. Happy, healthy mitochondria with less oxidative stress can even help reverse some of the signs of aging

Mitochondrial Functions Overview 8] 9] 10] 11]

- Produces an estimated 90% of the body's energy
- Signals cell death and cell turnover
- Aids in the differentiation of types and function of immune cells
- Supports hormone production and balance
- A storage area for calcium needed for muscle movement

Let's Talk About Sex

One of my favorite books on the matter of the female sex drive is by hormone and sex researcher Dr. Emily Nagoski. Her book is called *Come As You Are: The Surprising New Science that will Transform Your Sex Life*. 12] It's a fascinating, research-backed exploration of how sex drive is unique to each individual—and that's completely okay. She offers practical tips on how to work with your body, not against it.

This book is not just for women, but for men as well. Both partners need to be educated to be fulfilling sexual partners for each other. It turns out that male and female sex drives are not the same. Of course, we've all known this for years, but it's still enlightening to understand how and why we experience our sex lives the way we do. While men and women are different, we share some common reasons why our sex lives may be negatively impacted. One major factor for both men and women with unfulfilling sex lives is stress.

In understanding female sexuality, it's helpful to view desire through the lens of a dual-action model for how sexual arousal is turned on and off. Dr. Nagoski uses an analogy for sex drive by describing both a brake and an accelerator. Of course, this is just an analogy. You can't literally find someone's sexual brakes and accelerator, but the concept of brakes versus accelerators is useful for psychologically framing our physiological and emotional motivations and inhibitions. Nagoski writes,

> *"There's a normal bell curve distribution of how sensitive the accelerator and the brakes are. Most of us are just heaped up in the average section. There are some people with extra sensitive or insensitive accelerators and extra sensitive or not sensitive brakes – most of us are just average. And, from the moment we're born, our brains are learning what to count as sexually relevant and what to count as a potential threat, and that's what we can change. It's learned. There's almost nothing that's actually innately sexual, so we learn that, and we can unlearn it and teach it something new."* 12]

According to Dr. Nagoski, as mentioned in the quote above, we can't really control our natural, baseline sexual drive. However, what is in our control is how we program our brains to respond to external stimuli. Many of us are walking around with an imbalance in what we perceive as sexually relevant input in our daily lives. If our brains start seeing everyday stressors—like traffic, work, or taxes—as existential threats, we might never feel free enough to fully enjoy a fulfilling sex life with our spouses. Raising kids, attending PTA meetings, juggling soccer practice, making dinner, and managing a career will never feel "sexy." But we can change how we emotionally relate to these responsibilities so they don't sabotage our sex lives.

On the other hand, for those whose sexual desire is expressed in unwanted or unhealthy ways, there's also the possibility of reprogramming what is and isn't sexually stimulating. After all, sex is one of the most intimate human experiences, and there's often a deeper, even spiritual connection to it. Yes, I know—sex and religion can be a tricky subject. But if you're facing challenges in this area, it might be worth sitting down for an honest conversation with God. Perhaps you feel shame, regret, or loneliness. Maybe you experience too much or too little desire, or perhaps you're angry at God for giving you urges and then making you feel guilty for acting on them. Honest conversations with God, where you express your frustrations and ask for help, can be an important step toward healing this deeply spiritual aspect of our lives.

One of the biggest inhibitors to healthy sexual expression is a poor relationship with stress. When we don't manage stress effectively, it lingers in our bodies and keeps our sexual brakes engaged. While this connection between stress and inhibited sexuality is evident in men, it's especially relevant for women. Biologically, this makes sense: for a man in constant danger, sexual risk-taking may feel necessary because he might not have long to live. But for women, chronic stress signals to the body that the world is too unstable to risk pregnancy and childbearing.

Dr. Nagoski's chapter on stress and sex drive resonated so deeply with readers that she co-authored another book with her twin sister, Dr. Amelia Nagoski, called *Burnout: The Secret to Unlocking the Stress Cycle*.13] Reading *Burnout* reinforced something we had already deeply integrated into our clinical practice: Your body must process the stressor before it can move on from the trauma. You might talk about it a hundred times, but until you clear it from your body, it will feel as if the stress is still with you—because it is. We can't just talk about the things that stress us; we must release the stress itself. Otherwise, those stressful events remain stored in the nervous system. For example, in *Burnout*, the authors describe exhaustion as the result of being "stuck." "Emotions are tunnels... Exhaustion is when you get stuck in an emotion, and your body is stuck in the middle of a stress cycle."

Given the importance of addressing our patients' emotional terrain, we also take steps to help the body release stress from the nervous system. Alongside balancing hormones physically, releasing past trauma is essential to helping people feel more grounded, safe, and hormonally balanced. We discuss this process in more detail later in the book. For now, just understand that proper adrenal function and healthy cortisol levels will require emotional, spiritual, and physical effort.

Restoring your Adrenal Function...it Takes a village

In *Burnout*, the Nagowski sisters conclude that recovery is not a single event, such as a massage or a day off. Furthermore, to truly recover from burnout, it takes changing the way the community you live in functions as a whole.

> *"We knew the answer to our exhaustion wasn't "self-care" --- self-care is the fallout shelter you build in your basement because the government says it's your responsibility, not theirs, to protect yourself from nuclear war. And revolution? We couldn't wait for a revolution; we needed help now."14]*

I like to use the term self-advocate instead of self-care. Taking care of yourself is more of a daily check-in—a moment to ask, "How am I doing?" And then, it's about having the permission to reach out to your community when you need support. Too often, we try to solve everything on our own, and that's when we start thinking, "How can I take on even more?" But maybe the better question is: How can I share some of this responsibility with others?

Adrenal recovery isn't just about rest—it requires action and a willingness to make changes. When someone's heading straight toward adrenal fatigue, the crash is coming. It could look like autoimmune disease, chronic illness, a major health crisis, a nervous breakdown, or damaged relationships. Honestly, some or all of these issues may already be brewing in people who are over-stressed. And illnesses often labeled as hormonal issues can have an underlying adrenal and mitochondrial dysfunction component, thyroid diseases included.

People over 40 often come into our clinic asking for bio-identical hormones—things like estrogen and testosterone supplementation. But what they usually need is to rebalance their blood sugar, correct thyroid imbalances, clear stress from their bodies, and, yes, get some proper sleep.

I Used to Sleep... Once Upon a Time

In his book, *Why We Sleep: Unlocking the Power of Sleep and Dreams*, Matthew Walker describes our cultural neglect of sleep as a "suffocating noose." The author goes on to state that "a radical shift in our personal, cultural, professional and societal appreciation of sleep must occur." 15] Ideally, things like schools and businesses would open later, and we'd work fewer hours so as to accommodate better sleep. But, given that we can't change the world until we change ourselves, we need to take the "noose" of inadequate sleep off our necks; we must choose to prioritize sleep.

In our clinical practice, we're big proponents of something called sleep hygiene. Do you really want more energy, a healthy sex drive, faster metabolism, and improved mood? Do you want to heal from chronic disease or recurrent infections? If so, you MUST get consistent, restful sleep EVERY night. There are many reasons why people have issues going to sleep, staying asleep, and waking in the morning feeling rested. But, until the foundations of sleep are established, we cannot tell what might be causing the sleep issues in the first place. When it comes to sleep, routine is key. Here are some simple guidelines we encourage ourselves, our families, friends, and patients to follow to help reestablish proper sleep. Of course, there are times when a medical issue makes healthy sleep difficult or even impossible to maintain. However, we can't diagnose these less common situations until we've first established proper sleep hygiene.

Ways to Improve Sleep

Stick to a regular bedtime. Go to bed and wake up at around the same time every day. With a reliable routine, your body will establish an internal clock. Regular rest/wake cycles reinforce a proper circadian rhythm. Your body will set a natural alarm clock if you're diligent about this routine. Shoot for at least 7.5-8 hours of sleep per night. According to the Chinese medicine organ clock, it's very important to get in bed before 10 PM to prepare for vital cleaning processes that take place overnight. Chinese medicine teaches that 1 AM to 3 AM is when the blood returns to the liver for cleansing; being in bed by 10 PM allows us time to prepare for this cleansing period during the night. Going to bed too late means you won't be prepared, and the liver will not fully cleanse the blood overnight. Over time, the liver will become less effective, making you more susceptible to illnesses and hormonal imbalances.

Establish a screen and technology bedtime. Begin to lower the lights and turn off all electronic devices 1 to 2 hours before bed. Let's say, by 8 or 9PM. Set your technology on wind-down mode, wear blue light-blocking glasses, and set light filters on your phone. Blue light from electronics can influence your sleep significantly. Keep the phones and bright lights away from your bedtime routine. I suggest plugging your phones in and putting them flipped upside down in unreachable areas. As another, more powerful option, consider charging your phones in the kitchen and using an old-fashioned alarm clock. Turn off your television. Don't use the TV to lull yourself to sleep. Better yet, remove the TV from the bedroom altogether. Make your bedroom a sanctuary for sleep, restful conversation, and intimacy. My husband and I do not have a TV in our bedroom, and we never will. Our bedroom is a place of restful time together.

Don't have stressful conversations right before bed. This is a big one for my husband and me. We tend to get fired up about some current topic or things we're working on in our businesses. We're both passionate people, so we have regular conversations about whatever we're learning or the ideas swirling around us. For this reason, we've had to put some serious boundaries around these topics at bedtime. If we're not careful, we can easily discuss various topics well into the night; of course, we pay the price the next day feeling groggy and sleepy. We limit ourselves to lighthearted, funny or happy topics before sleep. We often have to keep each other accountable to shift the conversation back to a more restful banter.

Establish a sleeping sanctuary. Sleep in total quiet and darkness. Yes, even the colored light from the smoke detector gets covered with electrical tape in our house. Of course, don't compromise safety, but do cover up any annoying light sources in your room. It always surprises me how many random devices have LED lights that just stare at us from the darkness. Speaking of which, get rid of all the LED bulbs in your bedroom—these emit blue light that keeps your brain awake and disrupts your sleep-wake cycle.

If you live in an area with city lights, invest in blackout curtains, and keep the room temperature cool. It's okay to spoil yourself a little: get comfortable sheets, a supportive pillow, and update that old mattress. Diffuse some essential oils at night to promote relaxation. I love a mix of juniper berry, frankincense, and lavender—just two drops of each in an oil diffuser. If it's allergy season, I recommend peppermint, cardamom, ravensara, and lemon essential oils.

Our bedroom is one of our favorite places to be at night. It helps lull us to sleep and makes waking up comfortable. A 2018 study of university students in Italy showed how room color affects studying, concentration, and mood. The study found a significant preference for blue—students in blue rooms studied better and felt a sense of tranquility and calm. Light green and light yellow came in as close seconds, likely because they mimic nature, offering both calmness and energy.

Whatever color you choose for your room, pick one that makes you feel relaxed, centered, and ready to catch some z's.

Establish stable blood sugar before bed. Eat a macronutrient and micronutrient-dense dinner. This means making sure you're eating enough protein, fats, fiber, and greens. A balanced dinner keeps your body satisfied. Too much sugar at night can cause blood sugar to crash later in the night. Sweets and alcohol in the evening may lead to unhealthy blood sugar fluctuations in the night. These blood-sugar fluctuations can lead to nightmares and sleep interrupted by the need to urinate. Ideally, have dinner at least 2 to 3 hours before bed, and don't have sweets or alcohol within a few hours of sleeping.

This gives your body enough time to start digesting so it can repair and cleanse during the night. If you eat a huge meal right before bed, your body will be overwhelmed with digestion and won't be able to focus on rest and repair. Sometimes, when I'm trying to help a patient re-establish balanced blood sugar, I need to get them to sleep better. Occasionally, I'll recommend a small protein-based snack before bed, but absolutely no sweets. Once we get better sleep established, we'll try to move the last meal closer to the three-hour window before bed. If you want better sleep, limit or better yet eliminate all alcohol, especially within 3 hours of bedtime. Contrary to popular belief, alcohol is not a good sleep aid. While it can help you fall asleep, it also causes serious blood sugar problems and prevents your body from going into the deep restful sleep. People who rely on alcohol for sleep interrupt the body's natural sleep patterns and end up feeling much less rested than they should.

Establish a bedtime routine. Bedtime routines should be boring and predictable. The point is consistency. When you make changes, do so carefully and intentionally. I always tell my body, "All roads lead to sleep" as I set my intention for the night.

Our routine starts around 7:00-7:30 PM. We finish dinner, clean the kitchen, and send our oldest upstairs for the bathroom, teeth brushing, and pajamas. We then follow with our youngest. We get her in her jammies, brush her teeth, and put her to bed. If it's not too late, we read one chapter of a novel, then say family prayers. After that, it's off to bed for the kids.

What we don't do is drag out their bedtime or tolerate arguments or misbehavior. Kids' behavior is all about motivation, and story time is something they really look forward to. They know stories won't happen if they're acting out. If you let them, kids can easily take over your entire evening. Instead, we give them focused attention during dinner and story time. The whole bedtime routine takes about 35 minutes from start to finish, and by 8:00 PM, it's my turn.

I wash my face, floss, brush my teeth, and get into my pajamas. My husband and I stretch and chat for a bit. Then, it's sex and sleep—or if I'm working early the next morning, just sleep. On my days off, I might deviate slightly from the routine, but I don't stray too far. Sleep is still a priority, even on the weekend.

Sleep is central to our health and ability to cope with stress.

Prioritize Sex in Your Marriage. The exact frequency of sex depends on how we're feeling, but no matter what, we prioritize it in our marriage. It happens because we make time for it and create opportunities for it. Sex and connection with your spouse releases oxytocin, helping you feel loved, connected, and ready for sleep. Like going to the gym, every parent knows it won't happen unless you schedule it. Yeah, I know what you're thinking: planning takes the sexiness out of sex. But hear me out.

When you were dating, dates and time together were often scheduled and planned for. When you're in love, you make an effort to be with your person. Married folks often long for the days of "spontaneity," but honestly, that's mostly a myth. That "spontaneous" moment happened after you picked out special clothes, took extra time to groom, cleared your schedule, and made sure you had interesting things to talk about. Maybe you lost a little weight, washed your car, or tidied up your house. That so-called spontaneity happened because you put time and effort into making it happen.

Don't fall for the myth of spontaneity. You planned dates when you were dating. You planned a wedding. You planned a honeymoon. So now, be intentional and plan time for romance and making love with your spouse. When I make time for romance with my husband, I'm ALWAYS glad I did. When we prioritize time together, we feel more relaxed, more connected, and more ready for sleep. And let's be honest: nothing helps you fall asleep faster than a good orgasm.

No, it's not always convenient or easy. But your marriage and your sex life are worth fighting for.

Herbs. Herbs and botanical medicine are powerful tools to restore function to the body. Herbal medicine comes in many forms. The most fundamental medicinal herbs we take are our food and nutrition. Avoid junk foods. Incorporate healing herbs, medicinal plants, and nutrient-dense food into your daily life. In cases of anemia, feeling cold and weakness, choose hearty cooked foods including bone broths, red meats and stewed vegetables seasoned with traditional herbs. I love soups, stews, and teas sipped throughout the day. Try incorporating ginger and licorice root when you can. I also love mushrooms, which are great for the immune system. Mushrooms are excellent for restoring people who are exhausted. If a person tends to be too hot and complains of lots of phlegm and excess body weight, we tend to also recommend cooked foods in the fall and winter and incorporate more fresh green bitter foods. These folks need to cut out sweet and starchy foods more than others. We love things like dandelion greens, arugula, lemon water, and cinnamon.

Nutrition. Nutrition is not just what we eat but how we eat. Making sure you have the correct macronutrients, protein, fats and yes, some carbohydrates. As simple as this is, following sound principles around our food is very powerful. Processed junk foods create stress on the body. If we don't consume enough of the basics, especially if our hormonal system is imbalanced, our body perceives it as stress. Stress, as we learned about earlier, Increases cortisol. Cortisol tells insulin to remain high because we're going to need to run from a wild animal very soon here, so get ready to need energy. Naturally, if your body feels like it may need energy to survive, it'll need to store more energy (in the form of fat). Simple reminders about how to eat to prevent a stress response.

Make time to eat. Many of us (including myself unless I continually become conscious of this) grab a quick bite on the run. In today's culture, we eat in our cars, we take a few bites as we walk from one scheduled obligation to the next. We fail to sit and breathe and taste the food and eat. Try putting your fork down between bites and taking a few breaths.

Chew your food. One study conducted on nearly 4,000 middle-aged adults correlated fast eating with increased incidences of obesity. 16] Yet another study showed, eating slower can reduce the calories consumed. This happens through the hormones related to fullness and satiety. 17] It turns out, that slowing down while eating will leave you more satisfied with a meal while eating less. One rule of thumb, without being obsessive about the number of times your chew is, chew your food until it is liquid. This may be 15 chews for something soft like peaches or melon or 40 chews for something like steak or your mother-in-law's pot roast. Disclaimer: My mother-in-law is an excellent cook, and I genuinely love her cooking. I love you, T.L. This really is here as a humorous anecdote.

Don't drink water or any liquids WITH meals. "What? You may ask. But sometimes I need liquid to swallow my food." I've got two pieces of advice for that. First, maybe your food is overcooked—time for a new cook. Or second, see reminder #2: chew your food until it's liquid before swallowing. Drinking water with meals can dilute your stomach acid, which makes you more susceptible to acid reflux or GERD (gastroesophageal reflux disease)—we dive into this more in our chapter on antacids.

Here's the bottom line: without enough stomach acid, food doesn't break down properly, and you don't get the nutrients you need. And no nutrients = no bueno. We're talking constipation, diarrhea, gas, SIBO, IBS, skin issues, malnutrition, irritability, anxiety, headaches, nausea, cramps... the list goes on. Nutrients are essential for every cell in your body. Drinking a lot of liquid during meals can dilute your stomach acid, leading to poor digestion. And poor digestion equals poor sleep and messed-up hormone health.

No working while eating. I will admit this one is the most difficult for me. Sometimes, during lunch is the only time I have to make a work phone call or answer an email. I really need to focus on this one. Working while eating increases stress levels. When you're stressed, you don't receive the normal signals for digestion from your brain. Without the proper signals you do not make enough of the digestive enzymes and acids to break down the foods. No breakdown, no nutrients. You know how this one goes.

No screens while eating. For the same reasons as above, you become distracted and tend to over-eat and do not get the proper signals from the brain. It's so easy to become addicted to our phones and screens. But it's harmful to so many areas of life, including digestion and sleep.

No rigorous exercise after eating. Yes, exercise in itself is good. But, exercise places you into a fight-or-flight state. That does not work well when we want to rest-and-digest. Wait at least an hour or two after eating a meal to do strenuous exercise. A light 10-minute walk after each meal can be a good idea because it supports a balanced insulin response. If you've had a major meal, it's probably best to wait a few hours before strenuous physical activity.

No fighting while eating. Kids who had parents who fought at the dinner table are more likely to develop issues with digestion such as IBS. 18] Sometimes hard conversations must happen, but try not to have them at the dinner table. Use prayer and humbling yourself to God to realize that in any argument, you're partly right... but also partly wrong. Don't be so proud to think that your spouse's opinion is always wrong and you're always right. Don't argue or fight at dinner.

What can we learn here? Stress of any kind must be avoided while eating food in order for the signals of our digestive system to work properly. We are mammals. This means we are highly affected by various signals that are used to protect us. If we push this stress response system consistently for too long, disease and dysfunction will occur. Acquiring and digesting food is essential for long-term health and reversal of disease processes. Historically, things like famine, starvation and lack of nutrition have been scourges on society. For this reason, we have stress and strong emotions surrounding food hardwired into our DNA. If you don't have enough nutrients, your body becomes focused on surviving and will not have enough to heal let alone to thrive.

Oxytocin. In Dr. Ana Cebeca's book *The Hormone Fix*, she highlights the importance of the big "O" in your life. Oxytocin, that is. Oxytocin is a hormone that's released in the presence of emotional bonding, affection, and closeness. Oxytocin is also made when pregnant mothers give birth; it helps with muscle contraction but also plays a role in helping the mother bond with her new baby. Large amounts of oxytocin are released during orgasm from both male and female partners. So, I guess you can say the "O" in oxytocin does have a relationship to the other big "O."

Dr. Cabeca points out in her book, how vital regular oxytocin release is to heal from chronic stress. After the loss of her son, Dr. Cabeca completely reversed her early menopause by dramatically lowering her stress through a combination of mindfulness, clean nutrition, therapy, movement, and focusing on increasing oxytocin release. She suggests love, laughter, play, and experiencing joy as the key to her own recovery. Yes, I know the phrase *live, laugh, love* has become a vapid platitude for many of us. But we do need all of those things. Oxytocin is the hormone that's released with eye contact and breastfeeding an infant. When released properly and regularly between infant and mother, it teaches us how to connect and bond with others in relationships as we grow. Oxytocin builds healthy and sometimes unhealthy attachments, especially if we don't receive enough bonding time with our parents. Oxytocin counteracts the effects of cortisol and adrenaline; it helps the body let go of constant high alert. Oxytocin can be a powerful way to increase trust and bonding between people.

Research is looking into the development of an oxytocin drug that may treat anxiety. While developing this drug, researchers found that oxytocin isn't only responsible for the warm, fuzzy, and connected feeling we get, it also intensifies anxiety and fear in situations that are negative or stressful. 19]

Oxytocin is a powerful hormone and should be used wisely. Oxytocin is the hormone responsible for strengthening social memory in the brain. For example, if higher oxytocin levels exist between two people and that person betrays you, oxytocin is the hormone partially responsible for repeatedly reliving that event in your mind long after the event. If healing happens in trust and connection patterns, oxytocin is the hormone that needs to be re-released in a healthy relationship to heal from the previous betrayal. This is a perfect example of how hormones and neurotransmitters need balance. Not too much and not too little. Here are a few ways to increase Oxytocin to help counteract the effects of chronically high cortisol.

Get human contact. Prolonged eye contact, a 10 second or longer hug, a massage and regular orgasms are some of the best ways to increase oxytocin, reduce cortisol and feel calm. 20] – 26]

Hugs and snuggles with your favorite pet. If humans are not available, get a pet. Research shows that,

> *"Concentrations of beta-endorphin, oxytocin, prolactin, beta-phenylethylamine, and dopamine increased in both species after positive interspecies interaction, while that of cortisol decreased in the humans only. This occurred with as little as 5 minutes of physical touch with a pet."* 27]

Optimize your vitamin levels. This is especially true for cofactors of oxytocin production, such as vitamin D, Vitamin C, magnesium, and taurine. Consuming balanced nutrition full of proper macro and micronutrients is key to healing on every level. The above are very specific to the production and excretion of optimal oxytocin levels and have been researched to play a role in the stress response system. 29] – 31]

Practice loving kindness, meditation, and prayer. Any type of mindful breathing will help promote relaxation. However, this specific practice has been researched in regard to increasing oxytocin levels. If you have or want faith, meditation is a perfect time to clear off the harassing thoughts so you can connect with God's quiet and gentle voice. At times, I've heard some Christians express misgivings about some meditation practices being tied to other religions. If you're one of these people, meditate on God's love for you, turn off all distractions, and spend some time reading Psalms or Proverbs. Remember that Psalm 119 mentions meditation 8 times. 32] The research model to evaluate the effect of Loving Kindness Meditation (LKM) focuses on empathy towards oneself and others. The idea of practicing LKM is to build up your capacity to have compassion and empathy for both you and others.

> *"The model presented here proposes that empathy is composed of basic attentional, perceptual and motor simulation processes, simulation of another's affective body state, and slower and higher-level perspective-taking... At all levels in the process, neural systems are influenced by oxytocin and the pro-inflammatory immune system. Kindness-based meditation practices may influence each of these neural systems; however, to date the most consistent evidence supports the idea that LKM enhances the neural systems important for emotion regulation." 33]*

Meditation while bringing up love and kindness brings us closer to God and is universally beneficial. Here's an easy way to think about it.

Prayer is talking to God. Meditation is listening to God.

Get acupuncture. There's a reason why acupuncture is incorporated into many of our treatment plans. Acupuncture boosts oxytocin, dopamine, stimulates circulation and supports the vagus nerve. 34] We call acupuncture the easiest form of meditation. It's at least somewhat beneficial in just about every ailment and is a powerful system of health restoration.

Increase positive social interactions. Research shows that not only will being with people in a positive way boost your oxytocin levels, but it may also actually promote healing from injury. 35] We are social creatures, and we need positive human interaction to feel whole and well.

Try intermittent drinking. No, I don't mean alcohol. Intermittent drinking is where a person drinks large quantities of liquids at more spaced-out intervals rather than steadily drinking throughout the day. Here's the research:

> *"Intermittent bulk drinking should be defined as water (including tea and coffee) drinking up to a feeling of satiety and regulated by a mild feeling of*

thirst. *This would mean that people would not drink less quantity but less frequently, and that's how all animals, but also human newborns, behave." 36)]*

The same thirst receptors in the brain also trigger oxytocin receptors as well.

"Recent research shows that the homeostatic disturbances leading to the 'thirst feeling' not only activate specific substances regulating water and mineral household but also the 'trust and love'" hormone oxytocin, while decreasing the production of the typical stress hormone cortisol." 36]

End your hot shower with cold immersion. This is also called contrast hydrotherapy, and the benefits are quite remarkable. Cold immersion has been shown to increase oxytocin, reduce stress hormones, reduce muscle pain, calm the body, promote circulation, boost metabolism, help with mental clarity, and improve immune function. 37] The key is short immersions in cold water (no more than a few minutes), followed by gradually warming the body. I love using a sauna and then jumping into cold water. After repeating this hot-and-cold cycle, I can feel my body relax, and a warm sensation spreads through me—kind of like a nice glass of wine, but without the side effects. On nights after sauna sessions and a cold plunge, I sleep deeply.

Sing or hum every day. I love singing in the car on my way home from work, especially worship music. I highly recommend singing or even humming throughout the day. Not only does it boost oxytocin, but it also tones your vagus nerve and lowers stress hormones. "findings suggest that listening to slow-tempo and fast-tempo music is accompanied by an increase in the oxytocin level and a decrease in the cortisol level, respectively, and imply that such music listening-related changes in oxytocin and cortisol are involved in physiological relaxation and emotional excitation, respectively." 38]

Another study showed that oxytocin levels increased in both professional and amateur singers after a singing lesson, and both feelings of well-being and arousal were demonstrated in both groups. 39] Singing in a group has been shown to not only boost oxytocin but also lower blood pressure, increases the immune system, and lower the perception of pain. 40] Combining our need for human connection with song is powerful medicine. No matter where you are or who you're with, it's clear that humans love music and singing. This is a powerful natural tool to support your stress and overall health.

Try Aromatherapy. Aromatherapy sometimes gets a bad reputation because people tend to exaggerate the effects, but it's still a legitimate form of medicine. We incorporate therapeutic-grade essential oils into our treatments because they are fantastic plant-based medicine and also powerful natural antimicrobials, but they also have a profound impact on mood and the brain. Aromatherapy is a powerful tool that influences the limbic nervous system and supports parasympathetic tone.

The parasympathetic system is the "rest and digest" part of your autonomic nervous system, and it needs support in order to heal from chronic illnesses, particularly autoimmune diseases or long-term infections. Two oils specifically researched for supporting oxytocin levels are jasmine and clary sage.41] 42] We have over a hundred different essential oils and blends that we use at our office. We use these oils in custom blends for our patient's specific needs, including blends to help counteract the effects of stress.

Move, because movement is good. You must move your body. Stress is stored in the body; we'll discuss this in detail when we go over our emotional health. Trauma and stress stay in the body until you move it out. Stress is an emotion that demands physical action; it won't leave unless the body has a physical signal to do so. One of the most effective forms of movement therapy is resistance stretching or mindful movement. Personally, I don't like stretching; it's a necessary evil for me.

Yoga is tied to religious traditions that differ from my own, so I no longer practice it. However, stretching and moving our bodies isn't exclusive to any one faith. In fact, my church now offers a Christ-based mindful movement and flexibility class, which I attend when I can (though, I still don't love stretching). Mindful movement stimulates the vagus nerve and has been shown to increase oxytocin levels and help with facial emotional recognition in people with schizophrenia.

Let me back up for a moment and share something with you. I've been stretching for over a decade, and I'm still not flexible. I'm the one in class who looks like I'm related to the Tin Man. I have McArdle's disease, a muscle disorder that makes my muscles extremely stiff. Stretching is painful for me, and flexibility doesn't come naturally. But, if I don't stretch regularly, I'm even stiffer and in more pain. So, every single time I attend a movement class, I'm the angry troll for the first 10-15 minutes. I consider running, yelling, and crying. I make excuses about why I can't do it... and then, I do it anyway.

I always feel better at the end of a movement sequence. I feel calmer, and when I went through a tough divorce, the exhaustion of medical school, and chronic illness, mindful movement helped bring me back to life. With my tight schedule, I can only attend a live class once a week right now, but the energy of being in a room with like-minded people nourishes my body and soul.

My advice as a doctor—and as a human—is to find your version of movement, whatever that is, to get that release. You need to stretch, move, and meditate. I walk, lift weights, do HIIT (High-Intensity Interval Training), hike in nature, play with my kids, and use my body intentionally. Every. Single. Day.

- I find movements that feel good in my body
- I only stress my body for small intervals, then I rest in between
- I challenge myself physically, and then I rest
- I do movements that bring me joy (minus the first 10-15 minutes of any workout)
- I reinforce this joy in my nervous system
- I talk about how good the workout felt, how it feels so amazing to think better, build strength, and how calm my body feels after I have been able to move
- I let go of the idea that movement is punishment
- I stopped obsessing over how I move. Instead, I focus on the consistency of moving every day
- Some days, I have an hour to move. Most days, I have about 15-20 minutes

- Many days, I follow up movement with 5-15 minutes of mindful breathing, prayer, and meditation

The above disciplines reinforce my nervous system to remember how I can always become re-centered and calm even after vigorous movement.

Routine. The key to restoring the adrenal/stress system and recovery from chronic illnesses is routine. We talked earlier about the importance of restoring proper cortisol awakening response or CAR to increase your body's resiliency, to heal, and to reverse autoimmune processes. We are mammals, we are connected to nature, and we are subject to natural rhythms. We are affected by the moon, for goodness' sake. As author and speaker Rob Bell wrote in his book, *EVERYTHING IS SPIRITUAL: A brief guide to who we are and what we're doing here,*

"Her monthly egg-releasing cycle was influenced like every woman everywhere since forever, according to the sequential unflappable consistent movements of the moon...the moon I will say that again out of sheer admiration for the unexpected oddness of this particular relationship...the moon. To be clear, the female body has an intuitive synchronistic alignment with a rock floating in space 238,000 miles away." 43]

Strange as it seems, moon phases affect our circadian rhythm, energy levels, and hormonal cycles. No, this isn't astrology, it's logic. God designed us to take advantage of the extra light offered by the full moon by staying up later and having more energy. Conversely, if it gets dark outside super early, it is wise to just stay home and go to bed. We humans are tied to nature in ways we have almost forgotten about.

Taking back your rhythm

Get your body in nature. Multiple studies have highlighted the benefits of spending time in nature, including its ability to reset circadian rhythms and improve insomnia patterns after just a few days of camping outdoors. One early study by Yoshifumi Miyazaki, a forest therapy expert and researcher at Chiba University in Japan, found that people who spent 40 minutes walking in a cedar forest had lower levels of the stress hormone cortisol—linked to blood pressure and immune function—compared to when they walked for the same amount of time in a lab. "I was surprised," Miyazaki recalls. "Spending time in the forest induces a state of physiological relaxation."45]

Time in nature resets proper levels of melatonin. Some people who get depressed in winter have been shown to have higher levels of melatonin during the day due to a lack of exposure to natural sunlight. Exposure to natural sunlight first thing in the morning is key to resetting melatonin levels and restoring cortisol awakening response.

Food and Light. By now, most of us have heard that eating turkey makes you tired, but there's more to it. Foods that help boost melatonin contain an amino acid called tryptophan. Tryptophan is converted into 5-HTP, which can then be turned into either the mood-stabilizing neurotransmitter serotonin or melatonin. Foods rich in tryptophan or 5-HTP, such as salmon, poultry, eggs, spinach, and seeds, are all part of the nutritionally dense whole food diet we recommend. However, research shows that eating these foods may not be enough on its own.

"Melatonin is synthesized from tryptophan, an essential dietary amino acid. It has been shown that certain nutritional factors, such as vegetable intake, caffeine, and some vitamins and minerals, can influence melatonin production—but none as strongly as light, the most dominant factor in regulating melatonin." 46]

Nature for the win! It seems our bodies are more in sync with the outside environment than anything we put into them internally. Humans are meant to be in rhythm with the seasons and the natural cycles of day and night. To reinforce this, aim to sleep within 1-2 hours of sunset and wake with the sunrise whenever possible. Keeping a consistent sleep schedule—no matter the weekend—is key to getting your body back in sync with nature.

Living in a dark place for part of the year? No problem! Try a natural light alarm clock, full spectrum light bulbs or a Himalayan salt lamp that you turn on when you wake up. The goal is to get natural light into your eyes first thing in the morning, which has been shown to significantly increase cortisol levels.46]

Eat with your circadian rhythm. Just like our sleep is key to resetting our natural routine, so are eating patterns. Our brains love predictability.

When a person is under chronic stress and trying to recover, eating simultaneously every day is an excellent way to calm the nervous system and level out blood sugar spikes and dips. When our blood sugar surges, it leads to a feeling of over-excitement and physical signs of anxiety. When our blood sugar dips, we get irritable, confused, and experience lack of motivation.

The blood-sugar rollercoaster creates a miniature depressive state. One study showed the correlation between glycemic variants and an increased incidence of depression. 46] Managing these peaks and valleys on a physical level can help signal that our bodies are safe and stable on a mental-emotional level as well. I recommend eating at regular waking intervals and fasting after certain times of the day. The research backs up my position:

> *"Increasingly evident is that metabolic homeostasis at the systems level relies on accurate and collaborative circadian timing within individual cells and tissues of the body. At the center of these rhythms resides the circadian clock machinery, an incredibly well-coordinated transcription-translation feedback system that incorporates a changing landscape of mRNA expression, protein stability, chromatin state, and metabolite production, utilization, and turnover to keep correct time."* 47] 48]

This eating pattern with the sleep and wake cycle improves digestion, restores normal hormonal balance, and improves cognition and energy. 47] 48] Again, you can't outrun nature. Those who follow the natural patterns and rhythms of the seasons become restored, relaxed and have the power to heal from disease.

Case Study:

Meet Keisha. Keisha is a 48-year-old woman who came to see us, asking us to fix her hormones. She was about 30 pounds overweight and felt like she was "dragging herself through the day." Keisha owned a very successful business and managed over 40 staff members who constantly reported to her. On top of that, she still saw her private clients, whom she loved. But she was feeling pulled in too many directions—between running the business and serving her clients. She had built her business from the ground up and was in the process of expanding into a larger space where she could double her business capacity.

From the outside, it looked like she had it all together, but inside, she was barely holding it together. Keisha had always been an overachiever and believed she was capable of doing even more than she was already doing. So, when she found herself unable to keep up with everything without crashing, she was confused and frustrated.

We started by running some basic blood work to check her thyroid function, vitamin D levels, immune system, kidneys, liver, and cholesterol. The results were eye-opening. It was clear she wasn't absorbing nutrients properly, likely due to chronic stress and a "leaky gut". Her thyroid antibodies were through the roof, and she had very little nutrients available for repair. Despite being overweight, she admitted she'd been skipping meals a lot because she was so busy—and also trying to cut calories to lose weight.

We decided to run a functional adrenal stress panel, which revealed that her adrenal glands were producing high amounts of cortisol throughout the day. Her cortisol levels were also very high, showing that her body was trying to manage the inflammation caused by that constant stress. Essentially, she was making a ton of stress hormones but also breaking them down at an extremely fast rate to keep up with the unrelenting stress.

To address this, we started her on a low-dose compounded thyroid medication and several herbal adrenal support complexes. One of those contained licorice root, which is fantastic for people with dysfunctional adrenals. It helps slow the conversion of cortisol to cortisone and supports overall exhaustion. (Just to clarify, licorice candy doesn't do the same thing—unfortunately, it's not the same thing at all!) Licorice root also helps support the immune system, which was key for Keisha. Many times, people with autoimmune conditions like Hashimoto's hypothyroidism also have undiagnosed infections like Epstein Barr, parasites, mold exposure, or Lyme disease that resurface. So, restoring her immune function was critical.

We also suggested she begin a customized IV nutrition repletion plan which included the basic nutrients and vitamins her body desperately needed for repair.

Two weeks later, Keisha came in beaming, saying she felt "like a million bucks." While she was still a little tired, she felt like she was finally starting to come back to life. We were just getting started, but we were confident we were on the right track. We explained that we still had a lot of work to do—restoring her gut function, rebuilding her immune system, and bringing her mitochondria back online. Of course, we'd need to help her reset the way she processed stress so that she could feel even better than before.

The truth is, this part is never quick or easy. Restoring a system takes a lot more than just supplementing it. It takes time, patience, and consistency. But that's exactly the kind of commitment that leads to real, lasting change. We were in it for the long haul with Keisha, and we knew that this was going to make all the difference in her health and well-being.

TLDR: Too Long Didn't Read

Despite having unprecedented access to food and comfort, stress remains a widespread issue in today's world. It impacts our health on multiple levels, from the top down and the bottom up. At the top level, stress disrupts our body's hormone profile, which leads to long-term health deterioration. On a microscopic scale, ongoing stress forces our mitochondria to remain locked in the Cell Danger Response—a state that diverts energy away from vital functions and uses it to alert other cells about ongoing trauma. This process, along with oxidative stress, damages our cells and contributes to premature aging, disease, and even cancer.

In the past, stress was linked to physical dangers that often had a clear beginning and end. Think of defeating a predator or fending off an invader—stressors with tangible starting and ending points. Today's stress, however, is often intangible, poorly defined, and continuous. Modern stressors—such as traffic, work deadlines, constant distractions from phones and devices, or the chaos of national and global politics—don't come with clear start or end points, leaving us in a constant state of tension.

To manage this ongoing stress, it's important to unplug from excessive media consumption, ensure adequate sleep, nourish our bodies with proper nutrition, engage in physical movement, and cultivate emotional and spiritual well-being. For me, I believe that investing in a relationship with God is a vital part of managing stress. I find that turning to Him gives me strength, peace, and guidance, helping me navigate life's challenges. Along with this, I believe that healthy, supportive communities—real-life relationships—are essential. If one area of our life is out of sync or unhealthy, it inevitably creates stress that spills into other areas, affecting our overall well-being. Finding balance and centering my life around my faith has been key to managing stress and restoring peace in my heart and mind.

Chapter 11
Your Emotional Body

> *Then the eyes of both of them were opened, and they realized they were naked; so they sewed fig leaves together and made coverings for themselves. 1]*
> —Genesis 3:7

We humans stand with a foot in two worlds. The human spirit can imagine, love, contemplate the past, hope for the future, and even reach out toward the infinite. Paradoxically, this indomitable spiritual nature is contained within a physical body bound by natural laws. Clothing is physical protection and concealment from a hostile environment, but it also symbolizes the persona that we wear to mask our vulnerability. Some clothing is thin, even revealing; other garments are protective against harsh environments and injury. Trauma victims often feel at risk of being exposed, vulnerable, or defensive in situations that are not generally threatening.

It's tempting to cope with past trauma by rationalizing, learning, and over-spiritualizing. But it doesn't work. We can cognitively understand our body's fight-or-flight reactions and still be completely at the mercy of these physiological rollercoasters. Unfortunately, rationalizing and "head-knowledge" are often just useless platitudes, empty words swept away into the yawning gulf of human tragedy. In the wake of experiencing evil, our coping strategies become flimsy fig leaves that will never truly protect us. In the Garden of Eden, Adam and Eve felt dangerously exposed after learning the painful reality of good and evil. They tried to clothe themselves with fig leaves.

Even with the leaves, they still felt exposed and vulnerable. Similarly, victims of trauma experience a profound understanding of good and evil in a uniquely painful way. While physical injuries may heal, deeper wounds often remain. As psychiatrist Bessel van der Kolk aptly said in the title of his book, *The Body Keeps the Score*, trauma leaves an indelible mark on the nervous system. 2] Until the body receives a signal otherwise, it stays on high alert, ready to react to any perceived danger. A constant state of alertness often leads the nervous system to shift into emergency mode prematurely and frequently.

This heightened response creates a person who's highly skilled at navigating danger, full of grit and determination. Trauma survivors often develop a remarkable ability to face challenges fearlessly and rise through adversity, climbing the ladder of success one step at a time. However, it's not all about grit and success. Trauma can also cause people to lash out or emotionally withdraw when anyone tries to get close. Without emotional healing, this can evolve into a pattern of mistrust, where the mind is constantly racing and unable to find peace.

Trauma survivors may also struggle with addiction, emotional numbing, or isolating themselves from others and situations. Sometimes, people fall into a mix of these coping strategies. Adverse Childhood Experiences (ACE) are strongly connected to a range of health problems that continue to impact individuals throughout adulthood. Researchers describe ACE as:

> *"Potentially traumatic experiences and events, ranging from abuse and neglect to living with an adult with a mental illness. They can have negative, lasting effects on health and well-being in childhood or later in life. However, more important than exposure to any specific event of this type is the accumulation of multiple adversities during childhood, which is associated with especially deleterious effects on development."* 3]

Individuals who have experienced ACEs have a higher incidence of depression, anxiety, autoimmune disease, heart disease, and premature death. 4] 6] In the US, roughly 10% of children experience three or more ACEs, with some regions and demographics being higher. 3] Things like divorce and marital instability have long-term negative consequences for society over time. While ACEs are often associated with social and psychological hurdles to overcome, traumatic events during childhood are so significant that there is also a direct correlation between childhood trauma and physical health problems in adulthood. Common ACEs include abuse, neglect, parents' divorce, drug abuse, alcoholism, parent with mental illness, parent incarcerated, poverty, domestic violence, gangs, and violent crime.

The pain of growing up in a home touched by divorce or abuse may even go so far as shortening life expectancy and diminishing quality of life. The echo of past familial harm also plays out in our finances also. A 2019 meta-analysis on estimated costs of ACEs and ACE-related illnesses across Europe and North America found that a 10% reduction in ACEs would save 3 million DALYs (disability-adjusted life-years) and save $105 billion in cold hard cash. 7] Improving the quality of life for children by reducing the impact of trauma isn't just humanitarian; it's also good fiscal policy. It's logical that reducing ACE would improve the economy by at least $100 billion if we could get even a 10% reduction.

"One of the most sobering findings regarding ACEs is preliminary evidence that their negative effects can be transmitted from one generation to the next. Toxic stress experienced by women during pregnancy can negatively affect genetic "programming" during fetal development, which can contribute to a host of bad outcomes, sometimes much later in life. Infants born to women who experienced four or more childhood adversities were two to five times more likely to have poor physical and emotional health outcomes by 18 months of age, according to one recently published study." 3]

We discuss genetics in greater detail elsewhere in this book. But for now, what I want you to realize is that early childhood experiences matter, even experiences before birth. This is one thing in which epigenetics plays a major role. The effects of trauma can be passed down through generations genetically and through the home environment.

Your Body Remembers

Psychotherapist and teacher Dr. Peter Levine has been describing the experience of recovering from trauma for over 30 years. He has been an advocate for using the body as a way to process trauma through his system called *Somatic Experiencing* ®. Dr. Levine began by learning how animals process stress and trauma. We commonly call the stress response *fight-or-flight*, but this isn't quite complete. There's a third way to respond to stress called *freeze*. Dr. Levine discovered some interesting things about fight, flight, or freeze that we humans need to understand. Freezing or "playing dead" when you can't defeat or outrun a predator is useful in the animal kingdom so long as the freezing response is allowed to run its course. 8]

Let me say it more clearly: the freeze response to stress must be allowed to play out, or the stress reaction can become a lingering phenomenon. According to the research, the stress reaction commonly known as fight, flight, or freeze must play out in the body, or our physiology may end up perpetually in that state. In our bodies, the emergency alarm was tripped. We must physically do an activity (or even freeze for sufficient time) to match the level of the emergency. Or else we experience stress that never seems to go away. When our body's emergency response is repeatedly stifled in this manner, the body interprets this as a danger that is never resolved. Many people find emotional relief through strenuous physical activity like working out, running, and martial arts. These physical activities give our bodies an outlet to release the pent-up energy of our accumulated stress responses. Let's revisit an example from the chapter on adrenal fatigue. I know it's the same idea, but it really serves as an effective way to anchor the concepts of stress and trauma. Suppose a caveman is attacked by a tiger. Option one is that the caveman defeats or eludes the predator. Option two is that the caveman is dead, and long-term stress is no longer an issue for him. A caveman's stress was probably based on physical things that he or she could directly control.

Prehistoric stress was driven by tangible problems—things that could be physically solved. In contrast, modern stress often centers around intangible, societal issues that can't be solved individually. However, this doesn't mean we have to be passive victims of our circumstances. To better understand how we can resolve trauma patterns in the body, let's turn to Dr. Levine and his research for some valuable insights.

Dr. Levine discovered that deep trauma often involves the third survival response to a perceived life threat: freeze and collapse. He found that "playing dead" or collapsing was the most effective way for an animal to stop an ongoing violent attack. Immobility also decreases natural pain signals, which can further support survival in some cases. According to Dr. Levine, this response is a natural tactic our bodies use to cope with overwhelming danger.

Dr. Levine's understanding of trauma is informed not just by his research, but by his personal experiences. He discusses these in his book, *In an Unspoken Voice: How the Body Releases Trauma and Restores Goodness*, where he shares how trauma can be healed through understanding and releasing these deeply ingrained body responses.10]

His personal experience with trauma began when he was struck by a car while walking to a friend's birthday party. In his book, he describes having an out-of-body experience, seeing his "limp and twisted body" from a third-person perspective. What's even more striking is that a doctor, who happened to be a first responder, helped kickstart his trauma recovery by holding his hand and staying with him as his "self" returned to his body.

He vividly recalls the physical shaking, tears, and a rush of cold and heat as his body processed the overwhelming emotions of being injured. At the time, he had already trained thousands of people in somatic trauma release. But the life-threatening accident brought him face-to-face with the deep, personal nature of trauma recovery in a way he had never experienced before.

In his own words, Dr. Levine reflects, "I know what to do, but I don't know if I could have done it alone. I would have needed this other person, this empathic witness, to be there and to help hold that space."9]

So much of our humanness can only come to life in shared experience. For Dr. Levine, just having someone there to hold his hand while he went through personal suffering was meaningful and constructive. At our clinic, the role of empathic witness is one that we take very seriously. Corroborating Dr. Levine's experience, we also find that having an empathetic witness is crucial to the healing process. He continues, "You don't have to know the facts of your story to be able to reprogram the symptoms or the outcomes." 9]

Likewise, we also believe that trauma doesn't have to be stuck and stagnant; if we take the right steps in the right environment, we can let go of past trauma so that it no longer controls our present and future. Improving the way our patients process stress and trauma is an important part of almost every treatment plan that we create. The research shows that animals respond to stress through intense physical activity (fight-or-flight) or by deliberate inactivity (freezing). When animals act out their natural response, they recover from trauma better than many people. Contrary to popular belief, humans have the capacity to do the same; we just don't know how. In modern times, we've mastered the art of masking, ignoring, or self-medicating our stress. But, in my clinical experience, I've found that these coping strategies are not healthy solutions to our negative emotions. Suppressing or denying our anger, fear, or shame leads to more serious consequences in the long run. You don't have to be a doctor to know that you can't hide from your own feelings.

My parents divorced when I was around 18 months old. My older sister and I found ourselves caught between their shared custody. Their disagreements often made my sister and I feel like we were caught in the middle. As I've grown older, I've come to realize that my parents were both very young when they had us, and they were still navigating their own lives when they started a family. With this perspective, I can see that they were doing the best they could, even though they were both still growing themselves.

My dad has always worked very long hours and values work above most things in life. For better or worse, I can relate to this because, in my own life, valuing my work is central to how I operate. On an otherwise typical Wednesday after the divorce, it was my dad's turn to pick me up from daycare. I remember the details vividly, even though I was only three. The brain is like that sometimes; our memories fade unless strong emotions are attached to them. In this case, I vividly remember waiting at the gate in the back of the playground. I watched all the other kids leave one by one. I watched my favorite teacher leave.

Finally, after some time, I remember another teacher asking me, "Where is your dad, Danielle?" The painful reality was that my dad was always late; this time was just worse than usual. The teacher informed me that it was well past the time that my dad was supposed to pick me up; my mom was not answering the phone (this was long before cell phones were common). With the sun going down and the daycare past closing time, the teacher told me she was going to call the police. My small, 3-year-old spirit was crushed; seconds felt like minutes, minutes felt like hours, and I was waiting for the police to come to take me away. To my horror, the teacher made good on her word, and the police finally did arrive. As the police were about to take me into custody, my dad came barreling into the parking lot and proceeded to engage in a shouting match with the officers. I watched him yell back and forth with the cops, shouting out his excuses to the officers. At three years old, I didn't know much, but I knew that cops arrested bad guys and threw them in jail. Now, the cops were here for me and ostensibly on the edge of arresting my dad as well. I thought I was going to jail because I did something wrong.

As the situation unfolded, I was terrified that my dad was going to jail. If he got arrested, the police would take me as well. I remember crying and screaming at the back gate, begging the police not to take my daddy. This memory is so visceral in my body that I can still feel it in the center of my chest as tears well up from deep within. This feeling of being left and forgotten was often reinforced throughout my life. I was mostly the quiet kid in the family. After both my parents remarried, I was passed back and forth between two blended families. I was not usually causing the problem, so there was not much reason to pay attention.

Instead, I tried to get love by being perfect. I got perfect grades and tried to do the right thing all of the time. I took responsibility for everything I could. It made me very capable. I was also very lonely. I learned how to care for others and found my personal identity in being the responsible one. The incident at preschool and many others like it led me to believe that I would be abandoned. If something went wrong, it was my fault, and if I asked for anything, I was "too much." On the surface, I was clingy, and I lacked self-awareness. But underneath that, I was unconsciously reliving my childhood trauma by picking men who would never truly commit or connect with me. I was left chasing the attention of men who emotionally and even physically kept me at arm's length. I chose men who had "commitment issues" or who I thought were "better than me." I accepted all this as normal and resolved to just work harder to make these doomed relationships succeed. It's also possible that I unconsciously picked my later boyfriends as a defense mechanism because, deep down, I knew they could never truly connect with me. That way, when my fears came true, and they left me, it would hurt a little bit less because they weren't that close anyway. Within this framework, I tried to love them enough to make them stay. I settled for men who did not have the capacity to love me and see me on a deep level. Perhaps I even unconsciously sought out doomed relationships to avoid being hurt if true love failed. Nobody would be surprised to learn that these boyfriends lied to me and cheated. Ultimately, I blamed myself.

My painful relationship pattern finally reached its peak when my first husband's infidelity was exposed, leaving me divorced with an infant son. I was completely devastated and uncertain about how to move forward. In that moment, I made a vow to myself to break every pattern that had led to this repeating cycle in my life. Seeking clarity and healing, I turned to professional counseling to help me understand and heal my broken way of finding love.

During our sessions, my counselor recommended that I study and understand adult attachment theory, which explains the predictable patterns that influence romantic relationships. This concept has been life-changing for me, and I'll dive deeper into it later. For now, I want to mention it here because if you've ever struggled with finding or keeping love, I highly recommend the book *Attached* by Amir Levine and Rachel Heller. 10] It offers profound insights that helped me shift my perspective and begin to understand the dynamics that shaped my relationships.

My childhood trauma unconsciously programmed me to fail at love. Breaking this pattern, I now realize, involved what I call repentance and humbling myself, though at the time I wouldn't have used those terms. The word repent has a negative connotation in modern society, but in the Bible, it simply means to change direction. If what you're doing repeatedly fails, maybe it's time to try something new. In my case, I had to admit that the way I chose relationships had played a role in the negative outcomes. Then, I had to decide to turn in a different direction. We've all known someone whose "picker" was broken—well, in my case, I had to humble myself and admit that I was the one with the broken picker. It was my fault.

To be clear, most of my past boyfriends were not great, and my first husband did betray me. But I had picked those relationships. It was time to try something different. Even though I didn't yet know God, I still found myself crying out to Him, asking Him to remove anything in me that had led me down the path of broken relationships.

Humbling myself meant letting go of everything I thought I knew about relationships. I began to seek counseling with the goal of learning a new way of being. As I let go of my old beliefs, learning new patterns became much easier. The relationship strategy I had used as a coping mechanism had perpetuated a cycle of trauma in my life. This is why I want to emphasize that there's never one solution for healing trauma.

Looking back, I thank God for setting me apart early and protecting me, allowing me to eventually grow and process my trauma. After my divorce, and after the painful process of relearning how to love, God blessed me with a wonderful husband, Richard, whom I met at the age of 34.

Before meeting Richard, I learned I was a somatic processor—someone who processes emotions through the body rather than through words. This means I had difficulty verbally expressing my feelings and instead stored them in my body, which would manifest as pain or dysfunctional patterns. I learned to process the trauma stored in my nervous system using a technique called *Neuro Emotional Technique* (NET®).

One of the original stressors stored in my nervous system was the trauma from when I was three years old in preschool. Using NET, somatic talk therapy, and a lot of crying out to God, I began to heal deep emotional wounds. Therapy and NET helped me break free from the patterns that had influenced the choices I made in relationships, teaching me how to see things differently. I discovered that I'm not very good at externally revealing my internal emotions. Years of keeping a stiff upper lip and being *the responsible one*—making sure everyone around me had what they needed—had built a defense mechanism around my heart. I was always *the strong one*, *the adult*, *the counselor*, and *the listener*, but I was terrified of letting anyone get too close. I was afraid that if someone got too close, they'd leave me, forget me, or abandon me.

When I met Richard, I asked him if he would be willing to practice secure attachment with me, so that we could build a relationship that would allow both of us to heal from our past traumas. He's shown me love, compassion, and patience as I've navigated through patterns of loneliness, anxiety, and fear.

When we started dating, Richard told me he wanted to create a metaphorical garden for me—a space where I could feel protected and free to grow into the person God had called me to be. Richard's love has truly exemplified what the apostle Paul writes in the Bible: "Husbands, love your wives, even as Christ also loved the church, and gave himself for her." 11] This is no small thing. Jesus sacrificed His life for the well-being of humanity, and Richard has made that kind of sacrificial love a reality for me and our family. Even now, he's helping me bring this book to life. Thank you, Love.

As my story shows, making life decisions from a place of unprocessed trauma leads to painful outcomes. Trauma hijacks our decision-making, steering us toward emotional reality rather than historical reality. Emotional reality is the story we tell ourselves—the story that says, "You were too much." Historical reality, however, is that "this other person was not capable of consistently showing up for you." Trauma gets stored in our bodies, and we unconsciously wait until we feel safe enough to process it.

On Brené Brown's *Unlocking Us* podcast, she interviewed Tarana Burke, who shared her own healing journey. Tarana said, "We are not seen until we are heard." She carried the shame, fear, and anger of being molested and sexually abused when she was just six years old. She went on,

> *"The reason I have such a terrible memory is because I have spent every day for the last 39 years trying to forget… our only hope is to get this pain out of our bodies someday, and we never really can."* 12]

When trauma continues to hold on in our nervous system, it feels as though it is still present, even if the traumatic event happened years or decades ago. Healing requires engaging the mental, physical, and spiritual aspects of ourselves to free our nervous systems, minds, and souls from events that occurred long ago. If the nervous system doesn't receive the safety signal, trauma continues to play on repeat in the body, like a broken record.

In the chapter on stress and adrenals, we discussed how the *Cell Danger Response* (CDR) must complete all its phases in order to reach resolution. Otherwise, the CDR continues indefinitely. Similarly, when stress isn't fully processed, it doesn't go away. The nervous system runs a background program of destructive hyper-vigilance, even if we're not consciously aware of it. Psychologist Bessel A. van der Kolk explains this in his book *The Body Keeps the Score*. He writes:

> "*Traumatized people chronically feel unsafe inside their bodies: The past is alive in the form of gnawing interior discomfort. Their bodies are constantly bombarded by visceral warning signs, and in an attempt to control these processes, they often become experts at ignoring their gut feelings and numbing awareness of what is playing out on the inside. They learn to hide from [themselves]… Trauma victims cannot recover until they become familiar with and befriend the sensations in their bodies. Being frightened means that you live in a body that is always on guard. Angry people live in angry bodies. The bodies of child abuse victims are tense and defensive until they find a way to relax and feel safe. In order to change, people need to become aware of their sensations and the way their bodies interact with the world around them. Physical self-awareness is the first step in releasing the tyranny of the past.*" 14]

The journey of healing trauma is not linear, but as we learn to process it, we begin to experience freedom from its grip. It takes time, patience, and often a deep surrender, but it is possible to heal and thrive.

I'm biased, but being biased doesn't make me wrong. I think the first step is surrendering all of your terrifying trauma to God. I didn't always believe in God. Although I was raised as a cultural, casual Catholic, I soon put such ideas aside as superstition when I entered adulthood. My religious views were shapeless and without structure; at times, I felt like the spiritual world was real, that maybe God was a force, but I also felt like humans were just here by some natural accident, and it was up to each human to define reality. In those days, I'd pursue spiritual experiences but didn't care to be burdened by defining them or having those experiences affect the way I chose to live. Like many in the natural health space, I predictably drifted toward a vaguely New Age buffet of Eastern religious ideas that I was always considering but never truly committed to. I traveled the world, practiced yoga, attended tea ceremonies, consulted with shamans, and even saw an astrologer. No matter what I tried or where I went, there was no arresting the anxiety that always seemed to creep back in. New Age practices reduced my symptoms for a bit, but the fear always came back stronger than ever. Although therapy, NET and getting my body in shape helped considerably, anxiety and trauma always remained in the shadows, lurking until just the right time to pounce.

Then there was Jesus, and everything changed for me. Eventually, I repented of all New Age practices. I no longer practice yoga. I have thrown away or burned all of my New Age items and books. I no longer use astrology. Instead, I now rely on the Holy Spirit because the Lord has not given us a spirit of fear. God's word reminds us,

> *"Fear not [there is nothing to fear], for I am with you; do not look around you in terror and be dismayed, for I am your God. I will strengthen and harden you to difficulties. Yes, I will help you. Yes, I will hold you up and retain you with My [victorious] right hand of rightness and justice." 15]*

If you don't know Jesus, you might want to. He patiently waited for me to seek him and ask for his peace and love. If you truly seek Jesus, you'll find him, and he will do the same for you.

To reiterate, our bodies are both physical and spiritual, so we need to address both. How do we begin to do this, Doctor Dani? Pray, then witness. If you don't believe in God, your first prayer might be to sincerely ask the Creator of the Universe to reveal himself to you. Keep asking God to reveal himself in a sincere and respectful frame of mind. Then, witness. Witness how you feel internally and what happens in your body on a physical level when you feel certain experiences or entertain certain thoughts and memories. Next, let another person witness your feelings and emotions. Trauma has a way of severing our spiritual and emotional lives, cutting them off from our physical experience. Witnessing our physical sensations while getting in touch with emotions rebuilds these bridges. Van der Kolk says,

> *"The mind needs to be reeducated to feel physical sensations, and the body needs to be helped to tolerate and enjoy the comforts of touch. Individuals who lack emotional awareness can connect their physical sensations to psychological events with practice. Then they can slowly reconnect with themselves." 14]*

One of the most important things we can do as doctors and healing professionals is to **believe the experience that our patients**

tell us about. As care providers, we must be reliable, empathetic, and consistent witnesses to a person's emotional experience. Without this, trust between patient and clinician will never form, and the patient will never reach their full health potential.

Our Negative Minds

Our bodies are fine-tuned machines on a constant lookout for danger. We're wired to react to negativity. This means we utilize negative information far more often to make decisions than we do positive information. Why? Negativity keeps us safe. This means once we have an experience where someone has disappointed or let us down, we store that as a truth. Then, our nervous system tags this person as dangerous and looks for all the ways this person is messing up. Think about it: you're a caveman walking around and living amongst animals. Wouldn't you like to distinguish a bird from a lion as quickly as possible?

In order to survive, we'd rather avoid trauma rather than gain a potential upside. When balancing a risk versus a reward, a risk might kill you; a reward would be nice but is unnecessary for survival. What does this look like in modern relationships? Here are some ways that negative bias will show up in everyday life.

- Recalling unpleasant or critical information more than compliments
- Physically and emotionally responding more readily to negative actions or conversations
- Narrowing your focus on negative information more than positive
- Ruminating on harmful, unpleasant, or traumatic events more than joyous interactions

There was a meme floating around the internet recently that really stuck with me. It said, *Ask yourself, was it a bad day, or was it a bad five minutes that you milked the whole day?* It got me thinking about how often we get caught up in that emotional reaction. Same goes for relationships—are they truly a bad partner, or are they genuinely trying to grow and make positive changes? Sometimes, the answer is clear: Nope, they're still a bad partner. But other times, the answer is simply patience. At other times, people hang onto negative experiences because they gain power or provide a convenient excuse. For example, a wife may avoid feeling guilty for being verbally abusive to her husband by recalling how he used to be an alcoholic 10 years ago. In this case, the wife is using her husband's past as fig-leaf to hide her current issues.

The truth is, our brains are wired for pessimism. That old reptilian part of us is always on the lookout for danger, and it's quicker to focus on the negative than the positive. This is why our emotional reality often doesn't line up with the truth. When we're feeling upset, it's important to pause—pray, question, research, and then decide. This applies to everything; from the news we consume to the arguments we have in our relationships.

We're taught these biases from a young age, and many of them are tied to our survival instincts. For example, toddlers learn that fire is dangerous so they don't burn themselves. The negative wiring in our brains helps us navigate harmful versus safe situations. This tendency gets passed down through generations. Unfortunately, this same negativity bias is often exploited by advertising and media by manipulating us with fear.

But here's the thing: this bias also makes us complacent, negative, avoidant, and, frankly, not the best parents or spouses. One study found that the more attention we give to an event, the more firmly it gets locked into our memory.16] So, when your spouse forgets to pick up their socks, the more you focus on it, the more you forget all the times they did remember to pick them up. And then we start saying things like, "You ALWAYS forget to…" Sound familiar?

It's easy to fall into that trap. But the more we can step back and look at the bigger picture, the easier it is to let go of these tiny moments that don't define the whole relationship. Signs of a negative bias in a relationship:

- Assume the worst. We set ourselves up to be offended, disappointed, and angry.

- We spend time dwelling on the worst possible outcome. Then, we unconsciously look for ways to make that negative outcome true.

- We put weight on negative interactions with others as more important than any positive interactions we might have.

- We will look for evidence of them becoming someone we do not want them to be. For example, "You are just like my (parent, ex, etc.) who had issues with his temper, just like you."

How We Attach and Why It Matters

Research shows that, if left to our own devices, we marry people who are like our caregivers because we marry what is familiar. Especially if we came from trauma, we would choose someone who subconsciously allow us to work out the trauma we had from our childhoods. We marry someone who will give us a "second chance" to do it right. Granted, sometimes you luck out and end up with a person who has stable, loving caregivers with great boundaries. These are the people who can help integrate your nervous system in a more healthy and balanced manner. The problem is that the dating pool is disproportionately filled with people who have issues with healthy attachment. Emotionally healthy people get married and stay married. As we age, the dating pool ends up with a concentration of people with unhealthy attachment styles. In Dr. Sue Johnson's book *Hold Me Tight*, she says,

> "To achieve a lasting, loving bond, we have to be able to tune in to our deepest needs and longings and translate them into clear signals that help our lovers respond to us. We have to be able to accept love and to reciprocate." 17]

We must first be transparent about what those needs are and communicate them clearly and in plain language with our partner. In my marriage, we've adopted a technique called "Can you say this another way?" It's a simple but powerful cue that helps us rephrase what we're saying so we can better understand each other's true intentions. It's been a game-changer for our communication, and it's something we're still working on—because, like most couples, we're always learning how to better connect. At the heart of it all is understanding how we're each wired to attach to others.

After my ex-husband's infidelity reached a breaking point, I asked for a temporary separation. In response, he asked for a divorce, eager to continue his lifestyle of partying and affairs. As our marriage came to an end, I realized I needed to get to the root of why I was choosing love that wasn't truly reciprocal. This realization led me to seek therapy, where a colleague of mine helped me dig deep into the layers of stress that had built up in my nervous system over the years.

That's when I was introduced to Neuro-Emotional Technique (NET). The process of using NET felt like peeling away the layers of an onion—each session revealed more about the emotional stress I had been carrying around. The first time I experienced NET, something shifted inside me. It was like an inner voice I'd never quite been able to hear before started to make itself known—quiet, but clearer than it had ever been; you might describe it as the "still, small voice (of God)."

After each session, I would process emotions very viscerally and felt like I needed to talk through what I was experiencing, so I also began to see a therapist with a somatic focus. The somatic focus was important for me because I am the type of person who has a difficult time recognizing that I am stressed to begin with. I am what you call a "stuffer of emotions." Through NET and somatic counseling, I began to take responsibility for my role within my past relationships and began to see there was a different way to be. In the past, I chose men who could be accurately predicted to leave and/or be emotionally distant. My therapist encouraged me to read a book called *Attached* by Amir Levine and Rachel Heller, which I spoke about earlier in this chapter. 18]

This book has quickly become one of the most recommended reads in our office because effective communication and understanding how we behave in relationships are crucial for growth and healing. *Attached* introduced me to a deeper understanding of attachment theory, which explains how we bond with others. Our attachment patterns are shaped by the way we connected (or disconnected) from our primary caregivers growing up, and they are also influenced by the relationships we form as adults.

When I first read *Attached*, it felt like an explosion in my mind—everything suddenly clicked. This book is so transformative that I believe it should be required reading for anyone entering the dating world. In fact, I think it should be part of the sex education curriculum for teens and young adults. It's also one of the books on our clinic's reading list for patients who are struggling in their relationships, as it gives us a common language for discussing healthy needs and desires within the context of human bonding.

Here's a brief breakdown of the four major attachment styles we form as humans:

Secure Attachment. This is the goal for healthy relationships. Secure attachments create a foundation of trust and emotional intimacy, where partners can be close while maintaining their individual identities. Affection is expressed confidently, without fear of abandonment or betrayal. Both spouses feel free to express their needs and emotions in a loving, supportive environment. This attachment is built on love, mutual respect, and meeting each other's needs—not driven by fear or anxiety. Often, people with anxious or avoidant attachment styles mistakenly believe they are secure when they are not.

Anxious Attachment. Those with an anxious attachment style are highly sensitive to rejection and often develop co-dependent patterns in relationships. They seek intense intimacy and constant reassurance from their partners, driven by a deep fear of abandonment and betrayal. The anxious person is often drawn to avoidant individuals, even though they may know deep down that it's not a healthy choice. This dynamic can lead to a cycle where the anxious partner's need for closeness pushes the avoidant spouse further away. The best path for those with anxious attachment is to seek relationships with other anxious individuals, as there is a strong mutual understanding. However, it is equally important for them to work on healing, building trust, and developing a solid relationship with God and others, so that fear and jealousy don't harm the connection.

Avoidant-Dismissive Attachment. Individuals with an avoidant-dismissive attachment style often seem oblivious to emotions and can pull away or shut down when someone seeks more intimacy or when they've been hurt or rejected. They may pursue someone intensely in the early stages of a relationship but will gradually become emotionally or physically distant once the relationship settles into routine. Avoidants may become "busy," spend extended periods away, or just emotionally withdraw. They sometimes idealize past relationships or hold a previous lover on a pedestal, making it difficult for their current partner to measure up. If threatened with the end of a relationship, the avoidant may temporarily shower their partner with affection to regain control, but once things return to normal, they revert back to emotional disconnection.

Avoidant-Fearful/Disorganized Attachment. This attachment style is characterized by mixed signals. One moment, the individual pulls away, and the next, they are desperate for reassurance. They embody both anxious and avoidant traits and often express confusion about their feelings. They may say they are "not sure" how to feel about their spouse. Healthy emotional connections are critical to development, and it's encouraged for this style to spend time alone to understand their attachment tendencies. This period of self-reflection helps them navigate their needs and desires, as well as heal from past relational trauma. Eventually, they must enter into relationships with others, as this provides a path to healing and growth.

For individuals with an anxious attachment style, healing these patterns is crucial, as they often find themselves in unhealthy, unbalanced relationships. Their nervous system remains unsettled until they find emotional security in a relationship. As Dr. Levine explains, anxious individuals tend to react with extreme emotions when they sense something is wrong in a relationship. They often expect their partner to respond negatively, believing the relationship is fragile and on the verge of collapse. This thought process can make it difficult to express their needs effectively.

Healing and growth in relationships—whether through friendships, work associations, or marriage—are essential for all attachment styles. Through these connections, we learn how to express and meet emotional needs, and work through unresolved patterns.

Boundaries & Bonding Are Central to Growth

Healthy boundaries are key to secure relationships. Boundaries aren't walls; think of them as membranes—like the ones in biology class. Membranes decide what enters and exits. If they let too much in, they become bloated and self-destructive. If they let too much out, they shrink and shrivel. The goal is balance—allowing some things in and some things out, creating harmony.

Weak boundaries can lead to unhealthy, even abusive relationships. For example, people with an anxious attachment style often gravitate toward relationships where they are emotionally starved, absorbing all the feelings and working harder for love and affection. This pattern mimics their early caregiver relationships. Dr. Levine explains that abuse isn't just physical or sexual; it can also be emotional manipulation, especially in a stressed nervous system.

The goal in every relationship is secure attachment. Secure attachment is vital both in raising children with healthy boundaries and for an intimate marriage. To build a secure bond, increasing oxytocin is key. Oxytocin, often called the "cuddle hormone," plays a huge role in attachment, boosting trust, cooperation, and emotional connection. It's released during moments of intimacy, like cuddling or orgasm, counteracting stress and strengthening bonds.18] Oxytocin plays a key role in reducing conflict. When we skip quality time with our spouse due to other demands, we miss the oxytocin boost that makes us more agreeable and less prone to conflict. In parenting, oxytocin is released through actions like breastfeeding, hugs, and eye contact, forming secure attachment bonds with children. When our actions align with our words, children learn to trust, setting the foundation for healthy relationships.

Making time for family and loved ones strengthens social bonds and fosters emotional security. EQ is a play on IQ, where IQ is the Intelligence Quotient, EQ is the Emotional Quotient. Emotional intelligence is our ability to manage our emotions, especially when triggered. EQ also involves recognizing emotions in others through facial expressions, tone, and cues.

Daniel Goleman, author of *Emotional Intelligence*, explains that people with high EQ are more effective and content in life. Negative emotions like anger, anxiety, and depression can be as harmful as smoking if improperly managed. High EQ can prevent illness and improve overall well-being.19] One way we might begin to develop EQ is through what psychologist and author M. Scott Peck calls discipline. Discipline is made up of 4 parts: delaying gratification, acceptance of responsibility, dedication to truth, and balancing. 20]

Here are some ways to cultivate discipline in your life.
Delay gratification: Do your hard work up front, then do the fun stuff. For example, doing your homework before you can watch TV.
Accept responsibility: Take responsibility for how your actions and choices have led to a certain outcome.

For example, understanding that your constant unavailability has led to the demise of a close relationship. You can do this in simple ways like making your bed, practicing daily hygiene, cleaning your house, and paying bills early instead of procrastinating.
Dedication to the truth: Giving voice to the full reality of your emotions and speaking with clear intent. You must learn to distinguish between your historical and emotional reality. For example, you may have an emotional reality that the reason your parents divorced was because of you when in historical reality, it was because they had completely different values that became obvious when they attempted to raise children together. M. Scott Peck says,

> *"Our view of reality is like a map with which to negotiate the terrain of life. If the map is true and accurate, we will generally know where we are, and if we have decided where we want to go, we will generally know how to get there. If the map is false and inaccurate, we generally will be lost."* 19]

It is not that we have the wrong map; it's that, at a certain point, we fail to update the map. I often say to patients,

> *"You are loving the 1.0 version of your partner's software, when they are operating a 3.0 and vice versa. It's time to update the software on your relationships."* 20]

Balance: The ability to have emotional flexibility. This is the art of learning how to say what needs said, and when it is appropriate to say it. Blurting out in anger during the middle of the dinner, when something your spouse did that frustrated you, is not a good idea. Scheduling time to talk after you have had a chance for people to leave so you can more calmly express your disappointment is a much better tactic. However, there are times when expressing your anger immediately is more appropriate, such as protecting your child from immediate physical danger.

Practicing these forms of discipline cultivates emotional intelligence. The best way to build these skills is to get comfortable with being uncomfortable. Especially if your goal in life is to grow, M. Scott Peck writes,

"So if your goal is to avoid pain and escape suffering, I would not advise you to seek higher levels of consciousness or spiritual evolution. First, you cannot achieve them without suffering, and second, insofar as you do achieve them, you are likely to be called on to serve in ways more painful to you, or at least demanding of you, than you can now imagine." 20]

Instead, he finds love to be the only way to heal from the trauma of the past but makes it clear that love is an active process and distinguishes it from the chemicals of love or lust at first sight. He says,

"Similarly, loving spouses must repeatedly confront each other if the marriage relationship is to promote the partners' spiritual growth. No marriage can be judged truly successful unless husband and wife (partners) are each other's best critics...I define love thus: The will to extend oneself for the purpose of nurturing one's own or another's spiritual growth...When we love someone, our love becomes demonstrable or real only through our exertion – through the fact that for that someone (or for yourself), we take an extra step or walk an extra mile. Love is not effortless. To the contrary, love is effortful." 20]

To develop healthy boundaries, you first need to recognize your role in the dynamic. It begins with asking yourself, "What am I feeling?" Then, explore "Why am I feeling this way?" Finally ask, "Where did I learn to feel this way?" Once you can answer these three questions, the emotions buried in your subconscious, which drive repetitive patterns, can be released. When you align with the truth, and your subconscious and conscious minds are in agreement, real change can happen. Then, those old patterns can be broken.

This is why I'm confident that anxiety and depression aren't just chemical reactions in the brain. Research, such as a meta-analysis by Bair et al., shows that around two-thirds of patients with depression report distressing, painful physical symptoms, highlighting the connection between emotional and physical health. 21]

Mentally healthy people will suffer in the growth process. Depression and anxiety can be a clue that you're stuck in the middle of a growing pain. At Terrain, we believe that the mind is much more complex than just a chemical signal. Yes, balance the chemistry and give the body what it is deficient in. At the same time, we must also clear the emotional signals in the body. This gives the brain the "all is OK" signal and allows the body to fully integrate. Without addressing what the body is trying to "say," you are missing the "we are going to be all right" signal so desperately needed in order to leave behind old patterns that have been locked in the nervous system.

Case study: Gabby

Gabby, a 32-year-old woman, came to our office at the suggestion of her mom and sister, who were both patients of mine. She'd been struggling with severe stomach aches for years, and despite seeing multiple specialists, no one could pinpoint the cause. Gabby was meticulous—she brought in a neatly organized folder with lab results, imaging reports, and dates. She was taking maximum doses of over-the-counter pain relievers daily and had started self-medicating with alcohol to numb the pain.

When Gabby first came in, she shared that she'd been having persistent night terrors, which kept her from sleeping. She was gaining weight and struggling to lose it. She'd started seeing a counselor and was ready to make some changes.

We ran several functional lab panels, including a GI panel and a comprehensive thyroid test. The results were eye-opening: Gabby had a low-functioning thyroid, pre-diabetes, elevated cholesterol, liver enzyme issues, and significant nutrient deficiencies, particularly in B vitamins. Her GI panel showed some minor digestion issues, including difficulty processing fats, and she needed probiotics to repopulate her gut bacteria.

We started by asking Gabby to become aware of her alcohol use. At first, she wasn't ready to quit, so we respected that and focused on

IV nutrition repletion, neuroemotional technique, and acupuncture. After three weeks, Gabby was sleeping through the night for the first time in years, and her nightmares had stopped. She felt more hopeful and agreed to cut back on alcohol. We also began a hormone-reset nutrition plan and started her on natural thyroid replacement medication.

Two weeks later, Gabby had dramatically reduced her alcohol intake and was 90% compliant with the nutrition plan. We also worked on releasing trapped emotions in her stomach area, using muscle testing to identify and process stress stored in her body. With each emotional layer cleared, her physical pain began to lessen.

Six months later, Gabby had lost over 30 pounds, stopped drinking (except on holidays), landed a new job, and started repairing relationships with her family. Her lab results improved, and her stomach pain has gone from a 7-8/10 at its worst to 2-3/10 on average. The pain is still there, but we're making progress.

Gabby's case highlights the importance of a combined therapy approach, addressing both physical health and emotional well-being. Her humor and energy are shining through, and we're excited to continue helping her take back her health and live a pain-free, whole life.

Conclusion

Our relationships—with others, with God, and how we engage with the world—are all influenced by past trauma, which can sometimes show up in physical symptoms. Healing from trauma requires addressing all three parts of who we are: physical, emotional, and spiritual. In today's world, there's a temptation to lean into a vague spirituality that lacks structure or accountability. Without that accountability to God, we lose our personal boundaries, making emotional and spiritual growth feel impossible after a certain point.

The truth is, our emotional health directly impacts our physical well-being. This isn't just self-help fluff—it's a fundamental truth that we need to grasp if we want to be healthy and live fulfilling lives. Healing requires us to make peace with God and be honest about where we are emotionally. It's not just about understanding trauma intellectually—it's about how it impacts our biology and stress response. Science may not fully understand all the connections, but we know that emotional trauma can manifest physically.

TLDR: Healing from trauma goes beyond just knowing about it. Many physical issues clear up when we uncover and address the emotional or traumatic memories tied to them. Stress and trauma can get trapped in the body. To release stress, we must align our physical, emotional, and spiritual selves by being truthful, honest, and integrating our logical and emotional minds with our bodies. In this way, we can release past trauma and move forward, free to live our best lives.

Chapter 12
Living in a Toxic World

"Behold, I am going to feed them wormwood and make them drink poisonous water." 1]

In ancient prophecy, people were collectively punished for the corruption and evil running rampant in their societies. Not all were guilty, but all suffered the punishment. Modern culture tells us that these writings from thousands of years ago are barbaric and cruel. In the 21st century, we're tempted to discard God as a petty and vengeful superstition. We dismiss the God of our ancestors because He punished people for breaking rules that don't seem to matter. Many such prophecies describe a tipping point where all of society is punished for the collective wrongs of some, which our modern sensibility rejects as unfair. But what if the forgotten lore scrawled on archaic scrolls was still relevant today?

In an echo from the past, we've reincarnated old mistakes in our own futuristic way. In the modern world, the poor choices of some and the inattention of most have contaminated our food and poisoned our water. Prophecies describe God as punishing evil. But in modern times, our problems are self-inflicted at the societal level. Maybe God's so-called punishment is simply allowing people to experience the consequences of their own choices. We are the ones poisoning ourselves through our own human character flaws. We choose taste and convenience over health. We see these human flaws played out at every level of analysis. At the top, we have corporate greed colluding with corrupt politicians; at the bottom, we have an insatiable population-wide demand for *more*. We want pampering, pleasure, and personal praise. It's easy to blame banks, billionaires, and bureaucrats for our problems. But to be brutally honest, we all have some small part to play. The nebulous *they* who bring about society's collapse only make the products that we consume. The result is that everything from plastic byproducts to pharmaceutical drug residues are being pumped into our environment worldwide.

We're all partly responsible. Nobody likes pollution, but we all like free same-day shipping; everything we desire is available online at a discount. In this world of unprecedented luxury, even the most level-headed individual could easily fall into a toxic mentality of entitlement. Most of us don't wake up in the morning and see ourselves as arrogant, but it's easy to spot inflated egos in the people we don't like. We dislike ego in others but are blissfully blind to our own hubris. We are all human. Even the best of us has a background level of egotistical entitlement: the American zeitgeist wants *more* and demands *better*. We want to eat *more*, we want to own *more*, we want it to be *easier*, we want to feel *better*. The problem is that *more* and *better* are fueled by chemicals in the form of plastics, pesticides and pills.

Elsewhere in this book, we discuss the impact of medications, processed foods, and artificial ingredients on our health. But much like unresolved emotional wounds, these chemicals don't just disappear once they've entered our bodies. Whether you eat clean or not, we're all exposed to toxins in some form. Our body's ability to eliminate these toxins plays a significant role in how and when we get sick. While we can limit exposure to a certain degree, there are still things beyond our control. For example, even if you live far from modern conveniences, your water could be contaminated by a distant uranium mine that closed decades ago (yes, this happened with one of my patients). Toxic exposure can feel unavoidable, like prophecy; it's part of our environment. But even so, there's always something we can do to improve our situation. As Alexander Pope once said, "Hope springs eternal."

Conventional vs. Naturopathic Medicine

Since the Industrial Revolution, two things have happened simultaneously: global exposure to chemicals that don't naturally occur in the environment, and a surge in health issues tied to these substances. While it's true that correlation doesn't always mean causation, we can still use these patterns as clues. What do we do when someone is sick and we can't pinpoint the cause? Or when a person isn't improving and we're unsure why?

In naturopathic medicine, we look for these clues. While there's no definitive proof, the link between increased toxic exposure and certain diseases is worth considering. When we can't find a clear reason for an illness, we often explore past toxic exposure as a possible culprit. In contrast, conventional medicine tends to conclude that if they can't identify a cause, then there must not be one. This mindset is defined by: *if we don't know it, it doesn't exist*. Though often well-intentioned, this way of thinking feels prideful, dismissive and, frankly, lazy. We humans can be so unaware of our own limitations, and the more I grow in my faith, the more I realize how easily I can fall into these traps myself.

Conventional Medicine's Responses to Unsolved Health Problems:

- You're making up the problem
- You're lying about the symptoms
- It's your genetics
- It's an autoimmune condition

In my integrative medicine practice, I try to take a different approach. When we have a chronically ill patient who isn't improving as expected, and we can't establish a direct cause, we start looking for indirect causes. One of the principles of naturopathic medicine is to remove the obstacle to cure. This principle means that if a patient is not responding to treatment, there must be factors to the illness that have not been identified. Of course, we investigate other causes that may explain the symptoms. We look deeper if we can't find a proverbial *smoking gun* that explains the illness and why the patient is not recovering. Exposure to certain chemicals, toxins, or mold can increase one's susceptibility to illness. This is part of the reason I'm suspicious of autoimmune disease. Yes, of course, autoimmune diseases are real. Genetic predisposition to certain ailments is also real. But I don't believe that autoimmune comes out of nowhere, and it's scientifically lazy to just blame genetics.

Lifestyle does play a significant role in triggering autoimmune disease. Unfortunately, where you live and the environment you're exposed to are part of that lifestyle. To say your autoimmune condition has no cause outside of genetics is misleading. It essentially lets everyone off the hook: your doctor, chemical companies, the food industry, pharmaceuticals. Even worse, calling everything autoimmune unfairly blames God for giving you bad genes. The reality is, it's not just about genetics, and blaming autoimmune disease solely on that misses the bigger picture.

If only it were so simple. In my practice, a common pattern is that a patient had a toxic exposure that put an excessive load on their immune system and detoxification organs. **"Autoimmune" is not a diagnosis; it's a symptom of a body under constant duress.** Here's an example. If the liver or the kidneys are overloaded with trying to cleanse the body of a toxin, then your body is far less able to process and eliminate normal waste products. This background toxicity lowers your ability to fight off infections and can also lead to a vague cluster of symptoms centered on feeling "unwell." Parasitic infections also increase the toxic load on the body and cause generally reduced health, but here we're focusing on toxic exposures. Industrial processes like mining, commercial farming, and manufacturing routinely involve a host of harmful substances. As an example, fine particulate matter like fly ash from coal-burning power plants contains lung-damaging silica and calcium oxides. 3]

Yes, we still burn coal in the US, and there's also oil and natural gas extraction, refining, transportation, and burning. While many of these chemicals are technically natural, they were never present in the environment in the quantities we see today. There's a big difference between the occasional silica dust on a beach and the constant output of a cement factory.

While substances like lead and uranium do occur naturally, they usually don't pose major health risks unless disturbed by human activity. These dense materials naturally sink to low points in the earth, away from where people live. However, activities like strip mining and river dredging bring these carcinogenic chemicals into the human environment. Without human involvement, substances like lead and uranium remain trapped under sediment. Radon gas, another naturally occurring toxin, does seep into the air, but it wasn't likely to build up to harmful levels before homes were tightly sealed with recirculating air systems.

As with most things in life, it's complicated. Are energy-efficient homes bad? No, but these new homes mean that we now need to pay attention to radon gas buildup. There are also competing human factors at work with regard to pollution. Areas like the state of Wyoming rely heavily on natural gas extraction for their economy, and other areas benefit from affordable energy. In the Green River Valley, a hotspot for natural gas exploration, Wyoming recently recorded ozone levels at 124 parts per billion, worse than Los Angeles' 114 parts per billion during the same year. 4] As a reference, the maximum recommended healthy limit for exposure is 75 parts per billion. However, it's not just ozone and smog that pose risks. Natural gas drilling (hydraulic fracturing) also exposes workers to harmful silica dust. Crystalline silica, found in materials like quartz and granite countertops, can cause silicosis—an incurable but preventable lung disease—when inhaled by workers cutting or drilling stone. Recent air samples from several drilling sites have shown unsafe levels of crystalline silica dust in the air. 5]

Wyoming is not an isolated case. In 2011, oil companies reported over 1,000 oil spills in North Dakota, with many more going unreported, as state officials admit. 6] The Associated Press also reported that the amount of chemically tainted soil from drilling waste increased by nearly 5,100 percent over the past decade, reaching more than 512,000 tons last year. 7] Water pollution is another growing concern. As an example, Poplar, Montana is an area affected by unsafe drinking water linked to fossil fuel drilling. 8] In Poplar, oil companies are required to pay fines and provide alternative water sources due to ongoing contamination of the town's drinking water supply. While the situation in Poplar is significant to the people who live there, it was soon overshadowed by the more widely publicized water crisis in Flint, Michigan. 9]

Residents in Flint had complained about foul-smelling, rancid water leading to illness. These repeated public complaints were denied and ignored by politicians and local leaders. Outbreaks of skin rashes, hair loss, itchy skin, and lead poisoning finally forced the ongoing issues into the public eye. Apparently, the Flint River had been a de facto dumping site for numerous commercial industries for around a century. City sewer systems had also periodically dumped raw sewage into the river. Chemical residue from agricultural runoff and leaching landfills also took a toll on water quality in the area.

During the 1980's car makers closed production plants, local industry shut down, and the money left. With half the residents leaving the city, the remainder of Flint was left impoverished, and the city government was broke due to declining tax revenue. The cash-strapped city of Flint began using river water as a way to save money, and that's when all hell broke loose. On at least two occasions, the pollution in the river was so bad that the surface of the water actually burned.

Poverty and pollution go hand-in-hand. Even still, we're all at risk of toxic exposure regardless of economic status. Researchers studying chemical exposure found hundreds of toxins in the umbilical cord blood of newborn babies both in the US and abroad. Carcinogenic materials found in plastics and pesticides such as polychlorinated biphenyls (PCBs), organochlorine pesticides (OCPs), polybrominated diphenyl ethers (PBDEs), hydroxylated PBDEs (OH-PBDEs) and perfluorinated compounds (PFCs) were found in alarming rates in a 2010-11 study conducted on women in urban areas of San Francisco, California. 10]

Study after study has shown the same information: everyone in the world today is at some risk for toxic exposure regardless of their personal health decisions. Logically, we tend to only think about known exposures that we've directly had based on life choices that we've made. But toxic chemicals can sometimes be found even in safe and healthy foods and supposedly clean drinking water. Plastic food containers, prepared food eaten at restaurants, and even organic produce and livestock may be contaminated by unethical dumping that happened miles away back when our grandparents were young.

The Valley of the Drums

Environmental medicine was one of the most depressing classes I took in medical school. After learning just how much toxic waste has been released into the environment, Sometimes, I'm surprised that we don't all have cancer already. Maybe I'm exaggerating, but then again, maybe I'm not taking it seriously enough. If you want to read a scary story, look up a place called *The Valley of The Drums*. On this single 23-acre plot of land out in the woods near Louisville, Kentucky, over 5.5 million gallons (100,000+ barrels) of polychlorinated biphenyls and dioxin-like compounds were dumped. 11]

Some 27,000 barrels were buried or thrown out in the open. The remaining 73,000 barrels were poured out into open trenches. Infamous "superfund" dumping sites are the ones we know of, but what about all of the somewhat smaller industrial dumping sites that were never discovered? From superfund sites like Love Canal and The Valley of The Drums, to the chemical residues common to 21st-century domestic life, our water supply is becoming more contaminated daily. Heavy metals, pesticide runoff, pharmaceutical drugs, and industrial waste don't just go away once we're done using them. One study conducted by the Minnesota Pollution Control Agency evaluated streams and rivers for medical waste:

> *"Among the pharmaceuticals detected, iopamidol, an X-ray contrast agent, was the most frequently detected, found at 78% of the locations sampled. The antidepressants sertraline, amitriptyline, and fluoxetine were detected in water at 48%, 44%, and 10% of the locations, respectively, and the antibiotics sulfamethoxazole and erythromycin were detected in water at 24% and 14% of the locations, respectively. Metformin, a medication used to treat type II diabetes; triamterene, a diuretic; and carbamazepine, an anticonvulsant medicine, were detected at 18%, 16%, and 14% of the locations, respectively. The insect repellent DEET, the plastic component bisphenol A [or BPA], the corrosion inhibitor benzotriazole, and benzotriazole breakdown products were also widespread."* 12]

Could rampant exposure to harmful chemicals be behind the rise of mysterious illnesses? Many of the contaminants we discuss have been found in treated and filtered water, including trace amounts of pharmaceutical drugs and pesticides. These drugs don't disappear after they leave the body; millions of people take antidepressants and birth control. Where do those drugs go after the person takes them? Drugs, and drug biproducts are excreted as waste in urine and feces. This drug residue accumulates in sewers every time we flush the toilet. Over time, this buildup impacts wildlife, causing birth defects and infertility. The widespread use of birth control has even been linked to chemically induced transgender frogs, and similar effects have been observed with the pesticide atrazine, causing chemical castration in male frogs. 13][14]

The amount of pharmaceutical waste in our environment is staggering. To combat this, some government agencies have started drug take-back programs. But honestly, a better solution might be for people to get healthier and reduce reliance on prescriptions. We've only begun to scratch the surface of the damage caused by the Industrial Revolution. A prime example is the Love Canal disaster, where toxic waste was dumped by unethical companies, and a school and neighborhood were built on top of it. 16]

The Love Canal disaster caused leukemia, miscarriages, birth defects, and intellectual disabilities. What's chilling is that the dumping began over 80 years ago, but the area wasn't evacuated until nearly 40 years later. Even seemingly pristine areas may have hidden chemical exposures from decades ago. Imagine living downstream from Love Canal or getting your water from a river affected by chemical dumping. The truth is, we've all been exposed to toxins, and some of us may have unknowingly had large exposures.

Wealth, Poverty & Toxic Exposure

It would be easy to blame industrial manufacturers and fossil fuel companies for the pollution we face today. But simply pointing fingers at these industries won't solve the problem. If we all switched to electric cars, we'd still face the issue of mining the toxic minerals needed for their batteries, like cobalt, often mined in brutal conditions by child laborers in the Congo. 17] Furthermore, even if we went green, we'd still need to deal with how to charge those electric cars. The truth is, pollution and poverty are deeply linked. 18] Wealthy nations are often out of touch with the realities of pollution faced by the poorest areas, where people burn garbage simply to survive. Poor countries don't have the luxury of recycling or waste management systems. They burn trash for heat, to cook food, or because there's either no garbage service available, or they can't afford to pay for it. Poverty is likely the largest contributing factor for air pollution. Across the world, 14% of adults burn garbage in the open.

The stark reality is that as global per capita income rises, pollution levels drop massively. 20] Logically it follows that lower-income populations are more exposed to toxic chemicals. For example, a study of infant umbilical cord blood showed that 95% of participants showing toxic exposure came from households earning under $40,000 a year, and many were from ethnic minorities exposed to environmental toxins like flame retardants. 10] Toxic exposure often reflects class, with wealthier individuals having access to cleaner environments and safer homes.

It's a hard truth: living in a less toxic environment costs more. Pollution affects everyone, but the poorest suffer the most. And while pollution is often framed as a luxury issue for the wealthy, for those in developing nations, it's a matter of survival. The best way to address global pollution is not just with solar panels and electric cars, but by fostering peace and economic opportunity for the millions living in poverty.

The focus on "going green" by the ultra-wealthy can sometimes feel more like a way to ease personal guilt, rather than tackling the deeper issue of pollution, which often stems from poverty. Erecting solar arrays or driving luxury electric vehicles doesn't address the systemic issues that cause pollution, especially when millions still live without basic utilities. It's easy to forget that even the most eco-friendly lifestyles still rely on oil for things like food production and transportation. Whether we like it or not, our current infrastructure depends on fossil fuels—diesel for farm equipment, commercial trucks, ships, trains, and even fertilizers.

In short, going green is important, but we can't ignore the fact that the real solution to pollution lies in reducing global poverty. The wealthy can afford to be environmentally conscious, but for a world in poverty, survival matters more than pollution.

Solving environmental pollution and worldwide poverty is beyond the scope of this book. What I'd like you to realize is this:

- Toxic exposure is everywhere

- Pollution & poverty are strongly linked

- Helping impoverished populations in the developing world is fundamental to solving pollution

How Does Subclinical Toxic Exposure Hurt Us?

In a world where warning labels are everywhere, the culture seems to respond with either terror or an indifferent shrug to the dire warnings of invisible toxins lurking in every shadow. As if running from the inescapable specter of our own shadows, we've switched from cow milk, to soy milk, to almond milk, to oat milk. At the same time, we went from tap water, to bottled water, to filtered water, and now distilled water. The only constant in this struggle is a growing sense of futility. The spirit of the times is increasingly nihilistic: nothing's ever organic enough, green enough, or healthy enough. Sadly, people seem torn between becoming neurotic about their health or just giving up and eating junk food because everything is toxic anyway.

In the wake of all this, some people are tempted to just give up. The problem is that toxins are mostly invisible and in small amounts. The harmful actions of toxins are very gradual and hard to pin down. The solution is to ground ourselves in reality. Let's examine one tangible, easy-to-see way that toxins have harmed us. This will give a clear starting place on the map toward a solution. One clear way that ongoing micro-exposure to toxins negatively affects your health is in how your genes are expressed. Epigenetics is a branch of science that studies how lifestyle and environment affect gene expression. The discovery of DNA told us that our physical bodies and even our temperament are preordained from conception. We see this in nature; the family dog inherited his looks and quite a bit of his personality from his parents. Later on, epigenetics discovered that your genes may stay the same, but which of your genes dominate your life is very open to influence.

In a 2012 study published in the *Journal of Environmental Science*, the connection between toxic exposure and epigenetics became obvious. 21] The researchers looked at various toxins and showed how they influence our genetics. Everything from alcohol, heavy metals, plastics, and pesticides influence our genetic expression. Let's look at the plastic additive bisphenol, or BPA for short. BPA increases the risk of specific types of breast cancer and alters human reproductive capacity. These harmful effects are genetic in nature and hard to define. Some people get cancer; some couples can't get pregnant, so there's a frustrating ambiguity.

Even still, BPA is tied to hormonal changes, infertility, and generational diseases that may affect the children of those exposed. Exposure to BPA puts you at risk for nutrient deficiencies of important compounds like folate, selenium, and other B vitamins. 22] Folate and certain B vitamins are known as methyl donors, which is why supplementation with these can help counteract the toxic effects that BPA has on fertility and hormonal imbalances that lead to cancer. These substances are critical for the production and replication of DNA. Research is ongoing, but this much is already clear: although BPA toxicity is subtle, the harm is real and insidious.

How about the heavy metal cadmium? While cadmium is found in nature, burning coal, garbage, plastics, and metal smelting release a lot of this harmful element into the air. 24] We either breathe it in from the air, or it's absorbed into our water, plants, and soil. Then, people consume cadmium-storing plants like tobacco, potatoes, wheat, grains, nuts, seeds, and nut-based oils. Cadmium has been connected to prostate, liver, kidney, bladder, and testicular cancer. It also suppresses the immune system and stops natural DNA repair. 25] People who have higher cadmium levels have decreased amounts of B vitamins, selenium, and folate. I could go on and on about these connections, but the point is that toxic exposure leads to an overwhelming burden on the body.

Aside from acute poison control and ER visits, modern medicine doesn't seem to pay enough attention to the negative effects of chronic exposure to toxins.

Diseases related to toxins:
- Cancer
- Infertility
- Nutrient deficiencies
- Lowered immune function
- Inflammation
- Diabetes
- Hormone disruption
- Autoimmune diseases

Many chronic diseases are linked to toxic exposure and deficiencies in key nutrients like water-soluble B vitamins and trace minerals. For example, one study found that
"Methyl deficiency accelerates toxin-related toxicity and carcinogenesis through DNA hypomethylation" 26].

This suggests that nutrient deficiencies, particularly in methylation pathways, may speed up cancer caused by environmental toxins. Understanding the connection between epigenetics, food, and nutrients is crucial to addressing the long-term impacts of toxic exposure on our health.

When the body becomes overwhelmed by toxins, it has to store them in fat cells, organs, bones, and even the brain. This chronic toxic load places a significant burden on the body's detoxification systems. As a result, cell repair and immune function are compromised, leaving the body vulnerable to conditions like cancer, autoimmune diseases, and other health issues. In my clinical practice, we always prioritize identifying and eliminating the source of toxic exposure while also educating patients on how to reduce or avoid these harmful substances going forward.

One key factor in detoxification is the GST/GPX enzyme system, which plays a central role in the body's ability to detoxify. People with genetic variants in the GST/GPX complex (a specific SNP/variant) have a reduced ability to handle toxins like industrial chemicals, pesticides, heavy metals, and mold. These enzymes help bind toxins to glutathione, a powerful antioxidant, making the toxins water-soluble and easier to eliminate through urine. Without proper functioning of these enzymes, the body struggles to detoxify, leading to a higher toxic burden.

Interestingly, individuals with these genetic variants may act as "early warning systems" for their communities. In the past, these genetically unique individuals might have been more attuned to harmful environmental conditions, like bad food or air quality, allowing them to detect and avoid dangers. Additionally, chronic stress can increase the production of hydrogen peroxide in the body, leading to oxidative damage. This oxidative stress is one reason for visible signs of aging, like gray hair.

I've seen firsthand how improving detoxification pathways, reducing environmental exposures, and managing emotional stress can have a noticeable effect on the body. In some cases, patients have even reported a reduction in gray hair as their natural detoxification processes are restored. This is just one example of how addressing the root causes of toxic buildup can promote overall health and vitality.

The winning formula seems to be:

Less stress (both physical and mental) + more glutathione + more available nutrients + spiritual growth = less damage to the body.

People with impaired GST/GPX SNPs may be very sensitive to smells and chemicals; they gain weight easily regardless of what they eat and have a family history of cancer or autoimmune conditions. While genetics play a factor, you don't have to have a genetic SNP/variant in order for your GST/GPX system to be compromised. With enough stress, environmental exposure, and nutrient deficiencies, you will have all the same symptoms as a person who was born with a gene variant such as GST/GPX.

Getting Your Home and Work Environment Less Toxic

With toxins found literally everywhere, cleaning up your home and your environment is a daunting task. I've been aware of these risks for years, and I still don't consider my home to be perfectly non-toxic. We all know pesticides are bad, but when hornets viciously swarm your 6-year-old's birthday party and attack little kids, we're all tempted to reach for a can of bug spray even though we know it's wrong. But let's all commit to taking incremental steps over time. I love my house out in the Pacific Northwest forest, but every year, aggressive yellow jackets and hornets are an issue. Instead of spraying the eaves of my home with poison, it's better to put out traps early in the year. For household products, use up what you have and switch to safer versions of items such as cleaning products and laundry soaps when they run out.

Ask yourself,

- How safe is my water supply?
- How clean is the air?
- What's in my food?

Go down the list below to help you narrow down where to focus. **Fresh air from the outside is (almost always) much cleaner than inside air.** This may be problematic if you have seasonal allergies or live near freeways or active wildfires. For the most part, however, opening your windows at least once a day for a few minutes helps improve indoor air quality.

Avoid scented products and air fresheners. We have a joke in our family that conventional air fresheners are a great way to "spray cancer all over the house." A lot of people are accustomed to high levels of artificial fragrances, colognes, perfumes, and scents in cleaning products, dryer sheets, lotions, shampoos, hair products, and cosmetics containing VOCs (Volatile Organic Compounds). These artificial scents are unnatural, and a lot of them are terrible for the body.

"The negative impact of fragrance chemicals on human health includes cutaneous, respiratory, and systemic effects (e.g., headaches, asthma attacks, breathing difficulties, cardiovascular and neurological problems) and distress in workplaces." 27]

Toxins in the home come from things like furniture, paints, flooring, and even new clothing.

Common in-home pollutants include formaldehyde, Volatile Organic Compounds (benzene and trichloroethylene or TCE), airborne biological pollutants, carbon monoxide and nitrogen oxides, pesticides and disinfectants (phenols), and radon. These compounds cause asthma, allergies, headaches, fatigue, nervous system disorders, and cancer. 28] If you need new carpet, furniture, painting, or mattresses, consider having it done in the springtime so you can open plenty of windows to air out your house. Instead of air fresheners and deodorizers, we use natural plant-based products with high-grade essential oils as the fragrance.

Avoid non-stick cookware and pans. Non-stick chemicals get in your food, and it's bad. I write more about this in the exposure to heavy metals section. Seriously though, just say *no* to non-stick.

Avoid plastics for food and drinks. Studies have linked plastic exposure to metabolic conditions (obesity and diabetes), hormonal issues, and even infertility. The common plastic additives Bisphenol A (BPA) and chemicals called phthalates seem to be of particular concern. 29] Especially avoid heating food and storing food in plastics as much as possible. Drink out of glass or surgical-grade stainless steel instead of plastic cups. Look for foods that have not been packaged in plastic whenever possible. Microwave TV dinners and other prepackaged food are specifically heated up in plastic, which is bad news.

Purchase a good air filter to improve indoor air quality. Choose a filter that is HEPA-certified. If the air quality in your area is bad, consider moving. But also consider an upgraded cassette-type air filtration system for your home HVAC for added protection. Fresh air from the outside by opening windows is also needed.

> *"Indoor environment conditions contribute greatly to human well-being, as most people spend around 90% of their time indoors, mainly at home or in the workplace. According to the World Health Organization (WHO), indoor air pollution (IAP) is responsible for the deaths of 3.8 million people annually. IAP can be generated inside homes or buildings through occupants' activities, such as cooking, smoking, use of electronic machines, use of consumer products, or emissions from building materials. Harmful pollutants inside buildings include carbon monoxide (CO), volatile organic compounds (VOCs), particulate matter (PM), aerosol, biological pollutants, and others."* 30]

Purchase house plants that capture off-gassing. Studies conducted by NASA have identified over 50 house plants that help remove harmful pollutants and gases from the air. Here are the top ten plants that were identified in the study. These house plants removed toxins like carbon monoxide, benzene and formaldehyde from the air. 28]

- Areca Palm (Chrysalidocarpus lutescens)
- Lady Palm (Rhapis excelsa)
- Bamboo palm (Chamaedorea seifrizii)
- Rubber Plant (Ficus robusta)
- Dracaena "Janet Craig" (Dracaena deremensis)
- Philodendron (Philodendron sp.)
- Dwarf Date Palm (Phoenix roebelenii)
- Ficus Alii (Ficus macleilandii "Alii")
- Boston Fern (Nephrolepis exaltata "Bostoniensis")

- Peace Lily (Spathiphyllum "Mauna Loa")

Get your home and workplace inspected for mold. I live in the Pacific Northwest, and due to the heavy rainfall, toxic mold exposure is an issue. We live in a very damp environment much of the year, and a lot of the homes are older and less sealed up against moisture. Dampness causes mold. Mold can cause asthma, bronchitis, brain fog, fatigue, headaches, chronic body pain, sneezing, runny nose, skin rashes, chronic sinus infections, loss of taste, numbness or tingling, weakness or tremors, and much more.

One patient of mine couldn't get well after a traumatic head injury until we started simultaneously treating and addressing her mold exposure. Before we started seeing her, she thought maybe she was getting what she called early-onset Alzheimer's. Her ability to think, reason, and remember was impaired. She had difficulty sequencing her actions, and she would forget basic words. We tested her home for mold and found 1,000 times the healthy level of mold spores present. The technicians found that her water heater was leaking, spreading warm water inside her home's interior and creating a mold explosion. Similarly, her workplace was a large corporate building that had a leaking roof that had been improperly repaired. Once these environmental mold factors were solved, I prescribed supplements to detoxify her body from mold exposure, and she recovered. She said it was like "waking as if she had been in a dream." In cases where people just aren't getting better, it's always a good idea to test for mold.

Get your gas appliances assessed for leaks, or consider switching to electric. Gas appliances release carbon monoxide gas (CO) as well as nitric oxide gas (NO) and nitrogen dioxide. All of these toxic gases have been linked to serious side effects such as neurological conditions, heart problems, behavior issues, and even death. One study found that buildings with gas stoves had CO levels 5-30 times higher than those without. 30]

Nutrition as DETOX. We often think that we need expensive and exotic means to heal ourselves from chronic illness and toxic exposure. But, there are times when simple lifestyle changes in the foods we eat can significantly help us to both nourish and detoxify our bodies. Here are some easy ways to get started.

Limit foods high in heavy metals and pesticides. Figure out what's in your food. Eliminate processed foods and foods known to have high levels of toxins. While we can't avoid everything, and there are otherwise healthy foods that carry some exposure risk, we can limit our risk factors by how often we eat certain foods and what food combinations we enjoy routinely. 20% of women over age 45 are at higher risk of osteoporosis due to exposure to Cadmium. 31]

Common toxic metals include:
- Aluminum
- Antimony
- Arsenic
- Cadmium
- Lead
- Mercury
- Nickel
- Uranium

Toxic metals are inorganic elements that more readily bind to tissues in our bodies and are difficult to eliminate from the body. In chemistry, aluminum is classified as a metalloid and not a heavy metal. However, due to aluminum's known toxic effects, it is sometimes listed in the heavy metal category even though its atomic mass is 8 times lower than lead. Toxic (heavy) metals overwhelm our natural detoxification system and are difficult for the body to remove, especially in patients low in minerals like zinc and magnesium.

Research published in the journal *Interdisciplinary Toxicology* found that these harmful metals:

"(Toxic Metals) sometimes act as a pseudo element of the body while at certain times they may even interfere with metabolic processes. Few metals, such as aluminum, can be removed through elimination activities, while some metals accumulate in the body and food chain, exhibiting a chronic nature. Various public health measures have been undertaken to control, prevent, and treat metal toxicity occurring at various levels, such as occupational exposure, accidents, and environmental factors. Metal toxicity depends upon the absorbed dose, the route of exposure, and the duration of exposure, i.e., acute or chronic. This can lead to various disorders and can also result in excessive damage due to oxidative stress induced by free radical formation." 32]

It's more challenging to eliminate heavy metals when your body is also low in glutathione. Glutathione is a major antioxidant produced by our cells, essential for detoxification. If the body can't eliminate heavy metals, they start to accumulate in organs, bones, and even the brain, crossing the blood-brain barrier. This buildup affects the nervous system, immune system, and our ability to detoxify other substances, like medications and alcohol.

Most healthy individuals can recover from a brief, one-time heavy metal exposure. By "healthy," I mean having low body fat, toned muscle, balanced blood sugar, good cardiovascular endurance, balanced hormones, high energy, optimal nutrient levels, no autoimmune conditions, and stable moods. Unfortunately, many people fall short of this standard. The average person experiences fatigue, nutritional deficiencies, metabolic issues, and constant toxic exposure. As we age, face increasing exposure, lose bone density, or suffer from illness and poor nutrition, our systems become overwhelmed.

Heavy metal accumulation can lead to premature aging, memory problems, nervous system dysfunction, and autoimmune diseases. Naturopathic physicians refer to heavy metals as "obstacles to cure." In some cases, the burden is so great that we need to use chelating agents to help remove them from the body. Chelation, derived from the Greek word chēlē (meaning "claw"), uses compounds like EDTA, DMSA, and

DMSO to bind to heavy metals and remove them from tissues. However, these agents are only effective if the body's detoxification systems are functioning properly. The chelators pull metals from organs, bones, and the brain, but the body must be able to excrete them through urine, sweat, and bowel movements for the process to succeed.

Chelating agents must be used under the supervision of a trained professional, as they can also deplete vital minerals like zinc, magnesium, and iron. Chelation can be done orally or via IV therapy, with IV chelation requiring close monitoring through blood tests and heavy metal urine screenings. IV chelation works, but is often a very harsh treatment, because it leaves patients depleted of vitamins and minerals. Furthermore, the chelation process brings toxins that are sequestered in fat, bone and brain tissue out into the bloodstream, where they can cause unpleasant symptoms for the patient. At our clinic, we rarely use traditional chelation methods because we prefer the more gentle advanced oral binders. These oral binders, which contain carbon compounds, selectively remove harmful metals and pesticides while preserving beneficial minerals. Another alternative to chelation are IV Alpha Lipoic Acid (ALA) and glutathione. These compounds are helpful in detoxifying but are much easier than IV chelation.

Our focus is always on safety, and patients undergoing chelation process can expect to spend several months in the process. While chelation isn't part of our routine protocol, we reserve it for cases where other methods haven't worked. Now, let's look at ways you can start reducing your exposure to heavy metals.

Limit the following high-toxic metal foods:
- Swordfish
- Tuna
- Sea bass
- Sunflower seeds
- Rice, especially brown rice
- Potatoes, especially sweet potatoes
- Processed cereal grains

Type the following into your favorite search engine. "Food sources of ...cadmium, lead, mercury, arsenic, aluminum (choose a toxic metal)" to understand your exposure risk.

Drink Clean Water. Heavy metals can also be found in drinking water (yes, even "clean" city water can contain heavy metals, it's not something that is typically checked). A report conducted by the U.S. Geological Survey found large amounts of heavy metals contaminating the mighty Mississippi River. Due to its immense size, the Mississippi provides drinking water and crop irrigation for a large section of the country. Remember when we talked about the Valley of the Drums, the Flint Michigan water crisis, and Love Canal? These toxic waste dumps all leached out into their respective major waterways. With all of the industrial manufacturing and farming along the Mississippi, I'd be surprised if the city-water was truly safe to drink.

According to a 1986 publication by the U.S. Environmental Protection Agency (EPA), the primary sources of toxic metals in wastewater are industrial and domestic activities. The EPA estimates that around 81% of the metals entering wastewater treatment plants come from regulated industries, which dispose of waste into municipal sewer systems, while the remaining 19% comes from household products used by consumers. In industries along the Mississippi River, metals such as cadmium, chromium, copper, lead, and mercury are frequently used. Municipal wastewater treatment plants generate two main by-products: solid waste and treated wastewater. Typically, 70 to 90% of these heavy metals, including cadmium, chromium, copper, lead, and zinc, are removed as solid waste during treatment. However, 10 to 30% of these metals remain dissolved in the water that is discharged back into the river. 33] Over 18 million people depend on water from the Mississippi River, so we need to do more to protect our precious water supplies. Heavy metal removal can be expensive, and some municipal water treatment facilities don't have the technology to remove toxic heavy metals adequately. Wells are not always safe either, but they're often much better than city water, so long as you test them yearly.

Currently, my family drinks well water. I once had a patient who also relied on well water but was experiencing various health issues. After testing her water, it was discovered that arsenic levels were over 10 times the supposedly safe limit! Well water can be contaminated by upstream agricultural activities, mining, earthquakes, and pesticide runoff. However, there is some hope on the horizon. A 2018 study revealed that a safe, environmentally friendly polymer called Fe-BTC/PDA can effectively remove lead and mercury from drinking water. While this technology shows promise, it is not yet available commercially. If the results can be replicated and the product proves safe, it could become a valuable tool for filtering heavy metal contaminants. This method is selective, targeting only specific metals, and could potentially be cost-effective. 34] Of course, we must remain cautious to ensure that any solutions we implement don't come with unintended side effects.

Recycle old paint. Depending on what they're made of, older paints, especially those used in arts and crafts, still contain trace amounts of lead and other toxic metals. Even many modern house paints, primers, and thinners contain at least some harmful VOCs. If you must paint, open all windows and doors and allow plenty of time for the house to air out before staying there.

Move away from airports. In the past, lead was added to gasoline used in cars and trucks. Unleaded gas was introduced in the 1970s, but it wasn't fully phased out in the US until the mid-1990s. 36] However, leaded gas is still used in aviation fuel today. 35] A study found that children living within half a mile of airports using leaded gas had elevated lead levels. 37] Currently, about 75% of private planes in the US still use leaded gas. 38] While commercial jets run on kerosene (a highly refined diesel), small propeller-driven planes use aviation fuel, or avgas, which contains tetraethyl lead—an additive banned in automobile fuel since the 1990s. Avgas remains the leading source of airborne lead pollution in the US, and despite the availability of lead-free alternatives, the switch has been slow. 39] The EPA estimates that 16 million people live within one kilometer of airports where this fuel is used, with 3 million children attending schools in the same area. 39] These planes also fly overhead, contaminating fields and food supplies with lead.

Throw away certain cooking pans, ceramics, cooking utensils, and microwave popcorn. My husband Richard nearly gasped when I told him how much I wanted to spend on our cooking pans—maybe he had a point. But after reading a few too many studies about the dangers of certain cookware, I felt it was worth it. Research shows that heavy metals can leach into food from most pans, especially those made in countries with lower product safety standards, like China. 38] Non-stick pans are a big culprit and should be tossed right away, especially if they have cracks or scratches. The main ingredients in non-stick coatings are perfluorooctanoic acid (PFOA) and polytetrafluoroethylene (PTFE), marketed as Teflon® or the supposedly safer GENx coatings. These coatings are also found in microwave foods like popcorn. When heated, they release toxic fumes that can seriously affect our health, especially in kids. 40] One study even found that exposure to PTFE doubled children's risk of developing certain serious but preventable health conditions. 41] These non-stick surfaces are linked to everything from increased cholesterol and infertility to higher cancer risks. Women who struggle with infertility, for instance, are more likely to have perfluorooctane sulfonate (PFOS) and perfluorooctanoic acid (PFOA) in their blood. 42] These chemicals are also used as flame retardants and are found in non-stick cookware, carpets, and many other household items.

It's not just cooking pans—coffee mugs and utensils can contain heavy metals too, due to certain ceramic glazes and high levels of aluminum in some "stainless steel" products. 43] Not all stainless steel is created equal, so it's important to choose brands that test for harmful substances like heavy metals. The problem is that many products are only tested for a short period before hitting the market. It's just not economically viable to test cheap products for decades, so we often don't know the risks until much later. Non-stick pans and flame retardants are meant to make our lives easier, but unfortunately, we usually only learn about their long-term consequences years down the line.

Only use rigorously tested supplements and herbs. Some herbs and supplements contain unsafe levels of lead and other toxic heavy metals in their preparations. One study found the following:

> *"We discovered that a maximum permissible level (MPL) of Pb (lead) is exceeded in 21 plant medicine species, Cd (cadmium) in 44 species, and Hg (mercury) in 10 species." 42]*

For this reason, I'm very careful about what I allow into my clinical practice. We use supplement and herbal companies that do extensive testing for pesticides, heavy metals, and other harmful compounds to ensure you get the benefit of the plant without the downside of needless toxic exposure. That being said, all supplements that contain the root of the plant will have trace amounts of lead and other toxic metals found in them. It cannot be avoided. The key is to use companies that keep that number well under the allowable rate and continually batch-test each supplement, especially because herb suppliers differ greatly worldwide. Not all supplements, herbs, and natural medicines are created equal.

Check your personal hygiene products. The Food and Drug Administration in the US has guidelines for the amount of heavy metals that may be present in cosmetics. 44] I'll give you a hint: that number isn't zero! Cosmetic exposure is one of the main ways people are exposed to toxic metals, because these items are worn daily over several decades. Cosmetics are applied to the face; a certain amount is going to be eaten, inhaled, or fall into the eye, where it's absorbed by mucous membranes.

The trouble is the FDA does not require companies to tell you about heavy metal content, so you won't see it on the label. Even though the FDA publishes acceptable levels for heavy metals found in cosmetics, they don't enforce these standards on companies or test to make sure they meet the standards! Cosmetic companies are only required to list ingredients. Use companies that openly publish data on heavy metal content and concentrations in their products. Choose a deodorant over an antiperspirant. Most antiperspirants use aluminum to inhibit sweating. Several studies have shown that daily exposure to aluminum caused elevated levels to show up in breast tissue.

Other studies have tied aluminum exposure to a higher likelihood of developing cancers. 45]

Use caution with vaccines. Here, we only concern ourselves with openly published vaccine additives. Many vaccine makers put in adjuvants, which are additives that increase the immune response. The idea is boosting immune response will make a more "effective" vaccine. 46] The issue is *how* adjuvants boost the immune system. Adjuvants increase immune response by irritating, inflaming, or otherwise putting stress on the body. Adjuvants produce irritation, inflammation, and stress because they are harmful toxins. Their logic is that a little bit of a toxic substance may have a beneficial effect. But that little bit of toxin may build up over time when you consider the 150 vaccines on the current schedule. Adjuvants often contain toxic metals. Yep. That's right, the thing we are trying to avoid and get out of our environment is being injected into us through certain vaccines.

The most concerning adjuvants are aluminum and mercury. Mercury-containing thimerosal was removed from children's vaccines in the US in 2001. But, mercury (thimerosal) is still found in multi-dose vials of vaccines such as certain flu shots. 47] Mercury in vaccines is controversial, to say the least. 48] I tend toward being cautious when it comes to what I put into my body in general, especially when injecting mercury. Since I deal with the effects of heavy metal exposure with patients that I see, I err on the side of caution when it comes to vaccinations. For any medical treatment, including vaccines, I'm a strong advocate of informed consent. The problem with vaccines is that we're beaten with the mantra of *safe and effective* instead of being allowed to freely choose. During the Pandemic, people were fired from their jobs, kids were not allowed in daycares, private schools, and colleges if they didn't get the jab. This is coercion to the point that informed consent is not possible. I could say a lot more here, but if you know, you know. If you don't know, then even your child, spouse, or best friend dying suddenly wouldn't convince you. I digress.

Avoid Smoking. Tobacco contains heavy metals, including cadmium (Cd), chromium (Cr), lead (Pb), and nickel (Ni), which accumulate in the body through smoking. A study in the Middle East found that tobacco smoking is the primary source of cadmium exposure for the general population. Over time, even small amounts of cadmium can cause kidney damage, fragile bones, and stomach issues like irritation, vomiting, and diarrhea. Additionally, cadmium and lead in tobacco smoke significantly increase cancer risk. 49]

Consume foods high in polyphenols. Polyphenols, found in foods like turmeric, green tea, blueberries, and dark chocolate, help reduce damage from toxins and viruses. Some examples of these beneficial polyphenols include genistein, EGCG (Epigallocatechin gallate), curcumin, sulforaphane, and resveratrol. These compounds act as chemo-preventive agents by inhibiting DNMT (DNA methyltransferase), which can reverse harmful epigenetic changes, such as hypermethylation of tumor suppressor genes (TSGs). In simple terms, this means that polyphenols can help fix changes in our genes that might otherwise increase the risk of cancer. 26]

EGCG is found in high-quality organic green tea, but encapsulation is recommended to get the dosage needed to be effective. Green tea extract in the form of EGCG is used to treat exposure to the HPV virus as well. Certain strains of HPV cause cervical, throat, and anal cancers and therefore are known as "oncogenic" or cancer-causing viruses. **No, supplements won't cure cancer.** Even still, sound fundamentals with your food, supplement, and lifestyle choices can significantly lower the risk of all diseases and improve your health and vitality, too.

Curcumin, also known as turmeric, has a wide variety of uses as an anticancer, anti-inflammatory, and liver-support herb. It's found in foods like curry and should be eaten regularly and at the same time as a healthy fat, such as coconut milk or as a tea called "golden milk." Turmeric is also something we recommend consuming encapsulated, as it is difficult to consume a high enough quantity on a daily basis to get the full benefit. However, turmeric is also a root, so it can contain trace amounts of lead. It's important to source turmeric from supplement companies that do third-party testing for toxic elements.

Resveratrol is a potent antioxidant found in pistachios, grapes, and dark berries such as blueberries, cranberries, and dark chocolate. Not only has resveratrol helped with cancer prevention, but it also helps with cholesterol and blood lipid levels. Resveratrol may also have neuroprotective properties while playing a role in the prevention of neurodegenerative diseases such as dementia.

Sulforaphane is found in cruciferous vegetables like broccoli, kale, brussels sprouts, cauliflower, and mustard greens, with the highest concentration in broccoli sprouts. It helps reduce inflammation, has antimicrobial properties, and supports liver detoxification. Promising research suggests that sulforaphane may lower the risk of Alzheimer's disease and dementia, enhance body detoxification, and potentially prevent hormone-related cancers, such as breast and prostate cancer. 50]

Genistein is derived from soy isoflavones, this compound is found in soy products and supplements. As a phytoestrogen, it helps balance the effects of "bad estrogen" in the body. A derivative of it is even used in some cancer treatments, showing promise as an anti-cancer and anti-tumor agent. 51] Be cautious with chemically processed soy products, as they can contain high levels of pesticides. Also, since soy mimics estrogen, it's not ideal for those already high in estrogen or for men looking to avoid lowering their healthy testosterone levels.

Case Study: Lorraine

Lorraine, a 53-year-old woman, originally came into our clinic for help after a car accident. She had whiplash injuries and shoulder pain so severe that she could barely move her neck. As a secondary concern, she mentioned sometimes having trouble thinking. While treating her whiplash injuries, we also looked into her brain fog and forgetfulness. After 6 weeks of weekly care, her whiplash and shoulder pain had decreased by 75%. We used a combination of trauma processing, acupuncture, cold laser therapy, and prolotherapy in her shoulder joint and trigger points to completely clear the pain.

Two months later, Lorraine was back to practicing Pilates, walking daily, and spending time with friends and family. However, she was still struggling with brain fog. To dig deeper, we ran two tests: the DUTCH test (a hormone panel that checks for hormone imbalances and detoxification blockages) and a blood and urine panel that measured her nutrients, neurotransmitters, energy cycles, lipids, and heavy metals. Most results came back in optimal ranges, except for her detox pathways, which were blocked, and high levels of heavy metals, including mercury. Her mercury levels were 20 times higher than the average, according to the NHANES report from the EPA.

Upon further investigation, we realized Lorraine had two primary mercury exposures. The first was from the recent replacement of five silver amalgam fillings without proper mercury removal precautions. The second, more significant exposure came from her 1-3 times per week sushi habit, where she often ate ahi tuna, a fish known for high mercury levels.

We performed a second test using a combination of oral and IV chelation agents to "provoke" the release of heavy metals from the body and tissues. The results showed high levels of mercury, along with lead, arsenic, cadmium, and aluminum. Lorraine's lead levels, for example, were 34, whereas the NHANES report suggests an upper limit of 0.979!

We began a series of 10 IV chelation sessions, followed by nutrient repletion in between. Lorraine noticed that her brain fog worsened a few days after each session, but after a week, she experienced moments of mental clarity that she hadn't had in years. After the first 10 sessions, her heavy metal levels had decreased by half but remained in an unhealthy range. We proceeded with five more sessions, and after completing all 15, her heavy metals dropped to safe levels. While she still had occasional forgetfulness, she felt much sharper overall.

Today, Lorraine is feeling great, avoiding her weekly sushi habit, and even helping her husband run his company. She's able to make strategic, calculated decisions and solve complex logistical problems—proof of her restored cognitive function. Lorraine's case was a powerful reminder to our team of how crucial it is to remove obstacles to healing, like heavy metal toxicity, to allow the body to detoxify and restore proper function, especially in the immune system and brain.

Case Study: Mary

Mary, a sweet 7-year-old girl, came to us for help with behavioral issues and learning challenges. Although I never witnessed the outbursts in the office, her parents reported frequent anger and "full meltdowns" at home. We decided to run a urine test to check for metals and toxins, and the results were concerning. Mary had high levels of phthalates, a chemical used in plastics that can disrupt hormones and neurological function, as well as aluminum levels more than 10 times the safe upper limit.

After ruling out aluminum exposure from canned beverages, we suspected the source might be a combination of vaccines and contaminated water. To address this, we began Mary on carbon-based oral binders to help her body eliminate toxins. Over the next six months, we supported her detoxification process with healthy eating, herbs, supplements, and binders to help clear out the blockages. After retesting her urine, we were thrilled to find no detectable levels of toxic chemicals or metals.

The best part was seeing the positive changes in Mary's life—she was performing better at school and, most importantly, her meltdowns had stopped at home. It was a rewarding journey of healing, and Mary's progress was a great reminder of how powerful detoxification can be for the body and mind.

Conclusion

Toxins are everywhere, thanks to the Industrial Revolution. While issues like solar panels, electric vehicles, and trendy social media causes often steal the spotlight, one of the most effective ways to reduce environmental toxins might be to address worldwide poverty. Holding large corporations accountable is important, but government regulations are often slow and compromised, making meaningful progress difficult. Undiagnosed toxic exposure is a major, invisible barrier to healing, yet it's largely overlooked in conventional medicine. Conventional medicine often treats autoimmune conditions as the end of the story, while naturopathic medicine works to uncover why autoimmune conditions happen.

Though avoiding all toxins is impossible, there are steps you can take to reduce exposure. Start by testing your water, avoiding city water, steering clear of plastics, fragrances, chemicals, and non-stick cookware, and limiting high-toxin foods.

TLDR: Too Long Didn't Read

If you're dealing with persistent illness, autoimmune issues, or struggling to lose weight despite eating right and working out, toxic exposure could be playing a bigger role than your doctor realizes. Your body might be overwhelmed by hidden toxins, and instead of addressing the root cause, most regular doctors are just patching things up on the surface. It's like putting a band-aid on a broken leg—good luck with that!

Chapter 13
Your Genetic Landscape

Your genetics load the gun. But your lifestyle pulls the trigger. 1]
-Dr. Mehmet Oz

Google® attributes the phrase to Dr. Mehmet Oz, but as mentioned earlier in this book, I first heard it from one of my early medical mentors, Dr. Murzeck. Who said it first? I'm not certain, and honestly, I don't think it matters—but it's definitely worth repeating. In any event, it's a simple way to frame the concept of epigenetics. DNA was first identified in the 1860s by a Swiss chemist named Friedrich Miescher. 2] However, the DNA revolution truly began in the 1950s, when biochemist Erwin Chargaff discovered the now-famous DNA double helix. 3]

Since that time, genetics has become the fundamental way culture defines much of the human experience. The academic study of DNA became so widespread that scientists have famously declared that our genes determine much of our physical and biological fate. No, not your Levi's® jeans—I mean the genes you inherited from Mom and Dad. While this discovery marked a significant scientific breakthrough, it's only part of the story. Yes, certain diseases, cancer risks, and genetic traits are passed down through families, and understanding genetics has certainly advanced medical care in terms of diagnosis and prevention. But, as it turns out, our knowledge of DNA has also had some unintended negative consequences. These days, people unconsciously view genetics as a religious doctrine, sort of like predestination. Predestination is a philosophy that says that humans have a fixed outcome. In theology, it's the belief that certain people were always going to heaven, others to hell, and this was all pre-decided by God before the person was even born. Today, people treat DNA like some sort of scientific predestination.

"My dad had gout, so that's why I have gout. I guess there's nothing I can do about it." -Anonymous Patient 1

"Breast cancer runs in my family, so I'm taking precautions and getting a mastectomy." -Anonymous Patient 2

The downside of learning about DNA is that we might be tempted to treat genetics like the Word of God. In that worldview, our genetics become an inescapable fate. Some people make the mistake of learned helplessness with regard to genetics. Others bend their entire lives around genetic risks. Yes, some patients go so far as to have major surgeries in an attempt to prevent certain inherited illnesses. These types of patients make genetics the basis for their diet, lifestyle, and life decisions.

In the other camp, people use genetics as an excuse for their declining health, so they stop trying. Those who give up don't take responsibility for their poor lifestyle habits; they see weight gain, illness, and cancer as bad genetic luck. The logic of this camp states that since obesity runs in our family, we can't fight it, so why even try? Both of these ideological camps are based on observable facts. However, each side may use those true facts to reach a misleading conclusion. Genetics and a family history of disease are not the whole picture. In fact, without food, culture, lifestyle choices, medication/drug use, chemical exposure, and the sedentary lifestyles of modernity, I wager that far fewer inherited health problems would actually exist today. Remember, genetics aren't all you inherited. You also inherited your family's spiritual heritage, culture, habits, worldview, traditions, food choices, and moral values. Of these, which is truly more influential in your life outcome? Of course, you say it's the old nature-versus-nurture argument. Yes, but no. What I'm driving at is not nature versus nurture; it's more like nurture controlling nature. Epigenetics is a term that means above genetics; it means the study of how your environment and lifestyle influence your DNA expression. Because it's above the actual genetic sequence, epigenetics can simply turn genes on or off. In this way, DNA is the car, but your upbringing and current life choices are driving that car. Epigenetics can change how a gene is expressed.

Let's try a fun example. Storytime! Suppose we have twin unicorns (because who doesn't want to have a unicorn, let alone twin unicorns?) Sadly, the unicorns were separated at birth. Unicorn One was raised on a beautiful organic farm outside of the city. She roamed on fresh grass alongside sweet animal friends and was fed a diet of diverse organic fruits, vegetables, and grass. She was brushed and loved every day by her sweet, doting family. Unicorn One was adored and told how much they loved and appreciated her. She gave the grandkids rides on her back. She got plenty of exercise and fresh air. Unicorn One and her loving family laughed and played into the sunset.

Unfortunately, twin Unicorn Two led a much more tragic existence. Unicorn Two was sold to a traveling circus where they fed her junk food scraps left over from nights of partying: cotton candy, snow cones, pizza slices, corn dogs, alcohol, and soda pop. She was forced to perform in sweltering circus tents. When she wasn't young and fresh anymore, the circus sold her to a Las Vegas casino. There, she was caged up on display for the entertainment of tourists in smoky Las Vegas gambling halls, where she performed in windowless arenas. When she wasn't earning her owner's money, she was locked away in a high-security holding area that felt like a prison. One day, the sweet family who owned Unicorn One found out about the terrible fate of Unicorn Two. Eventually, they raised enough money to rescue her. On the day Unicorn Two arrived, everyone was shocked to see that the identical twins didn't look like twins at all. Unicorn One had a bright and shiny coat, she was muscular and had a brilliant rainbow tail along with a golden unicorn horn. Unicorn Two was a sad grayish color, she was overweight and had a wheezing smoker's hack when she woke up in the morning. She had a horn, but it lost its golden color, and her rainbow tail had faded to a dull purple color.

The unicorns seemed so different that the family thought they'd rescued the wrong unicorn. Being curious, the family ran a genetic test. In time, the results came back confirming that, yes, indeed, they were genetically identical. The test revealed a genetic family history of cancer, obesity, asthma, and heart disease. Yet, Unicorn One looked amazing and her metabolic health was similar to unicorns half her age. Meanwhile, Unicorn Two was in the early stages of diabetes, high cholesterol, and high blood pressure. Which factor was more important in this story, nature or nurture? Of course, you'll agree that nurture was the most relevant factor in this story. The lives we lead are usually much more influential than our genes. Welcome to epigenetics.

Epigenetics, SNPs, and Histones...thanks, grandma.

The unicorn twins are a great example of the power of epigenetics. While unicorns are make-believe, the message behind the story is real. You are not bound by fate or an unfair God; using your own free will, you can transcend your genetic destiny through the influence of diet, movement, environmental exposure, and proper stress processing. This became much clearer to me after reading Dr. Ben Lynch's book *Dirty Genes*. Dr. Lynch's book really helped me frame how each of us can influence our genetic expression. In our DNA, there is an important combination called an SNP. Pronounce SNP as "snip," which is short for Single Nucleotide Polymorphism. 5]

About ten million possible SNPs have been discovered in humans so far. Each of us have over a million. 4] Although there are millions of these SNPs, many don't affect us much. Some SNPs, however, are influential. Dr. Lynch states:

> *"Some SNPs, however, can make a huge difference in our health--and in our personality, as well. For example, SNPs in the MTHFR gene can create a whole host of health problems--everything from irritability and obsessiveness to birth defects and cancer....SNPs in the COMT gene can lead to workaholism, sleep issues, PMS, problems with menopause, and again cancer, along with boundless energy, enthusiasm, and good spirits."* 4]

These SNPs act above our genetic code regulators; they activate or deactivate certain genes within us. It's important to mention here that histones can also affect genes which control how tight or loose our DNA coils around itself. Genes that are loosely wound are expressed more. Histones act as a volume control knob, turning gene expression up or down. Each SNP is like a switch that turns a gene on or off. Histones and SNPs are found together in every cell in your body, giving direction to your DNA code. If you're a computer person (like my husband is), DNA is your computer programs, histones and SNPs decide which programs are active and what actions you do with those programs. By taking control of your epigenetics, you can deactivate unwanted genes, remove them from your desktop, and eventually put them in the trash. At the same time, you can activate beneficial programs instead. In this way, we're not slaves to bad genes. We can choose which genes are helpful and which aren't. How do you accomplish this intentional control of your genetics? Practice what we recommend in this book and you'll be off to a good start. SNPs are a way for our bodies to adapt quickly to changes in the environment, especially if an environment is toxic or dangerous. It's tempting to call certain genes good or bad, and when speaking within a context, I occasionally do it, too. Reality is more complicated, though. In the US, we usually view genes related to obesity as bad. But what if you found yourself in a world of supply chain problems and food shortages, aka famine?

In times of scarcity, people who can store extra fat when rare treats become available might have an advantage. In a tribal setting, a person with a SNP called GST or GTX may have been able to sense when a food was poisonous and warn the group. Today, these same people can be extra sensitive to toxic exposure. These patients might be very sensitive to smells and chemicals or get daily headaches from being exposed to certain irritants. SNPs are a valuable part of our human genome because they have positive protective attributes.

People with the MTHFR SNP are able to concentrate for long hours at a time and are great at problem-solving. These same people also have a higher rate of alcoholism, cardiovascular diseases, autism, and depression. This is all possible with these gene SNPs, but remember, it all depends on whether these SNPs are turned up or down. This ability to "change the volume" of gene expression is influenced in part by what you're exposed to through nutrition, supplementation, activity level, and your environment. Epigenetic code is not permanent; it can change over time and is influenced by what you put in your body and what you're exposed to throughout your life. Epigenetics can also be inherited from as far back as your grandparents. For example, while your mom was a baby in your grandma's body, YOU were being influenced by what your grandma ate, drank, or smoked. Do the math. Your grandma could have been one of the ladies smoking and drinking while pregnant, like on the show *Mad Men*. As a baby, your mom already had eggs in her ovaries, one of which was you! Thanks, Grandma. How do you know if your genes are expressing poorly? Great question. Here are some common complaints associated with poor genetic expression (the shortlist). 6]

- Allergies, including food & environmental
- Skin issues: acne, eczema, rosacea & psoriasis
- Mood imbalances: anxiety, depression & aggressive outbursts
- ADHD, autism & learning challenges
- Gut complaints: constipation, diarrhea, gas, bloating & acid reflux
- Problems with losing weight or keeping weight on
- Obsessive behavior & workaholism
- Alcoholism & drug abuse or a family history of
- Cardiovascular disease, or a family history of
- Insomnia
- Cold hands & feet
- Headaches & migraines
- Achy muscles & joints
- Sinus issues such as repeated infections or chronic nosebleeds

The list above covers most things I treat at Terrain Wellness. This shouldn't be surprising. Most people have poor gene expression. Most people would benefit from cleaning up the way their genes are expressed, which leads to our next question: what messes up your genes? The answer is deceptively simple but generally involves an imbalance in some or all of the following core areas.

- Nutrition
- Movement/exercise
- Circadian rhythm and sleep issues
- Environmental toxins
- Parasites
- Spiritual health, stress, emotional processing & relationships

So, what do we actually restore when we treat people with chronic health issues? You guessed it—the basics! Many people come to us after reading about genetic SNPs like MTHFR and ask for treatment. [7] And we totally get it, we'll get there, don't worry. But here's the thing: before we dive into those specific genes, we need to start with the fundamentals.

Why, Dr. Dani? I'm so glad you asked! No matter what genes you have, a few key factors need to be in place for them to function properly. Dr. Lynch refers to poorly expressed genes as "dirty." When one SNP isn't working right, it can mess with the expression of others. Instead of chasing every SNP, trying to fix them one by one like a game of whack-a-mole, we start with a solid foundation.

Once we've got your nutrition dialed in, movement and exercise on track, sleep optimized, toxins and parasites eliminated, and you've made peace with your spiritual health, THEN we can get into the deeper work. Only then can we focus on the specific SNPs that need extra support.

Genetic Testing:
The Good, The Bad & The Unhelpful

In my practice, genetic testing can be quite helpful, especially when it comes to giving people insight into their bodies and motivating them to take their health more seriously. For example, a patient might come in and say, "Heart disease runs in my family, so I need to make changes before it's too late." While this is great motivation, the real challenge is that genetic testing often doesn't provide clear instructions on what exactly needs to be done. Companies like 23andMe® or Ancestry® offer generalized health reports, but after multiple lawsuits, they now limit the amount of medical information they share with customers.

If you want the real in-depth information, you'll need to access your raw genetic data. And let me tell you, this data can look a lot like a jumbled computer error screen! When I dig into a genetic sequence, it feels a bit like peeking behind the curtain of the matrix. To make sense of it in a clinically useful way, I use programs like Strategene®, Opus 23®, or MTHFR Report®. 8], 9],10] These tools help translate that raw data into something actionable, but it's only the parts of your genetic code that can be influenced by nutrition and lifestyle changes that are clinically relevant.

When genetics are understood properly, they can offer insights into more complex risk factors. For instance, genetic testing can reveal if someone is at a higher risk of complications from surgery due to reactions to anesthesia, or how efficiently they metabolize B vitamins. This helps guide decisions on which nutrients will work best for that person. I see genetics come into play particularly when working with kids who have learning challenges like ADHD and dyslexia. Often, these kids struggle with processing B vitamins and the cofactors needed to make neurotransmitters like serotonin, dopamine, and GABA.

However, current genetic testing still has limitations. It can't tell you exactly which vitamins to take or what dosages are needed. Sometimes, reports might suggest a certain amount of a specific vitamin, but these are often vague, computer-generated recommendations that have been sanitized to avoid legal issues. Relying on these generalized suggestions could lead to spending money on a bunch of supplements that don't solve the problem.

For genetic testing to be truly helpful, you first need a solid foundation: clean nutrition, a non-toxic environment, and the elimination of factors that hinder processes like methylation (such as alcohol or certain medications). Without this, targeting specific genes can be frustrating and ineffective. For instance, a person might have one genetic SNP that requires a specific nutrient, but also have another SNP that suggests they should avoid that nutrient—so which one do you prioritize? This is why it's so important to work with doctors who know how to navigate genetics. In most cases, establishing those healthy foundations first will get your genes moving in the right direction. Once that's done, we can get a much clearer picture of what's truly needed to optimize health.

SNPs, Methylation and Genetic Influence through Nootropics

If you decide to complete your genetic profile through a company like 23andMe® or Ancestry®, there are a few important things to keep in mind. Just knowing the genes you were born with doesn't tell you how active those genes are. As Dr. Lynch says,

"Most of the folks who send away for genetic testing are unaware that a gene born clean can easily become dirty. When they read that their MTHFR is normal, they celebrate instead of realizing that due to diet and even lifestyle—it might, in fact, be super dirty. Even if your MTHFR was born dirty, you don't want to make the common mistake of thinking that you can target it with a magical methylfolate supplement and all will be well." [4]

Let's talk about methylation for a second. Methylation is the process where a methyl group (one carbon atom with three hydrogens) attaches to receptor sites in your body. This process is crucial for regulating genetic expression, producing enzymes, hormones, neurotransmitters, and converting vitamins into usable forms. Essentially, methylation acts as the on/off switch for your genes. Many of my readers are already aware that methylation plays a huge role in health; methylation disorders are linked to a range of chronic diseases. People with poor methylation often struggle with low metabolism, fatigue, diabetes, headaches, skin issues, frequent miscarriages, and muscle aches. It's also associated with mood imbalances, such as depression and anxiety. These are just a few of the many symptoms seen in patients dealing with methylation problems.

Folic Acid is NOT your friend

Okay, hear me out first. So, how does methylation start to go downhill? Here's a hint: the Western Diet and culture have had a major impact on health over the years. The typical Western Diet is calorie-rich but nutrient-deficient. In other words, we eat way too much of the wrong stuff. The Western Diet often leaves us missing key nutrients like usable B vitamins, iron, magnesium, and amino acids.

Methylation is a simple yet complex process that requires both macronutrients—protein, carbohydrates, and fats—to be available so the methylation cycles can work properly. But it doesn't stop there. Methylation also depends on micronutrients, including trace minerals such as magnesium, copper, iron, choline, selenium, and zinc, just to name a few.

The US government, in its infinite wisdom, realized this and required that food be enriched with vitamins and minerals. The Food and Drug Administration (FDA) now mandates that most grains be fortified with synthetic forms of vitamins and minerals. Yes, when your body is lacking minerals, these additives are better than nothing. But for those with methylation defects, these cheap vitamin additives can actually do more harm than good.

For example, many processed grains like bread, cereal, rice, cornmeal, pasta, and white flour is fortified with folic acid, an artificial form of Vitamin B9. Here's where things get tricky: natural Vitamin B9 isn't folic acid—it's folate. You get folate from eating vegetables like dark leafy greens (spinach, kale, collard greens, etc.), and this natural folate is far superior because it's easily converted into the bioactive form called methylfolate.

But folic acid, the synthetic version found in processed foods, is problematic. Your body loves folic acid—too much, in fact. It floods your folate receptor sites, blocking your ability to absorb and process natural folate. When your body is overloaded with folic acid, it can't easily convert it into the usable form (methylfolate). Folic acid actually slows down methylation. And when methylation gets disrupted, it causes damage at the cellular level, which leads to major breakdowns in the body.

Methylfolate, on the other hand, is immediately usable. It gets the system moving, building, and repairing. If you don't have the MTHFR SNP (genetic variation) and rarely consume artificially enriched foods, you're probably fine. But here's the catch: even people with functional MTHFR SNPs can run into trouble if they eat a diet rich in processed foods. It's not just about the genes; it's about the overall lifestyle.

Sadly, even individuals with unexpressed MTHFR SNPs can still develop methylation problems if they eat a lot of processed foods. And when that happens, methylation imbalances can lead to chronic disease. 48], 49]

How to Clean Up Your Epigenetics

Movement

Once you've eliminated processed foods containing synthetic folic acid, moving your body is the next step toward improving your methylation cycle. Yes, we're back on diet and exercise. Physical activity is the circulation of blood, lymph, and fluid in and around your cells, removing debris and waste while also bringing in additional nutrients. Movement also increases the cell's mitochondria (the cells' power plants) and fosters healthy cell turnover and repair. Methylation is needed every step of the way along this process.

Being sedentary will slow down the process of methylation and make you more susceptible to injury, slow healing, illness, and exhaustion. **Dear super-athletes: over-training over a long period of time can be harmful to methylation as well.** Over-exercising causes a spike in stress hormones and a depletion of nutrients, leading to a disruption in the body's ability to methylate. Don't get me wrong, most people who are not highly dedicated athletes are not over-training. Physical activity is good. One study directly linked exercise to improved methylation and healthier gene expression. Furthermore, the study went on to say that:

> *"The response to exercise training (trainability) has been shown to have a strong heritable component. Growing evidence suggests that traits such as*

trainability depend not only on the genetic code but also on epigenetic signals." 12]

This means that your natural ability to exercise may have been passed on through epigenetic inheritance. But it goes further. Your ability to exercise and train can be passed on to your genetic offspring. Following this thought to its end, it's important to exercise for your children's health both as an example to your family and also to improve your children's genetics. This is why it's so important for us to exercise before, after, and during pregnancy. It seems our kids will benefit from movement as well, and it will set them up for success in the future.

Rest. After we emphasize movement and fitness, we also have to cover rest and recovery. Getting proper sleep is central to health, as we discuss elsewhere. Here's one more reason: sleep is necessary for proper methylation. The conundrum exists: methylation is important for melatonin production, and melatonin and rest are also needed to have proper methylation.

Put more simply, you need enough melatonin to go to sleep and stay asleep, which requires proper methylation. Ironically, you need methylation to make melatonin, and you need melatonin to methylate. Holistically restoring methylation often includes restoring sleep and supplementing melatonin. Once we restore these cycles, we see all symptoms change for the better. Sleep is so important; get good sleep!

De-stress. Chronic stress is insidious in how it erodes personal health. Being in a high-stress state uses up methyl groups at a faster rate than can be replenished. In modern times, we think of stress as an emotional state. But medically, stress also includes physical fatigue. Stress can also be physical stress from over-exercising and from chronic infections that need to be cleared from our bodies. At times, these stress-inducing infections may be unknown and undiagnosed. When it comes to your body chemistry, any type of stress will decrease the amount of methyl donors available to run your methylation cycle. Without methyl donors, you begin to feel tired, and methylation slows.

Once we see this, it's more likely for a person to start developing chronic disease symptoms that eventually damage DNA. Damaged

DNA = premature aging, diabetes, and eventually cancer. 12] 13] When DNA lacks the ability to replicate consistently, you end up with rogue cells that do not function properly, producing even more dysfunctional cells that are not up to the task of performing normal bodily functions. The moral of the story? We need adequate methylation and time to chill.

Avoid Toxic Exposures. Exposure to toxic chemicals is another major disruptor of your body's ability to methylate. Common culprits include artificial fragrances, paint, carpet fumes, gasoline fumes, pesticides, heavy metals, mold, hormones, and antibiotics in meat. These harmful chemicals slow down methylation and make it harder for your body to detoxify. It's a classic catch-22: you need methylation to detoxify, but toxins mess with methylation, creating a vicious cycle.

Many patients come to me complaining about sensitivities to one or two specific chemicals. But from my experience, those few chemicals are usually the last straw—an already compromised methylation system has been struggling under the weight of multiple exposures. Research has shown that chemical sensitivities can slow methylation, and when testing individuals with diseases seemingly unrelated to chemical exposure, alterations in methylation patterns have been observed. A 2009 study in *Current Opinions in Pediatrics* highlights this, stating,

> *"For several exposures, it has been proved that chemicals can alter epigenetic marks and that the same or similar epigenetic alterations can be found in patients with the disease of concern or in diseased tissues"* *[14].*

The good news is that some studies also suggest that proper nutrition can help eliminate or even reverse the harmful effects of DNA-altering exposures. We dove deeper into this in our chapter on toxins.

Repeat. To keep your methylation cycle—and your body—running like a well-oiled machine, you'll need to turn these recommendations into daily habits. Once they become routine, they're just part of your lifestyle. And honestly, when you get into the groove, living in a way that supports your genetic health won't feel like a chore—it'll feel good. You'll start to love how you feel, and on the rare occasion that you fall off the wagon, those uncomfortable symptoms will pop up fast. And that's okay.

A lot of people worry about this, thinking their bodies are getting "too sensitive" to the world around them. But here's the thing: recalibrating your body is actually a great thing. It helps prevent serious diseases down the line, like cancer, heart disease, diabetes, and autoimmune conditions. The alternative? Feeling lousy becomes your new normal. You don't know why, but you walk around sluggish, tired but wired, frazzled, with trouble losing weight, dull skin, unhealthy hair, weak eyes, and low libido. People just chalk it up to "getting old."

But here's the kicker: I'm hearing these complaints from 30-year-olds! And last time I checked, 30 is not old. Meanwhile, I've got patients in their retirement years who feel vibrant, energetic, and, well—young.

This begs a much bigger question: despite having more conveniences than ever, why are we getting sicker and sicker? The answer? Some of those conveniences come with hidden costs. We're all part of nature, and we were made to live within its cycles and rhythms. But we've pushed past nature's laws in the name of ease. Of course there are going to be side effects.

Now, don't get me wrong—I love my modern conveniences, like washing machines and houses that stay warm in the winter. But I also believe we can keep the best of modern life while learning to reset from the things that don't serve us.

Case Study: Ben

Ben came to our clinic through his dad, Jack, a long-time patient who we helped with several issues. Jack's main concern, though, was Ben. His 12-year-old son was causing significant stress at home, despite Jack's own struggles with ADD, for which he was medicated. Even with the medications, Ben struggled in school and at home—unable to stay organized, focused, or motivated. Jack, a highly organized professional, didn't understand why his son couldn't complete simple tasks. Ben's issues were draining the family's time and patience.

When I started working with Ben, I listened carefully. I asked clarifying questions, not just to understand what he said, but to grasp his perspective. What I learned was eye-opening. Ben felt that "everything" in his life was hard. His brain felt "broken," and he was constantly overwhelmed by noise in his head. He feared making mistakes and falling behind his peers. His apathy was a defense mechanism, and he would avoid tasks just to buy time to give his parents answers they wanted to hear. At home, his older sister seemed to do everything effortlessly, leaving Ben feeling inadequate. His compulsive nail-biting, fidgeting, and severe digestive complaints—gas, bloating, and alternating constipation and diarrhea—were signs of deeper issues.

I ran some tests—a comprehensive stool test, heavy metal screening, and a test to measure nutrient absorption. The results were telling. Ben had serious methylation problems, as he couldn't properly absorb or process certain B vitamins, and had trouble detoxifying. He also had high levels of aluminum and mercury, which further complicated his condition. Interestingly, Ben had been put on a methylated B-complex months earlier but was still low in B vitamins. The test results were so abnormal that I recommended Jack get tested too, and sure enough, they both had almost identical patterns.

This stumped me for a bit, but it also pushed me to dive deep into research, scouring obscure studies and textbooks. In the meantime, I knew I had to start with the basics: gut health. I focused on restoring Ben's digestive system, which is crucial for brain function. We put him on an anti-inflammatory nutrition plan, removing gluten and dairy (known to negatively affect ADD/ADHD patients) and incorporating nutrient-dense vegetables like kale, broccoli, and carrots to support liver detoxification and brain health.

Ben's mom was nervous about his weight loss, worried that cutting out carbs would make him lose more weight. While I agreed that Ben was underweight, I believed the weight loss was more related to stimulant medications suppressing his appetite than diet. We agreed to monitor his weight closely and trial the new plan for 60 days.

Within a week of the new diet and supplement regimen, Ben was able to reduce his ADD medication by half. Jack, fully supportive, made sure Ben ate well and took his supplements. By the end of the 60 days, Ben had eliminated all his ADD medication. To his mom's surprise, he gained 10 pounds, his appetite was back, and he was on track for a growth spurt. With cleaner digestion, a better routine, and the right herbs and supplements, Ben thrived.

He became more open, engaged, and his grades improved. He even started noticing which foods and habits triggered his symptoms, allowing him to take control of his health. We didn't stop there—Ben also took to acupuncture, which helped calm his nervous system and reduce anxiety. Over time, anxious behaviors significantly declined, and his family reported that he was more independent, handling homework and chores with greater ease.

And all of this happened without medication. It's a reminder that there is hope for ADD/ADHD beyond stimulants. The path isn't always easy, but the rewards are worth it. When we identify and correct imbalances, kids with ADD/ADHD can truly thrive. These kids think differently, and that's something to be celebrated. When we give their bodies the right support, they're free to soar.

Conclusion

People often view genetics as either an excuse to give up on their health or as something that requires them to fight against the diseases that "run in the family." I used to think this way too, but I've learned that when we approach healthcare with a holistic mindset and build strong support, genetics become a canvas for us to work with, not a curse set in stone. Even those with the best genetics can still sabotage their health if they take their genes for granted.

Epigenetics, which refers to the influence above our genes, shows us how much control we actually have over our genetic expression. By taking ownership of what we eat and how we live, we can protect our genes from harmful factors like poor food choices, toxins, chronic stress, and a sedentary lifestyle. As biologist and author Heather Heying wisely says on her podcast, "Get outside, eat good food, be good to the ones you love." 15]

TLDR: Too Long Didn't Read

Genetics play a role in our health, but they aren't the whole story. Epigenetics shows how lifestyle and environmental factors can influence gene expression, meaning we have a lot of control over our health than DNA might suggest. The foods we eat, our activity levels, and how we manage stress can turn certain genes on or off, affecting our well-being.

We shouldn't make our genes or family history into God. Just because a condition runs in the family doesn't mean it's inevitable. While genetics may increase risk, they don't dictate our fate. The choices we make every day can have just as much—if not more—impact on our health and longevity. We're not powerless; we have the ability to shape our health through the decisions we make.

Chapter 14
Body Freedom: Living The Terrain Way

> *Order can become excessive, and that's not good, but chaos can swamp us, so we drown — and that is also not good. We need to stay on the straight and narrow path 1]*
> - Dr. J B Peterson

Throughout this book, I've been pretty critical about how the larger medical system can be way too rigid. Too much structure stifles creativity, crushes innovation, and breeds stagnation. Take the recent COVID pandemic, for example. The bureaucratic systems that make up institutional medicine failed (or refused) to adapt effectively. Instead of listening to the doctors who were successfully treating patients on the front lines, the system punished any kind of innovative thinking and demanded blind obedience. Even as the system was repeatedly proven wrong, they kept pushing the same flawed approaches.

- Ventilators were never a good idea.
- People who *took the jab* still got (and spread) COVID.
- Masks never really stopped the spread.
- The vaccines never stopped transmission.
- Forcing people to get *the shot* was always a mistake.
- Closing grade schools for a year or more did irreparable harm to our children.
- The virus was man-made in a lab.
- Many people who "took the jab" now have Long COVID.

To my knowledge, nobody in authority has ever really owned up to their mistakes or offered an apology. However, we're starting to get glimpses of the truth. Recently, CNN anchor Chris Cuomo admitted to taking Ivermectin to treat his long COVID. 2] Just a few years ago, Cuomo was publicly shaming people who used Ivermectin for COVID. The aftermath of the Pandemic has certainly painted control and order in a negative light, but, as always, life's never that simple, is it?

The lesson from COVID isn't as clear-cut as "chaos good, control bad." If we tossed out all order and followed every whim, most of us would end up cold, hungry, and miserable. There are certain standards we need, like access to clean water and ethical behavior. The same goes for medicine; a standard of care is necessary. For example, if you're bleeding and go to a hospital, you don't want doctors wasting time debating what to do. You want them to have a plan in place: stop the bleeding, stabilize heart rate and blood pressure, check for other injuries, and refer to surgery if needed. These standards exist for good reason—they help streamline care and prevent costly mistakes. Think of them like guardrails that prevent you from going over the edge.

But an overly rigid standard of care can become more like a railroad track than a guardrail. While we need structure, medicine also requires room for innovation. Complex health problems demand both a solid standard of care and creative problem-solving. This is where the system often falls short—many patients find themselves in a loop of traditional treatments that don't resolve their issues. At Terrain Wellness, we specialize in delving deeper into these complex cases, where other doctors have failed to find answers. If there were a one-size-fits-all solution, the patient would have probably found it online or in a 15-minute virtual consultation.

In general, the standard of care is in place for good reasons. But there are instances where that standard doesn't solve atypical health problems. Like many things in life, it's not always that simple.

At Terrain Wellness, our standard of care starts with a discovery process where we listen to the patient's health concerns and what they want to improve. After that, we run in-depth lab tests to measure blood chemistry, toxic exposure, and metabolism. New patients sometimes ask why we don't use their old lab results. The answer is simple: our testing is far more accurate and thorough than routine labs. More accurate labs lead to more accurate diagnoses. This allows us to customize our standard of care to meet the individual's needs.

Our approach offers flexibility in treating patients. In contrast, the hospital standard of care was designed in a culture where emergencies were the priority. Modern medicine grew out of conflicts like the World Wars, where fast, rigid procedures were necessary to save lives under pressure. 3] But sometimes, it's better to slow down and be more mindful in our approach to health so that the emergency never even happens.

At Terrain Wellness, we practice what we call "slow medicine." Our standards exist, but we take our time, using the standard more as a base recipe. We then customize our approach based on the patient's history, lab results, season of life, temperament, and symptoms. The key is to treat the patient, not just the disease. We've developed a simple yet powerful system for evaluating and restoring the body to balance—especially for those whose complex health issues have been overlooked or misdiagnosed by others.

Listen to the patient

Learn from the patient

Know The Patient

Treat the Patient

Note that listening and learning comes before knowing and treating. When we know someone, that person becomes more human to us. Understanding each patient's humanity means that we can empathize with the patient. Empathy leads to better patient outcomes. When my husband worked as a nursing assistant in a skilled facility Alzheimer and dementia unit, one of the patients would call out from her room every night at bedtime, "Whatever, whatever, whatever... Everybody needs a little love." Over a decade later, these words still ring true.

Terrain Wellness' Rules for a Healthy Doctor-Patient Relationship

Too many times, doctors can develop a habit of not believing their patients. If the doctor can't find the illness, it's often easier to assume that the patient is lying or imagining it. Think about it: it's harder for people to admit when they're wrong or need help... especially when that person is a doctor who's supposed to be the expert. We doctors are people, too, though. And sometimes, our egos get in the way of admitting when we don't have an easy solution.

At Terrain Wellness, we go the other direction by believing our patients. Undiagnosed pain is still real pain! Let's think about this for a minute. Nobody I know would make an appointment, pay for stacks of expensive blood work, take time off of work, arrange time in their personal life, drive to my office, sit with me for almost 2 hours, and then pay actual money... unless there was truly something wrong. The overwhelming evidence suggests that the patient is truly experiencing real symptoms, even if we don't know why.

Conventional medicine tries to match your symptoms to what they already know about. If your case doesn't match anything that the conventional doctor is familiar with, the common response is something like, "Sorry, I guess it's all in your head."

At Terrain Wellness, we listen carefully, trust your experience, and commit to digging deeper when others might overlook the answers. Here are statements we live by:

- The patient is telling the truth as they know it
- We must identify what the other doctors missed
- The cause is real, it just hasn't been found yet
- The cause could be multifactorial
- The whole body MUST be treated
- Treat the cause and ease the symptoms
- Look at it from a different angle

How We Work Up a Case:
Beyond conventional blood labs

Functional Lab Testing

When you get lab work done at a conventional doctor's office, they measure your results against the average for people in your area of similar age and gender. If your results fall outside that "norm," your doctor may or may not take action. Seems reasonable, right? Wrong. This approach is flawed because it assumes that a "normal" person in your area is actually healthy. But we all know that at least half the U.S. population is unhealthy. In fact, around 74% of adults in the U.S. are overweight or obese. 4] This means, for a conventional doctor to treat you based on lab results, you have to be significantly unhealthier than the already unhealthy majority.

Forgive me for being blunt, but doctors are supposed to be the best and brightest of society. How can so many intelligent doctors make such an obvious error in their standard of care?

The reality is, people who come to Terrain Wellness don't want to be "sort of average" unhealthy. Our patients want to be above average—living in robust health. That's why we don't compare you to conventional lab guidelines, which are based on the average population within a 500-mile radius of where you live.

If you want to be truly healthy, you can't compare yourself to average. The average person isn't well. With heart disease, diabetes, and metabolic conditions on the rise, using an unhealthy population as our baseline for health is a problem.

At Terrain Wellness, we focus on helping our patients achieve their best health. That means we compare your lab results to those of truly healthy individuals, aiming for ideal ranges—not unhealthy averages. By the time your numbers fall outside conventional lab ranges, you're already looking at as much as 60% dysfunction. We're in the business of preventing disease and helping people live their best lives. "Average" just isn't good enough.

Comprehensive GI Panel

Much like with our blood labs, we go above and beyond with our Gastrointestinal (GI) panels. Yes, we know you've had an Ova & Parasite test from your conventional doctor, but we're doing better than that. Standard tests are too narrow, only looking for a small handful of pathogens that most doctors expect to find. The problem is, if you only look for what you expect, you'll only find what you expect—and you won't solve complex health issues. It's basic logic, really. Doctors often miss pathogens that are considered "uncommon." But what if those pathogens are uncommon simply because no one is looking for them? This oversight leads to bad patient outcomes. Doctors who can't find the problem may either ignore it or prescribe the wrong treatment, potentially doing more harm to the patient.

At Terrain Wellness, we run these enhanced tests when it's called for. If the patient's symptoms suggest gut dysfunction, or if conventional methods haven't yielded answers, we use our advanced protocols to dig deeper. We test for a comprehensive list of yeast, parasites, bacteria, and worms. We use highly sensitive, multi-week culture testing along with DNA scans. Additionally, we measure how your body is digesting food, what's growing in your microbiome, how your liver is eliminating hormones, as well as autoimmune and inflammation markers.

From this sophisticated testing, we can give you far more targeted recommendations on how to address any pathogens found. Our comprehensive GI testing is one of our most powerful tools, and if we suspect gut dysfunction, it's often one of the first tests we recommend. Remember, it all starts in the gut.

Comprehensive Nutrition Panel

Our nutrition panel goes far beyond the standard tests you might get from your conventional doctor. We measure nutrition through urine, and there's an important reason for this. Most doctors check nutrients via blood tests, but there's a key difference between what's in your blood and what your cells are actually using to keep you healthy. By testing urine for metabolites, we can see exactly what nutrients are being properly utilized inside your cells. Many patients may have plenty of vitamins in their blood, yet still be undernourished when it comes to what their cells are actually able to use.

Unlike typical blood screenings, our enhanced nutrition panels tell us more than just whether you're getting nutrients—they show us if those nutrients are being absorbed and properly utilized by your body at the cellular level. This test allows us to identify if your body is effectively processing vitamins, minerals, fats, and amino acids. It can uncover hidden nutritional deficiencies and gut absorption issues that your old doctor might have missed.

If we find that important vitamins and minerals are low and your digestive system is struggling to absorb them, we may recommend IV nutrient therapy to ensure your body gets the necessary cofactors for repair. Without those fundamental building blocks of nutrition—delivered in a form your cells can actually use—your body won't be able to heal properly.

Advanced Hormone Testing

Hormones are another area where good people unnecessarily suffer due to poor testing. At Terrain Wellness, we begin with baseline blood screening as part of our comprehensive blood panels. This gives us a solid foundation to understand your hormone levels. But if those results don't provide the full picture, we take it further with advanced hormone panels. We use sophisticated testing protocols measuring blood, saliva, and dried urine, which gives us a much more detailed look at how your body is processing hormones. This approach helps us determine whether the issue is with your hormones themselves, or if it's tied to something else, like your liver or methylation system.

The enhanced testing allows us to see not only the levels of hormones in your body, but also how and when they're being processed. We use saliva to measure stress hormones like cortisol, as well as sex hormones such as DHEA, estrogen, progesterone, and testosterone. Both saliva and urine offer a wider snapshot of how hormones fluctuate throughout the day, something that blood tests alone cannot provide.

And it gets even more specific. We can run these tests at different times of the day or, for women, at various points in their menstrual cycle. This allows us to identify patterns and pinpoint when and how hormonal issues may arise. Many conventional doctors rely on just blood tests for hormones, but this misses out on understanding the day-to-day fluctuations in your hormone levels. Without this broader perspective, crucial aspects of care can easily be overlooked.

For our patients with complex hormonal issues like PCOS or infertility, these advanced tests, including dried urine and saliva, are invaluable. They help us understand what's truly happening in your body and how best to rebalance your hormones.

As I always say, "The more we understand what's blocking your ability to heal, the quicker you can heal." – Dr. Danielle Lockwood

Toxic Elements & Heavy Metals

Our toxic element screening is a simple test that can be performed with or without a chelating agent to help pull heavy metals from organs, bones, and tissues. The test is collected at specific time intervals to provide a clearer snapshot of your situation. This protocol is a tool for diagnosing the problem and evaluating how a patient responds to treatment.

Mold Mycotoxins

We conduct urine-based tests to screen for mold exposure and mycotoxins—something many other care teams may overlook. Our advanced protocol allows us to identify these hidden issues. Here in the Pacific Northwest where we practice, we're surrounded by stunning natural beauty and frequent rainfall, both of which contribute to water damage and mold growth. Mold mycotoxins, in high levels, can severely impair the immune system's ability to respond to other stressors.

We routinely screen new patients with undiagnosed chronic conditions for mold exposure. Symptoms like dizziness, tinnitus, asthma, chronic allergies, brain fog, headaches, and vision issues—especially when linked to living in older homes or those with a history of water damage—are strong indicators. Mold exposure can go unnoticed for years, but it's crucial to address it to avoid long-term health issues.

Harmful Chemicals

Conventional medical testing often misses the mark when it comes to toxic exposure. At Terrain Wellness, we go beyond the basics with an enhanced protocol that includes a comprehensive urine screening for toxins like parabens, plastics, VOCs, and pesticides. These widespread but harmful chemicals disrupt hormone pathways, overload the liver, weaken the immune system, and hinder the body's ability to process everyday exposures.

We live in a toxic world, but we don't have to just accept it. Our testing helps us identify what you've been exposed to, and once we have that insight, we can guide you toward healing. Knowing the toxic load on your body is the first step toward reclaiming your health

Comprehensive Neurotransmitter Panel

Have you ever wondered what your brain chemicals are actually doing? Are you under-producing dopamine or serotonin? Do you have a history of learning challenges such as ADD or dyslexia? Do you have mood imbalances such as depression and anxiety?

If you answered *yes* to any of these things, you might benefit from taking a snapshot of what your brain chemicals are doing. When we see this information, we look for patterns that we can improve upon. By changing nutrition, supplements, and lifestyle, we can use the information from our comprehensive neurotransmitter panel to improve your health and well-being. We can combine this data with information about your genetics to help us understand when a person is having issues with B vitamin processing or methylation.

Genetic testing

We can also screen for genetic SNPs (pronounced "snips") that can be influenced by nutrition, lifestyle, or supplementation. We use these tests along with software that processes genetic data into models of how nutrition, toxins, supplementation, pharmaceuticals or lifestyle choices influence those particular genetics. The models can predict how supplements, foods, and lifestyles will work with a person's physiology. Genetic testing allows us to individualize a process called nutrigenomics, which is the science of influencing genetic expression through nutrition.

If you have issues with over-methylation, we need to know which B vitamins your genetics can process effectively. Some people seem to react to everything: foods, medications, and chemicals. Genetic testing may be key to understanding how to work with these patients individually.

Food Allergy panels

Testing for food allergies can be useful if you react to certain foods, but allergy panels aren't the best way to identify food intolerances. Often, these panels show strong reactions to foods that aren't true allergies. This happens because high levels of inflammation, particularly in the gut, cause the gut lining to become swollen and leaky. When this occurs, food particles can cross the gut barrier and trigger the immune system.

What this means is that you might be reacting to a food or substance now, but with the right treatment to resolve underlying health issues, you may not be allergic to it in the future. That's why we only recommend allergy panels as a way to fine-tune your diet and lifestyle, after we've addressed and lowered inflammation.

Advanced pathogen panels

When we suspect infections like Epstein-Barr virus, herpes zoster, bacterial overgrowth, or Lyme disease, we may run additional tests. We use specialty labs for rarer pathogens to increase our chances of identifying evidence of infection. These tests often provide relief for our patients, confirming that their symptoms are real and they're "not crazy."

However, these lab results may not drastically change how I approach treatment for chronic conditions. My primary focus is on restoring the immune system through proper nutrition, healing the gut, and re-establishing healthy immune signaling. That said, I don't recommend advanced pathogen screening for every patient, as it may not always be worth the cost, depending on the situation.

A Few Treatment Modalities at Terrain Wellness

People often ask me, "What kind of medicine do you practice?" But what they're really asking is, "What tools do you use?" Since most people are familiar with conventional medicine, there's often some confusion about how and why Terrain Wellness is different. In fact, even my own father didn't realize I was a "real doctor" until he found out that I can order labs and prescribe medications.

So, to set the record straight, yes, I can and do prescribe medications when necessary. I can also order labs, and when needed, I use them to guide treatment. But for many patients, other approaches are more effective and have fewer side effects. Let's dive into some of these now.

Botanical and Herbal Medicine

One of my teachers in botanical medicine, Dr. Jill Stansbury, introduced me to what she called the innate intelligence, or spirit, of plants. I know, the idea of plant spirit and intelligence may seem far-fetched to some, especially those with a more logical mindset. But let me break down what I mean. Everything in nature is part of a larger puzzle, each piece fitting perfectly with the others. Fungi and bacteria help plants grow, those plants then provide food for animals, and animals contribute to the soil, which in turn nourishes fungi and bacteria. The cycle continues, creating a seamless connection between all living things.

Every plant, animal, fungus, and bacterium is interconnected in this giant mosaic of life. When viewed as a whole, the harmony of this system looks like intelligent design. The wildness, beauty, and genius of life on Earth bear the fingerprints of God. My job as a doctor is to understand what God was trying to teach me through the plant medicines of the earth.

Dr. Stansbury is one of the smartest people I know. She can recite every constituent and chemical involved in studies where plants were used medicinally, off the top of her head. But more importantly, she helped me learn what plants were teaching me. Years later, I now understand that God is revealing lessons about creation through these plants. In the Genesis account, God called humans to name the animals and take dominion over the earth. Naming and having dominion means more than just calling a big cat a tiger. It means understanding its nature, seeing how it fits with its environment, and recognizing how it serves a purpose in the grand design.

In medicine, ruling and subduing nature means understanding the essence of medicinal plants and using them to improve the health of suffering people. In the modern world, we often use plants to develop pharmaceutical drugs. Specific extractions are used to isolate the "active ingredient" of a plant to achieve the most potent result. Once the desired effect is identified, the active ingredient is replicated chemically and altered for mass production, sold at a high profit, and labeled as pharmaceutical grade. The other substances in the plant are considered inactive. But here's the question: is nature, where everything fits together so seamlessly, really wasting most of its effort making inactive ingredients? Is God wasting 99% of his effort on plants that seem mostly "inactive," or are we just beginning to understand the true nature of nature?

The pharmaceutical industry doesn't like herbs because they can't be sold for profit in the same way that patented drugs can. But God gave us plants as medicine, and His fingerprints are all over the world of plants, animals, and fungi. Herbs, in particular, have a wide variety of uses. Take turmeric, for example, which has been studied for its ability to treat everything from brain fog to arthritis. Herbs aren't just one-trick ponies—they've grown and adapted alongside humans for as long as humans have existed. Plant medicine is a powerful tool that we use in our clinic to help people heal from disease, balance their emotions, and become more spiritually connected.

Homeopathic Remedies

Similar to plants, we use homeopathy to treat physical and emotional imbalances. It has been my experience that homeopathy has the ability to clear inherited trauma as well as physical ailments. The homeopathic system was developed by a German medical doctor named Samuel Hannamenn in the early 1800's. Hahnemann became frustrated with the conventional medical practices at the time, which included bloodletting and arsenic in the treatment of disease. He began cataloging the use of medications at smaller and smaller doses and noticed fewer and fewer side effects. In 1810, he published the *Organon of the Healing*

Art, a book that would be written in 5 total editions before his death in 1842 at the age of 88 years old. 7] *The Organon* outlined the principles for the use of homeopathic medicine in general medical practice.

The term homeopathy is derived from the Greek language, means "similar suffering." This idea refers to the basis of homeopathy in its ability to treat using what Hahnemann called the *law of similars*. For example, if a person develops a unilateral, burning red rash that feels better with warm and worse with cold, we will give them Rhus toxicodendron, homeopathic poison ivy. The rash is very similar to the rash you would get when exposed to the poison ivy plant itself. When given at a microscopically small dose however, it has the ability to stimulate the body's ability to heal by activating the body's defense systems. One of my teachers in homeopathy, Will Taylor, MD, would describe homeopathy as a great dance. At first you are dancing with the wrong partner, the disease. Once given the correct remedy, the disease moves out of the way and the dance becomes a beautiful flowing waltz instead of a clunky toe-crushing movement. Homeopathy is a powerful tool that we incorporate into most treatment plans we create. I'm still pleasantly surprised at how quickly homeopathy can work when chosen correctly and given at the right moment.

Chinese medicine

Chinese medicine is more than just an alternative treatment; it's an entire medical system with thousands of years of practice and wisdom behind it. The principles of Chinese medicine form the foundation of how we approach healing. It's not just about treating isolated symptoms—it's about understanding the body as a whole, connecting the mind, body, and spirit. This holistic perspective is something we've embraced at Terrain Wellness because it aligns with our belief in treating the whole person.

Let's dive into some of the tools Chinese medicine uses, which have been honed over centuries. These are not standalone treatments, but rather part of a comprehensive approach tailored to your unique health needs.

Acupuncture

Acupuncture involves the use of fine, hairlike needles placed at energetic hotspots on the body. Western medicine often dismisses Chinese medicine, partly because it tends to approach healing in a more literal, mechanical way. A typical Western surgeon might argue that they've cut open a cadaver and never seen an acupuncture meridian. To that, I'd respond that meridians and energetic hotspots are useful metaphors for interacting with the body's complex nervous system. Meridians are "real" in the sense that if you apply an acupuncture needle with the right technique in the right location, it triggers a predictable physiological response.

Whether or not modern science fully understands it, there's clear evidence that acupuncture produces real effects. Now, back to the meridians. In the acupuncture system, energetic centers are mapped along channels or meridians—these pathways were identified by Chinese medicine doctors over 3,000 years ago. When applied correctly, acupuncture can alleviate pain, reduce inflammation, support digestion, improve circulation, and positively influence mental health.

We often incorporate acupuncture (or non-insertive acupuncture) into our care plans because it's a powerful tool. It can help the body heal more quickly and with fewer side effects compared to other treatment methods. Acupuncture is especially effective when physical and emotional symptoms are present. In these cases, physical symptoms can be clues that unresolved emotions are being expressed through the body's tissues. By addressing both, acupuncture helps restore balance on multiple levels.

Moxibustion

This is the controlled burning of dried Chinese mugwort plants on or near the body. We use moxibustion (moxa for short) when a person is in pain but has trouble with being massaged or in people who are very cold and nutritionally depleted. As a nice follow-on effect, the warming action of the burning plants is also calming and comforting to people who receive this treatment.

Cupping

This is where glass or plastic suction cups are placed along muscles and moved slowly to release tight, stuck pain and constriction. Cupping helps release the fascia, which is the underlying web of tissue under the muscles that influences the nervous system, immune system, and supports the movement of lymph. The suction cups can cause painless bruises that disappear in a few days, but leave the muscles feeling soft and supple afterward. Many of our patients who sit and lean over desks all day really enjoy the benefits of regular cupping sessions.

Massage

This falls under the category of Asian bodywork, and I've been trained in various techniques to help release trapped energy in the muscles and tissues. I use a combination of stretching, twisting, and kneading to loosen contracted areas and restore flow. One of the methods I use is Tuina Amna, a Japanese form of guided muscle release that translates to "push and grasp." This technique comes from the shiatsu massage tradition and the broader philosophy of Eastern bodywork. It's a hands-on approach that helps balance the body's energy and promotes healing by targeting specific muscle groups and energy pathways.

Gua Sha

This technique is called Gua Sha, and it involves using a flat jade stone to gently scrape the skin. The purpose is to help release trapped energy, known as "xue qi," which can be heat or cold stuck in the body and may slow down recovery from illness. During the process, the stone is scraped quickly and firmly over the skin until it turns a bit pink or red. Afterward, the area usually feels warm. Gua Sha helps improve blood flow, reduce pain, and support the body's healing process. It can also be used when you're starting to feel sick, as it may help bring on a mild fever, which can speed up the healing process.

Tai Shen

This is a gentle acupuncture technique that involves the use of a blunt device, usually metal, which cannot pierce the skin. This is an effective non-insertion acupuncture technique that is great for kids, those with bleeding disorders, or for people who are fearful of traditional acupuncture.

Ear Seeds or Press tacks

Are small seeds or needles affixed to a small piece of adhesive tape. These devices are placed in the ear or other parts of the body. The press tacks can be retained for hours or days to deliver continual therapy. We call these "acupuncture to-go" at our clinic.

Spinal Manipulation and Mobilization

In medical school I was taught spinal manipulation and mobilization techniques by chiropractic physicians. Spinal manipulation involves high velocity and low amplitude thrust delivered to the spine or other joints in the body using hands or an adjusting device. Mobilization uses gentle movements to guide the joints back into the correct position. When the joints are in the correct position, this helps with nervous system conduction by interrupting the pain pathway. I use spinal manipulation often because it's a powerful tool to quickly deliver a signal to the central nervous system.

Cranial Sacral Alignment

This technique involves a small, gentle touch that is applied around the head and spine. This movement helps with the flow of fluid around the central nervous system. The movements are assisted through the breath of the patient, and there is no pop or click with this type of structure support. I use cranial alignment to treat persistent whiplash, traumatic head injuries, TMJ/jaw pain, and chronic headaches.

Low Level laser Therapy, Red Light Therapy and Various Helio Therapies (light therapy)

Certain wavelengths of light have different effects on the body. These various wavelengths will help support the body's ability to heal and restore optimal mitochondrial function. Some wavelengths such as red light can also produce heat and are incorporated into sauna treatments. In the office, we use a low-level laser called a "cold laser" to stimulate the tissue of injured or painful areas to heal more rapidly. This is a pain-free way to heal damaged tissue and reduce inflammation. Cold lasers have even been shown to stimulate the healing of broken bones and chronic injuries. 9]

IV Nutrition Infusion

IV therapy is a powerful way to address nutrient deficiencies that can undermine your health. When you're nutrient-deficient, it impacts everything from hormone production to your digestive system's ability to absorb essential nutrients, creating a vicious cycle of declining health. Even if you eat well and take supplements, you may not absorb enough nutrients to break free from this cycle.

Common nutrients administered through IV therapy include glutathione, vitamin C, minerals like calcium, magnesium, and various B vitamins. For more advanced cases, we offer chelation therapy, which can be used to address heavy metal exposure—but this is only recommended in specific situations.

By delivering nutrients directly into the bloodstream, we can quickly restore healthy levels, allowing us to focus on long-term solutions, such as improving gut health and optimizing nutrient absorption. IV therapy is also a valuable tool for supporting hormone health, ensuring your body is getting what it needs to function at its best.

Ozone IV (Major Auto-Hemotherapy), Ozone insufflations, and Ultraviolet Blood Irradiation

Ozone and UV therapy serve as powerful alternatives to antibiotics, supporting your body's natural immune defenses. These modalities have been shown to help with conditions like autoimmune diseases, cancers, chronic pain, Lyme disease, chronic Epstein-Barr, mold mycotoxin illnesses, and other persistent infections. Ozone therapy also supports healthy circulation and boosts natural antioxidants like glutathione. Additionally, it has various applications for healing wounds, joints, and dental infections.

Ozone has been used since the late 1800s and remains a popular treatment in Europe, particularly in Germany. With over 11,000 research papers supporting its use, ozone therapy is well-documented.

Ultraviolet Blood Irradiation (UVBI) is another form of light therapy where a patient's blood is drawn, exposed to UV light, and then reintroduced into the body through an IV. This process amplifies the benefits of ozone treatments and is particularly helpful for chronic fatigue, difficult-to-treat infections, and other complex medical conditions.

Regenerative Injection Techniques

Regenerative injections are a great alternative to surgery, painkillers, and cortisone shots. Instead of masking the pain, these therapies help the body repair itself, naturally reducing pain. Here are some of the main types:

Joint Prolotherapy: A mixture of a numbing agent and sterile dextrose is injected into the joint to reduce pain, increase mobility, and stimulate healing in injured joints and ligaments. This treatment mimics the conditions present immediately after an injury, continuously stimulating the body's natural healing response.

Neural Prolotherapy: Similar to joint prolotherapy, but injections are placed just beneath the skin along the dermatomes (nerve points). This targets subcutaneous nerves that transmit pain signals, helping to reduce pain.

Platelet-Rich Plasma (PRP): This process involves processing the patient's own blood to concentrate blood platelets, which contain proteins that promote cell growth and injury repair. When injected into the site of injury to the soft tissues—PRP can help accelerate the healing of ligaments, tendons, muscles, and joints.

Prolozone® is a variation of prolotherapy that incorporates ozone gas. Ozonation boosts the effectiveness of the treatment by disinfecting joint tissue, improving circulation, and enhancing the healing process. Prolozone also increases oxygen utilization in the damaged area, supporting normal joint and collagen function.

These regenerative injection therapies are all designed to help your body heal naturally, reduce pain and promote long-term recovery.

Compounded and Conventional Pharmaceuticals. I know I've been really hard on pharmaceuticals, but that's because drugs are usually over-prescribed and often used to mask deeper problems. Nonetheless, I can and do prescribe when necessary. When I do prescribe, I'll often go through a compounding pharmacy so that we can be more precise in the type of medication and dosage. Compounding is useful for thyroid medications, injectable nutrients, and low-dose naltrexone, which is a powerful drug that can be used to lower inflammation associated with autoimmune disease. We work with local compounding pharmacies to formulate truly beneficial medications for our patients.

Peptides and Peptide Bioregulators. Peptides are small groups of amino acids that signal your body to repair damaged tissues, organs or hormonal systems naturally. Peptides are often injected, but some can be used orally, as nasal sprays, or used topically. We prescribe peptides through compounding pharmacies for things like accelerated weight loss, recovery from injuries, hair regrowth, and reduction of wrinkles. Peptides are used as a tool to assist an already robust nutrition and detoxification program. Peptides are not a "magic pill" or a stand-alone solution.

Functional Diagnostic Systems:
Muscle testing is part of a system called applied kinesiology. It is a powerful modality that treats the body as an electrical system. Developed by Dr. George Goodhart in the 1960's, it uses muscle testing to assess

imbalances in the body. Each muscle is connected to an organ, gland, acupuncture meridian, and even an emotion. By testing muscle strength or weakness, we can identify physical and emotional imbalances trapped in the nervous system.

Muscle testing helps us tap into the central nervous system, revealing disruptions that may be caused by nutrient deficiencies, emotional blockages, or unresolved trauma. This approach allows us to address not only physical symptoms but also the underlying emotional and energetic imbalances affecting overall health.

In our practice, applied kinesiology and other muscle testing systems complements other healing methods, enabling us to restore balance and promote both physical and emotional well-being.

Pulse diagnosis in Chinese medicine goes beyond heart rate and blood pressure. Practitioners assess over 25 qualities of the pulse, such as its depth, speed, strength, and rhythm, which reveal information about different organ systems. Each pulse quality corresponds to specific organs or energy pathways in the body, helping identify imbalances or health issues. This diagnostic tool provides valuable insights into the body's overall condition, guiding more targeted treatments.

Microsystems are small, localized areas of the body that reflect the overall health of the entire system, with each part corresponding to specific organs or functions. These areas, such as the ear, stomach, forearm, eye, and tongue, serve as a map for practitioners to identify imbalances, guiding them to targeted treatments that can help restore harmony and promote healing throughout the body.

Functional vitals and physical exams. You're probably familiar with the vital signs typically monitored at a conventional medical office—blood pressure, temperature, and maybe the occasional lymph node check. At our clinic, we do those too, but we go a bit further. We check them in both sitting and standing positions, and may even assess for zinc deficiency or the pH of your saliva. Additionally, every new patient undergoes a comprehensive NET® vital check. This involves a muscle testing-based mapping system that helps us quickly identify any imbalances in the body.

Why do we do all this?
We use all of these tools (and more) to comprehensively view what might be off in your body. We use a multifaceted approach to our lab testing to build a much more detailed picture of your health. Then, we're able to deliver much better care using some of the modalities described above. We call this individualized care plan a Roadmap because it serves to guide our care toward our patient's desired outcome. Here are the steps we use at our clinic, Terrain Wellness when we suspect a complex disease process is involved.

Test. Don't Guess. We utilize conventional and advanced functional medical lab testing as a way to look for clues that other doctors have missed. We advocate for baseline testing so that we can measure our progress as we go along the wellness journey. We compare these baseline tests to what we're seeing in the office with functional muscle testing. We like to see the body change from weak to strong.

Establish Healthy Nutritional Foundations. We teach patients how to think of food as medicine. We start with plans that are simple and that generally help reduce inflammation. We teach patients how and what to cook and the importance of food quality over quantity. We utilize health coaches and nutrition experts to customize nutrition plans to meet each individual's needs.

Replete Missing Vitamins and Nutrients. We use supplements, injectables, and IV nutrients to help pull your body "out of the hole." These are active forms of vitamins and supplements, ensuring your body can effectively absorb and use them. However, IV vitamin therapy should only be used while you're still depleted. Vitamin repletion is essential, but it's also a signal that something deeper may be going on. Chronic nutrient deficiencies often point to underlying issues like parasites, toxic exposure, environmental mold, or other disease processes. Parasites, toxins, and lingering infections can all contribute significantly to nutritional imbalances and need to be addressed as part of the healing process. These nutrients are crucial for supporting detoxification, and without them, your body cannot repair itself. The next step is stabilizing your gut health and immune system. Once these systems are balanced, we encourage you to get most of your nutrients from clean, nutrient-dense foods.

Open Drainage Organs/Emunctories. Think of this as the preparatory work you need to do before completing the demolition phase of a home renovation. Your emunctories—the organs responsible for draining and cleaning out substances that don't belong in the body—include the gut, liver, kidneys, lungs, and skin. For example, when your immune system destroys a germ, the remnants of that germ—whether bacteria, virus, fungus, or parasite—remain in your body. No healing is truly complete without properly supporting and stabilizing these drainage organs so they can efficiently remove the toxic debris.

Remove What's Not Supposed To Be There. Over time and repeated exposure to toxins, the levels of these harmful substances can be cumulative. This toxicity can be from chemicals, medications, radiation, plastics, and heavy metals. But there's more than that, mold mycotoxins, and parasites all involve toxic byproducts that can remain in the body. Whatever the source, these toxins will inhibit your immune system and prevent detoxification organs from recovering. If these harmful substances are left there too long, it can lead to more serious diseases. Cancer, autoimmune diseases, and neurological conditions can all be caused by prolonged toxic exposure.

Clear Physical Trauma and Balance Emotions. We know from earlier in this book that the body will hold onto pain and sabotage progress if trauma is not resolved. If these unresolved stressors are left unchecked, they can manifest as chronic tension, inflammation, and emotional blockages that keep the body in a constant state of stress. You must complete the stress cycle and allow the body to move from fight-or-flight to rest and digest. When this shift happens, the body can begin to repair itself, releasing stored tension and enabling healing to occur more effectively.

Rebuild Your Body

After people have been suffering with chronic illness, they become weak, tired, and run down. Once the main pathogens have been dealt with, it's time to refocus on optimizing your health. At Terrain

Wellness, we don't stop at *good enough*. Going from good to great includes the following:
- Rebuild the gut and strengthen the immune system
- Rebuild and repair cells and improve mitochondrial function
- Restore muscle strength and flexibility
- Spiritual Balance and Health Reclamation

We are here to be free, and for some, that starts with freeing their body from pain, suffering, and disease. But there's more to healing than just physical health. On the other side of illness is spiritual awakening. As it says in Isaiah 61:1, "The Spirit of the Lord God is on me, because the Lord has anointed me to bring good news to the poor. He has sent me to heal the brokenhearted, to proclaim liberty to the captives and freedom to the prisoners."

For me, God has been with me through countless difficult moments in my life. I tell my patients this: If you don't have a God, you may believe that it's all up to you to make yourself whole. At that point, you've essentially become your own God. You can't be the most important thing in your own life. Strength of will and determination may get you 80% of the way there, but to reach 100% fulfillment and healing, you need to seek the ultimate Truth and understand what He has for you.

What God had for me (thank God) was way better than anything I could have ever asked for or imagined. God freed me from decades of anxiety, and now I live with a sense of peace and freedom that I never thought possible before. I broke through old church hurt and denial of God's existence. In my 20s and 30s, I was determined to seek the truth, but I found myself chasing after false deities and New Age beliefs in an attempt to fill the void. I searched in places that promised answers but only left me feeling more lost. Eventually, the search for truth led me full circle right back to God.

If you're going through a health crisis, it's the perfect time to seek your Maker and make space for Him to show up in your life. All I had to do was ask, and there He was.

Maintain Wellness

Just in case you're wondering, here's how we at Terrain Wellness define a well person:

- Seeks deeper spiritual growth and is dedicated to serving others.
- Exhibits vibrant energy, manages stress effectively, and maintains a healthy weight.
- Enjoys a healthy sex drive, clear skin, and sustainable, real food nutrition.
- Free from vices like smoking, drugs, or excessive alcohol use.
- Maintains restful sleep, nurtures spiritual growth, and fosters strong, meaningful relationships.
- Has a healthy, well-functioning digestive system.
- Moves their body intentionally, prioritizing physical activity for strength, flexibility, and balance.

Wellness isn't "set it and forget it." Just like your car needs regular maintenance, your body does too. Don't wait for the warning signs—make your health a constant priority. Whether it's acupuncture, pressotherapy, massage, IV therapy, or health coaching, regular check-ins are essential. And don't forget your 6-12 month visits to assess blood work and functional imbalances. Now that you've read this book, if your care team isn't willing to dive deep, explore every option, and fully support your healing, then it's time to find a team that's committed to going the distance with you. Your health deserves more than a quick fix—it deserves a team that's ready to roll up their sleeves and get to work.

Is it time to *fire your doctor*?

Epilogue

"When you keep searching for ways to change your situation for the better, you stand a chance of finding them. When you stop searching, assuming they can't be found, you guarantee they won." —Angela Duckworth 11]

Your journey back to health doesn't end here—it begins again each time you challenge what you think you know. My hope is that this book reassures you: if you're experiencing health symptoms but your doctor can't find the cause, you're not crazy. There are countless ways to find your way back to wellness. Every symptom, every part of your body, is connected—despite what you've been told about them being "unrelated" or "insignificant." We know now that's not true. No system in the body acts independently. The truth has always been that our bodies are far more honest than our thoughts.

Our minds are shaped by a narrative of deficiency, scarcity, and fear. If something feels off, we often assume we're broken. I invite you to move beyond this pattern and reconnect with your core truth. This truth has been passed down through countless generations of human existence. Your body has a built-in capacity to heal and repair. If there's one key takeaway from this book, it's that your body was never meant to be treated in parts. True health requires seeing the big picture. Along the way, we've uncovered many truths, but there's one more to share: your body is far wiser than any doctor.

Yes, I'm a doctor, but as I've said before, my role is simply to guide your body back to its healing path. The body does the real work. As a physician, I can help identify the obstacles keeping you unwell, support your natural detox processes, and recommend what you need to address deficiencies. But after that, I need to step aside. The best doctors know when to get out of the way. Once the body is set on the right path, it can heal itself. Too many medications and too much intervention can actually hinder progress. Great physicians meet their patients where they are, while gently challenging the patients' self-defeating narratives. And the best doctors are teachers—leading by example and advocating for their patients.

If you find yourself stuck in an unhealthy, hierarchical relationship with your doctor, it may be time to find a new one. If your doctor doesn't remember who you are, it's probably time to move on. If they've run out of options, a second opinion is worth considering. If you've ever been told that the issue is "all in your head," you're not alone. I, along with countless patients, have been told "there's nothing wrong" or "the problem is psychological." There's more to your story than you've been told. Your body has the power to heal when given the right support. Part of why I became a doctor is because I was once a patient searching for answers. That's when I fired my doctor.

ACKNOWLEDGEMENTS

First and foremost, I acknowledge God. Jesus, you came after me even when I wanted to hide. You are my rock and my firm foundation. You sat me down every day for one hour and poured this book through me; thanks for trusting me with this medicine and your people.

Family

Next, thank you to my HUSBAND Richard. He's been a true partner to me from the day we met. Thank you for feeding me nourishing food that's made with love. You bring love, adventure, trust and stability in my life. Every day, I wake up deeply grateful for the love and friendship we share together. Thank you for always having my back, believing in me and holding me to my own benchmark of excellence. You are a gifted writer and you make my work outstanding. God truly sent you to me and I love living this life with you. Here is to more adventures with my best friend.

To my son Bennett; your light is so bright, love. Thank you for your enthusiasm and curiosity. You are one of my greatest teachers, and you bring love and depth to my life. Thanks for choosing me to be your mama, I am so glad God sent you to us. I am sorry this book is not about dinosaurs.

To my daughter Sophia Grace; you are my fierce warrior princess. You bring so much joy to our family. You are a gift from God and my life. You inspire me to be a great woman in this world.

To my mom Victoria: Thanks for learning how to love me even though I don't always make sense to you. Mama, your thoughtful gifts, support and love for my kids is more appreciated than you know. I love you Mama. Bubba, thanks for loving our crazy family.

To my aunt Donna Good - Auntie, you have always inspired me to trust my gut. You have always encouraged me to go out in the world and try things. What a gift you are to my life; you are always supportive and loving. Thank you for taking the time to know me. I love you Auntie.

ACKNOWLEDGEMENTS

To Uncle Chris and Aunt Denise: you have always been fun. I love your passion for life and continual learning.

To my dad Mike Beierschmitt: Thank you for loving me and always encouraging me to pursue education. You sat and did homework with me. By your own example, you showed me what it takes to get back up after the world has knocked you down. Thank you for "first grade lifestyle" and dinners together. I love you.

To my dad Jeff and my step-mom Debi: Thank you for showing me what hard work looks like. I love you both.

To my (wonderful) grandmothers, Jacki Smith Boardman, Kay Breceda, Patricia Freese (Nonie), my Great Grandmother Grace Conforti, and Grandma Eileen Beierschmitt- who are no-doubt watching over us now. Thank you for loving me and supporting me through the years, and inspiring me to lead.

To my (great) grandfathers who have passed on, Ross Smith, Jess Breceda (Papa), and Papa Chet, Grand-Pop B. We miss you and love you all. May God find you and keep you.

Thank you to my Smith family, my Beierschmitt family, my Breceda family, and my Lockwood family.

Theresa Lockwood: you are a lovely, creative and talented human. Thanks for your love and support over these years; you welcomed me into the Lockwood clan from day one.

Paula Lockwood: I greatly appreciate your passion for growth strategy, marketing know-how, and thank you for your love and support.

My Sisters and Brothers:

Ali: Thanks for getting to know me, the talks in the car on the way home from work, your sisterhood, and your friendship. You shine like the morning light, always know your worth. Ivan thank you for being so wonderful to my sis, do not forget how capable you are.

Nikki and my brother-in-law Elary- Thank you for loving my kids. Thank you for your love and support throughout my life.

Courtney: thank you for your love and support. You had the courage to trust me. Thank you for loving my kids.

Taylor: you have always sparkled. Please, keep shining. I love you.

Logan: you are such a hard worker.

To my brother, Brother JR: I love watching you grow to be a great man. Thank you for your support.

To my step-brother Adam: You rock, man. Never give up.

Mentors, Friends & Colleagues

I have deep gratitude to my teachers and mentors, both in medicine and in life. You have all influenced me greatly and taught me a new way of viewing the world.

Dr. Tony Mursak, Dr. Edwin Gibbs, Dr. Laysanji Edson, Dr. Steven Sandberg-Lewis and Kala Sandberg-Lewis, Dr. Paul Anderson, Dr. Rob Ciprian, Dr. Dick Thom, Dr. Jared Zeff, Dr. Deborah Francis, Dr. Sue Stoller, Dr. Pamela Jeane, Dr. Miller, Dr. Walter Schmitz, Dr Goodhart, Dr. Klinghart, Dr. Heather Zwickey, Dr. Tyna Moore, Dr. Ben Lynch, Dr. Randall Roberg, Dr. Carrie Jones, Dr. Mitch Ghent, Brandt Stickley, Ken Glawoski, Daniel Silver, Jim cleaver, Ken Glowacki, Cole Chaterrie, Dr. Son Lee Chen, Bill, Dr. Basil Ibe, Mr. Kempfer, Ms. Llapur, Mr. Paul Savaso, Ms. Yamaguchi, Dr. Pamela Wible, Tony Robbins, Ed Rush, Pastor Jack Hibbs, Pastor Vlad Savchuck, Rob and Kristen Bell, Dr. Heather Heying and Dr. Brett Weinstein.

Francey Marzicola- Thanks for always holding me to own being Dr. Dani; even when I didn't have the credentials to do it. Thank you for your unwavering support and vision for me. You are a sister, a mother and a friend all wrapped in one. Million$baby.

Dr. Abigail Ellsworth, thanks for always taking my call and knowing when I needed your sound advice. Thank you for being both a friend and inspiration.

Dr. Jade Dandy—thank you for generously sharing your wisdom and vision. Your words in the summer of 2015 gave me the courage to make the hardest—and best—decision of my life, and your presence continues to inspire me to live at my highest level.

Megan G.—your support, sharp questions, and clinical insight made this possible. I'm deeply grateful for your courage, passion, and heart for helping others. May God continue to refine and guide you.

ACKNOWLEDGEMENTS

Lindsay Zindell, thank you for years of friendship, love and laughter. Your friendship has been a staple in my life for over 20 years. Love you.

Kim Brahm: You are my sister from another mister. Thank you for being a strong voice and an awesome mirror in my life, here is to growth my friend!

To The Un-book club: Katie, Katy, Brie, Alycia, Chelsea, and Debbie A. Thanks for being the friends and fun in my life I love you all.

Noelle Hounshell: Thank you for tea, prayer, and truthful conversations. I love you, friend.

Shout out to Creature Keeper, Robin, and fam :) we all know who the real #1 is.

Dr. Sarah Dible: Thank you for being so smart and well-versed in this medicine. You're always willing to learn, laugh, and help people get better (despite themselves).

Erin Roest: Thank you for your steadiness, patience, and laughter. You keep the ship afloat. You are a powerful woman of God.

Dr. David Geller: Thank you for years of laughs and surviving med school with me. Hamilton Misses you. DRSL.

May Jackson: Thank you for being such an amazing spiritual grandmother to Rich and I. We love you and so does Jesus.

My Airway Collab buddies (especially Dr. Connie B & Jenny). Your vision to see people breathe better is spectacular.

My Mindmaster buddies - Dr Mary, Dr. Max, Dr. Judy, Dr. Donna, Annette and Dr. Katherine Minton, Dr. Bruce. Your love for kids and families, learning and thinking out of the box is how all doctors should think. I admire and appreciate you all.

To my *Church On The Rock, Lavish & Radiant* church families, thanks for being strong and courageous.

To Mary H., Carol B. & The Women's Basement Bible Warriors. Thank you for your generosity, wisdom and friendship.

To my incredible Book Review Crew—thank you for your encouragement and feedback. A special shoutout to Dani O. and Christy M.—your words and support helped bring this book to the next level.

To my patients—especially all the mamas learning to trust their instincts and fight like heaven for their kids. Your courage to pursue true wellness in a system driven by fear inspires me every day. You've walked through the fire, followed your gut, and proven that healing is possible. It's an honor to walk this path with you.

Lastly, to the heroes who are fighting for medical and religious freedom: Kathy S., Megan G, Scott M., Christina C., Chelsea N., Elizabeth P., Palmer D., Rob A, Misty R, Heidi S, Patriots United Washington, The Front-Line Critical Care Alliance, all the doctors, nurses, staff and first responders who lost their jobs standing against medical tyranny. I see you. I stand with you.

REFERENCE LIST

Citations From Chapter 1:

1. Qin Y, Roberts JD, Grimm SA, Lih FB, Deterding LJ, Li R, Chrysovergis K, Wade PA. An obesity-associated gut microbiome reprograms the intestinal epigenome and leads to altered colonic gene expression. Genome Biol. 2018 Jan 23;19(1):7.doi:10.1186/s13059-018-1389-1.PMID: https://www.nih.gov/about-nih/what-we-do/budget accessed: 6/16/21.

2. https://books.google.com/books/about/Fascism_Should_Rightly_Be_Called_Corpora.html?id=viCdzQEACAAJ accessed: 11/12/2021

3. https://www.statista.com/study/15826/health-care-and-social-assistance-in-the-us/ accessed: 12/7/23

4. https://educationdata.org/average-medical-school-debt accessed: 12/7/23

Citations From Chapter 2:

1. https://www.biblegateway.com/passage/?search=Revelation%2018&version=NIV accessed: 12/7/23

2. https://www.goodreads.com/quotes/8296220-the-line-separating-good-and-evil-passes-not-through-states accessed: 12/7/23

3. https://www.goodrx.com/drug-guide accessed: 12/7/23 Kines K, Krupczak T. Nutritional Interventions for Gastroesophageal Reflux, Irritable Bowel Syndrome, and Hypochlorhydria: A Case Report. Integr Med (Encinitas). 2016;15(4):49-53.

4. Mayer, EA. The neurobiology of stress and gastrointestinal disease. *Gut* 2000;47;861-869

5. Prescription Cholesterol-lowering Medication Use in Adults Aged 40 and Over: United States, 2003–2012 NCHS Data Brief No. 177, December 2014Qiuping Gu, M.D., Ph.D.; Ryne Paulose-Ram, Ph.D., M.A.; Vicki L. Burt, Sc.M., R.N.; and Brian K. Kit, M.D., M.P.H.

6. Functional Gastroenterology: Assessing and Addressing the Causes of Functional Gastrointestinal Disorders S Sandberg-Lewis - 2009 - NCNM Press

7. LAHNER, E., ANNIBALE, B. and DELLE FAVE, G. (2009), Systematic review: Heliocobacter pylori infection and impaired drug absorption. Alimentary Pharmacology & Therapeutics, 29: 379-386. doi:10.1111/j.1365-2036.2008.03906.x

8. Feldman M, Cryer B, McArthur KE, Huet BA, Lee E. Effects of aging and gastritis on gastric acid and pepsin secretion in humans: a prospective study. Gastroenterology 1996 Apr;110(4):1043-52. doi:10.1053/gast.1996.v110.pm8612992. PMID: 8612992.)

Citations From Chapter 3:

1. https://www.biblegateway.com/passage/?search=Matthew+12:43-45&version=NASB accessed: 02/02/24

2. https://emj.bmj.com/content/19/6/490accessed: 10/23/22

3. Buhner, SH. Herbal Antibiotics: Natural Alternatives for Treating Drug Drug-Resistant Bacteria. 2nd edition. North Adams, MA: Storey Publishing; 2012. 7-8, 25-27.

4. https://www.duffyfirm.com/blog/doctors-misdiagnose-deadly-fungal-infections accessed: 02/16/24

5. "Lack of new antibiotics threatens global efforts to contain drug-resistant infections" 17 Jan 2020. https://www.who.int/news-room/detail/17-01-2020-lack-of-new-antibiotics-threatens-global-efforts-to-contain-drug-resistant-infections. Accessed: 7/17/20.

6. Ter Kuile BH, Kraupner Graupner N, Brul S. The risk of low concentrations of antibiotics in agriculture for resistance in human health care. FEMS Microbiol Lett. 2016;363(19):fnw210. doi:10.1093/femsle/fnw210

7. Watkins RR, Bonomo RA. Overview: Global and Local Impact of Antibiotic Resistance. Infect Dis Clin North Am. 2016;30(2):313-322. doi:10.1016/j.idc.2016.02.001

8. Venter H, Henningsen ML, Begg SL. Antimicrobial resistance in healthcare, agriculture, and the environment: the biochemistry behind the headlines. *Essays Biochem*. 2017;61(1):1-10. Published 2017 Mar 3. doi:10.1042/EBC20160053

9. Aiello AE, Larson EL, Levy SB. Consumer antibacterial soaps: effective or just risky? *Clin Infect Dis*. 2007;45 Suppl 2:S137-S147. Doi:10.1086/519255

10. Allmyr M, Adolfsson-Erici M, McLachlan MS, Sandborgh-Englund G. Triclosan in plasma and milk from Swedish nursing mothers and their exposure via personal care products. Sci Total Environ. 2006;372(1):87-93. doi:10.1016/j.scitotenv.2006.08.007

11. Luby SP, Agboatwalla M, Feikin DR, et al. Effect of handwashing on child health: a randomised controlled trial. Lancet. 2005;366(9481):225-233. doi:10.1016/S0140-6736(05)66912-7

12. https://www.fda.gov/consumers/consumer-updates/antibacterial-soap-you-can-skip-it-use-plain-soap-and-water. Accessed 07/16/2020.

13. Petrelli F, Ghidini M, Ghidini A, et al. Use of Antibiotics and Risk of Cancer: A Systematic Review and Meta-Analysis of Observational Studies. Cancers (Basel). 2019;11(8):1174. Published 2019 Aug 14. doi:10.3390/cancers11081174

14. Rizzatti G, Ianiro G, Gasbarrini A. Antibiotic and Modulation of Microbiota: A New Paradigm?. J Clin Gastroenterol. 2018;52 Suppl 1, Proceedings from the 9th Probiotics, Prebiotics and New Foods, Nutraceuticals and Botanicals for Nutrition & Human and Microbiota Health Meeting, held in Rome, Italy from September 10 to 12, 2017:S74-S77. doi:10.1097/MCG.0000000000001069

15. Kostic AD, Gevers D, Pedamallu CS, et al. Genomic analysis identifies association of Fusobacterium with colorectal carcinoma. Genome Res. 2012;22(2):292-298. doi:10.1101/gr.126573.111

16. Mikkelsen KH, Knop FK, Frost M, Hallas J, Pottegård A. Use of Antibiotics and Risk of Type 2 Diabetes: A Population-Based Case-Control Study. J Clin Endocrinol Metab. 2015;100(10):3633-3640. doi:10.1210/jc.2015-2696

17. Zhu L, She ZG, Cheng X, et al. Association of Blood Glucose Control and Outcomes in Patients with COVID-19 and Pre-existing Type 2 Diabetes. Cell Metab. 2020;31(6):1068-1077.e3. doi:10.1016/j.cmet.2020.04.021

18. Cox LM, Blaser MJ. Antibiotics in early life and obesity. Nat RevEndocrinol.2015;11(3):182-190. doi:10.1038/nrendo.2014.210

19. Seganfredo FB, Blume CA, Moehlecke M, et al. Weight-loss interventions and gut microbiota changes in overweight and obese patients: a systematic review. Obes Rev. 2017;18(8):832-851. doi:10.1111/obr.12541

20. Yang JH, Bhargava P, McCloskey D, Mao N, Palsson BO, Collins JJ. Antibiotic-Induced Changes to the Host Metabolic Environment Inhibit Drug Efficacy and Alter Immune Function. Cell Host Microbe. 2017;22(6):757-765.e3. doi:10.1016/j.chom.2017.10.020

21. Yang JH, Bening SC, Collins JJ. Antibiotic efficacy-context matters. Curr Opin Microbiol. 2017;39:73-80. doi:10.1016/j.mib.2017.09.002

22. Zuccotti G, Meneghin F, Aceti A, et al. Probiotics for prevention of atopic diseases in infants: systematic review and meta-analysis. Allergy. 2015;70(11):1356-1371. doi:10.1111/all.12700

23. Lee YB, Byun EJ, Kim HS. Potential Role of the Microbiome in Acne: A Comprehensive Review. J Clin Med. 2019;8(7):987. Published 2019 Jul 7. doi:10.3390/jcm8070987

Citations From Chapter 4:

1. https://my.clevelandclinic.org/health/diseases/22700-cytokine-release-syndrome accessed: 09/04/2023

2. https://covid19criticalcare.com/wp-content/uploads/2022/08/MATH-Summary.pdf accessed: 02/29/2024

3. https://www.covid19treatmentguidelines.nih.gov/therapies/antivirals-including-antibody-products/remdesivir/ accessed: 07/21/2023

4. https://pubmed.ncbi.nlm.nih.gov/33340409/ accessed: 04/12/2023

5. https://www.whitehouse.gov/briefing-room/speeches-remarks/2021/12/16/remarks-by-president-biden-after-meeting-with-members-of-the-covid-19-response-team/ accessed: 02/29/2024

6. https://www.healthline.com/nutrition/6-foods-that-cause-inflammation#2.-Fried-foods accessed: 03/13/2023

7. https://www.ncbi.nlm.nih.gov/pubmed/7821339 accessed: 01/21/2023

8. https://archive.niams.nih.gov/newsroom/spotlight-on-research/long-term-benefit-steroid-injections-knee-osteoarthritis-challenged accessed: 12/21/2022

9. https://www.mayoclinic.org/tests-procedures/cortisone-shots/about/pac-20384794 accessed: 12/21/2022

10. https://archive.niams.nih.gov/newsroom/spotlight-on-research/long-term-benefit-steroid-injections-knee-osteoarthritis-challenged accessed: 10/17/2022

11. https://pubmed.ncbi.nlm.nih.gov/29304236/ accessed: 08/27/2022

12. https://www.ncbi.nlm.nih.gov/pmc/articles/PMC7958106/ accessed: 08/25/2022

13. https://www.cdc.gov/fungal/infections/immune-system.html- steroids and increase the chance of fungal infections accessed: 01/21/2021

14. Ali T, Kaitha S, Mahmood S, Ftesi A, Stone J, Bronze MS. Clinical use of anti-TNF therapy and increased risk of infections. Drug Healthc Patient Saf. 2013;5:79-99. doi:10.2147/DHPS.S28801

15. Stuck AE, Minder CE, Frey FJ. Risk of infectious complications in patients taking

glucocorticosteroids. Rev Infect Dis. 1989;11(6):954-963. doi:10.1093/clinids/11.6.954

16. Chen GL, Chen Y, Zhu CQ, Yang CD, Ye S. Invasive fungal infection in Chinese patients with systemic lupus erythematosus. Clin Rheumatol. 2012;31(7):1087-1091. doi:10.1007/s10067-012-1980-x

17. Cooper GS, Stroehla BC. The epidemiology of autoimmune diseases. Autoimmun Rev. 2003;2(3):119-125. doi:10.1016/s1568-9972(03)00006-5-more studies are needed

18. Roberts MH, Erdei E. Comparative United States autoimmune disease rates for 2010-2016 by sex, geographic region, and race. Autoimmun Rev. 2020;19(1):102423. doi:10.1016/j.autrev.2019.102423

19. Dinse GE, Parks CG, Weinberg CR, et al. Increasing Prevalence of Antinuclear Antibodies in the United States. Arthritis Rheumatol. 2020;72(6):1026-1035. doi:10.1002/art.41214

20. Bonafede M, Joseph GJ, Shah N, Princic N, Harrison DJ. Cost of tumor necrosis factor blockers per patient with rheumatoid arthritis in a multi state Medicaid population. Clinicoecon Outcomes Res. 2014;6:381-388. Published 2014 Sep 15. doi:10.2147/CEOR.S61445

21. Schmier J, Ogden K, Nickman N, et al. Costs of Providing Infusion Therapy for Rheumatoid Arthritis in a Hospital-based Infusion Center Setting. Clin Ther. 2017;39(8):1600-1617. doi:10.1016/j.clinthera.2017.06.007

22. Brinkhaus B, Roll S, Jena S, et al. Acupuncture in Patients with Allergic Asthma: A Randomized Pragmatic Trial. J Altern Complement Med. 2017;23(4):268-277. doi:10.1089/acm.2016.0357

23. Zhao SM, Wang HS, Zhang C, et al. Repeated Herbal Acupoint Sticking Relieved the Recurrence of Allergic Asthma by Regulating the Th1/Th2 Cell Balance in the Peripheral Blood. Biomed Res Int. 2020;2020:1879640. Published 2020 May 17. doi:10.1155/2020/1879640

24. Ohlsen BA. Acupuncture and a gluten-free diet relieve urticaria and eczema in a case of undiagnosed dermatitis herpetiformis and atypical or extraintestinal celiac disease: a case report. J Chiropr Med. 2011;10(4):294-300. doi:10.1016/j.jcm.2011.06.003

Citations From Chapter 5:

1. https://www.ncbi.nlm.nih.gov/pmc/articles/PMC6085824/ accessed: March 28th, 2024

2. https://www.nature.com/articles/nature.2016.19136 accessed: March 28th, 20244

3. https://www.ncbi.nlm.nih.gov/pmc/articles/PMC8452999/ accessed: March 28th, 2024

4. NIH Human Microbiome Project defines the normal bacterial makeup of the body. June 12, 2013. https://www.nih.gov/news-events/news-releases/nih-human-microbiome-project-defines-normal-bacterial-makeup-body accessed January 7, 2021

5. Nichols RG, Davenport ER. The relationship between the gut microbiome and host gene expression: a review [published online ahead of print, 2020 Nov 22]. Hum Genet. 2020;1-14. doi:10.1007/s00439-020-02237-0

6. Qin Y, Roberts JD, Grimm SA, Lih FB, Deterding LJ, Li R, Chrysovergis K, Wade PA. An obesity-associated gut microbiome reprograms the intestinal epigenome, leading to altered colonic

gene expression. Genome Biol. 2018 Jan 23;19(1):7. doi: 10.1186/s13059-018-1389-1. PMID:

7. https://advancedequinedentistry.com.au/articles/periodontal-disease accessed: March 28th, 2024

8. https://www.ncbi.nlm.nih.gov/pmc/articles/PMC9678577/ accessed: March 28th, 2024

9. Ohki T, Itabashi Y, Kohno T, Yoshisawa A, Nishikubo S, Watanabe S, et al. Detection of periodontal bacteria in thrombi of patients with acute myocardial infarction by polymerase chain reaction. Am Heart J 2012; 163: 164–167.

10. Olsen I, Yilmaz Ö. Possible role of Porphyromonas gingivalis in orodigestive cancers. J Oral Microbiol. 2019;11(1):1563410. Published 2019 Jan 9. doi:10.1080/20002297.2018.1563410

11. Olsen I, Yamazaki K. Can oral bacteria affect the gut microbiome? J Oral Microbiol. 2019;11(1):1586422. Published 2019 Mar 18. doi:10.1080/20002297.2019.1586422

12. Baker JM, Al-Nakkash L, Herbst-Kralovetz MM. Estrogen-gut microbiome axis: Physiological and clinical implications. Maturitas. 2017 Sep;103:45-53. doi: 10.1016/j.maturitas.2017.06.025. Epub 2017 Jun 23. PMID: 28778332.

13. https://healthmatters.io/understand-blood-test-results/beta-glucuronidase accessed: March 28th, 2024

14. Gershon, M. D. (1998). The second brain: The scientific basis of gut instinct and a groundbreaking new understanding of the stomach and intestine nervous disorders. New York, NY: HarperCollinsPublishers.

15. Strandwitz P. Neurotransmitter modulation by the gut microbiota. Brain Res. 2018;1693(Pt B):128-133. doi:10.1016/j.brainres.2018.03.015

16. Fadgyas-Stanculete, M., Buga, AM., Popa-Wagner, A. et al. The relationship between irritable bowel syndrome and psychiatric disorders: from molecular changes to clinical manifestations. J Mol Psychiatr 2, 4 (2014). https://doi.org/10.1186/2049-9256-2-4

17. Pennsi, E. May, 7 2020. Science Magazine Online "Meet the 'psycho-biome': the gut bacteria that may alter how you think, feel, and act" Accessed: February 12, 2021.

18. https://www.drugs.com/ritalin.html accessed: March 28th, 2024

19. https://www.drugs.com/adderall.html accessed: March 28th, 2024

20. Xavier JB, Young VB, Skufca J, Ginty F, Testerman T, Pearson AT, Macklin P, Mitchell A, Shmulevich I, Xie L, Caporaso JG, Crandall KA, Simone NL, Godoy-Vitorino F, Griffin TJ, Whiteson KL, Gustafson HH, Slade DJ, Schmidt TM, Walther-Antonio MRS, Korem T, Webb-Robertson BM, Styczynski MP, Johnson WE, Jobin C, Ridlon JM, Koh AY, Yu M, Kelly L, Wargo JA. The Cancer Microbiome: Distinguishing Direct and Indirect Effects Requires a Systemic View. Trends Cancer. 2020 Mar;6(3):192-204. doi: 10.1016/j.trecan.2020.01.004. Epub 2020 Feb 7. PMID: 32101723; PMCID: PMC7098063.

21. Wang Z, Klipfell E, Bennett BJ, Koeth R, Levison BS, Dugar B, Feldstein AE, Britt EB, Fu X, Chung YM, Wu Y, Schauer P, Smith JD, Allayee H, Tang WH, DiDonato JA, Lusis AJ, Hazen SL. Gut flora metabolism of phosphatidylcholine promotes

cardiovascular disease. Nature. 2011 Apr 7;472(7341):57-63. doi: 10.1038/nature09922. PMID: 21475195; PMCID: PMC3086762.

22. Velicer CM, Heckbert SR, Lampe JW, Potter JD, Robertson CA, Taplin SH. Antibiotic Use in Relation to the Risk of Breast Cancer. *JAMA*. 2004;291(7):827–835. doi:10.1001/jama.291.7.827

23. Picardo SL, Coburn B, Hansen AR. The microbiome and cancer for clinicians. *Crit Rev Oncol cvfc Hematol*. 2019;141:1-12. doi:10.1016/j.critrevonc.2019.06.004

24. Manzoor SS, Doedens A, Burns MB. The promise and challenge of cancer microbiome research. Genome Biol. 2020 Jun 2;21(1):131. doi: 10.1186/s13059-020-02037-9. PMID: 32487228; PMCID: PMC7265652.

Citations From Chapter 6:

1. HG Wells, *The War of The Worlds*, 1st published in The United States of America in Cosmopolitan Magazine in 1897

2. https://www.britannica.com/science/germ-theory accessed 04/29/2024

3. https://www.newscientist.com/article/2254471-the-microbiome-how-gut-bacteria-regulate-our-health/ accessed 04/29/2024

4. https://www.ncbi.nlm.nih.gov/pmc/articles/PMC10 022328/ accessed 04/29/2024

5. https://www.theatlantic.com/health/archive/2022/02 /covid-mask-mandate-washington-dc/622860/ accessed 04/30/2024

6. Translocation of a gut pathobiont drives autoimmunity in mice and humans. Manfredo Vieira S, Hiltensperger M, Kumar V, Zegarra-Ruiz

D, Dehner C, Khan N, Costa FRC, Tiniakou E, Greiling T, Ruff W, Barbieri A, Kriegel C, Mehta SS, Knight JR, Jain D, Goodman AL, Kriegel MA. Science. 2018 Mar 9;359(6380):1156-1161. doi: 10.1126/science.aar7201. PMID: 29590047.

7. Balakrishnan B, Taneja V. Microbial modulation of the gut microbiome for treating autoimmune diseases. Expert Rev Gastroenterol Hepatol. 2018;12(10):985-996. doi:10.1080/17474124.2018.1517044

8. Chandrashekara S. The treatment strategies of autoimmune disease may need a different approach from conventional protocol: a review. Indian J Pharmacol. 2012;44(6):665-671. doi:10.4103/0253-7613.103235

9. Kaminitz A, Mizrahi K, Yaniv I, Stein J, Askenasy N. Immunosuppressive therapy exacerbates autoimmunity in NOD mice and diminishes the protective activity of regulatory T cells. J Autoimmun. 2010 Sep;35(2):145-52. doi: 10.1016/j.jaut.2010.06.002. Epub 2010 Jul 16. PMID: 20638242.

10. Andrew W. Campbell, "Autoimmunity and the Gut", Autoimmune Diseases, vol. 2014, Article ID 152428, 12 pages, 2014. https://doi.org/10.1155/2014/152428

11. Schnorr, S., Candela, M., Rampelli, S. et al. Gut microbiome of the Hadza hunter-gatherers. Nat Commun 5, 3654 (2014). https://doi.org/10.1038/ncomms4654

12. Brett Weinstein, Heather Heying, *A Hunter-Gatherer's Guide to The 21st Century* | Diamond Creek Press, September, 2021

13. McFarlin BK, Henning AL, Bowman EM, Gary MA, Carbajal KM. Oral spore-based probiotic

supplementation was associated with reduced incidence of post-prandial dietary endotoxin, triglycerides, and disease risk biomarkers. World J Gastrointest Pathophysiol. 2017;8(3):117-126. doi:10.4291/wjgp.v8.i3.117

14. Jen-Min Huang, Roberto M. La Ragione, Alejandro Nunez, Simon M. Cutting, Immunostimulatory activity of Bacillus spores, FEMS Immunology & Medical Microbiology, Volume 53, Issue 2, July 2008, Pages 195–203, https://doi.org/10.1111/j.1574-695X.2008.00415.x

15. https://www.attachedthebook.com/wordpress/ accessed 04/30/2024

16. https://www.ncbi.nlm.nih.gov/pmc/articles/PMC4707391/ accessed 11/22/2024

17. Holy Bible | Philippians 3:19 New International Version

18. Holy Bible | Matthew 5:30 New International Version

19. Andrew W. Campbell, "Autoimmunity and the Gut", Autoimmune Diseases, vol. 2014, Article ID 152428, 12 pages, 2014. https://doi.org/10.1155/2014/152428

20. Ghaemi-Oskouie F, Shi Y. The role of uric acid as an endogenous danger signal in immunity and inflammation. Curr Rheumatol Rep. 2011;13(2):160-166. doi:10.1007/s11926-011-0162-1

21. Hasikova, L., Pavlikova, M., Hulejova, H. et al. Serum uric acid increases in patients with systemic autoimmune rheumatic diseases after 3 months of treatment with TNF inhibitors. Rheumatol Int 39, 1749–1757 (2019). https://doi.org/10.1007/s00296-019-04394-6

22. Liu Y, Alookaran JJ, Rhoads JM. Probiotics in Autoimmune and Inflammatory Disorders. Nutrients. 2018; 10(10):1537. https://doi.org/10.3390/nu10101537

Lin, L., Zhang, J. Role of intestinal microbiota and metabolites on gut homeostasis and human diseases. BMC Immunol 18, 2 (2017). https://doi.org/10.1186/s12865-016-0187-3

Citations From Chapter 7:

1. https://www.cdc.gov/obesity/data/obesity-and-covid-19.html accessed 05/24/2023

2. https://www.aclu.org/issues/national-security/privacy-and-surveillance/surveillance-under-patriot-act accessed 05/28/2024

3. https://www.nbcnews.com/news/nbcblk/joe-biden-didn-t-just-compromise-segregationists-he-fought-their-n1021626 accessed 05/28/2024

4. https://www.healthline.com/health/obesity-facts accessed 05/12/2022

5. https://www.nhlbi.nih.gov/health/metabolic-syndrome accessed 03/05/2023

6. https://www.cdc.gov/bloodpressure/facts.htm accessed 01/15/2023

7. Yeoh YK, Zuo T, Lui GC, et al Gut microbiota composition reflects disease severity and dysfunctional immune responses in patients with COVID-19 Gut Published Online First: 11 January 2021. doi: 10.1136/gutjnl-2020-323020

8. Behan PO, Behan WM. Postviral fatigue syndrome. Crit Rev Neurobiol. 1988;4(2):157-78. PMID: 3063394

9. https://pubmed.ncbi.nlm.nih.gov/30283076/ accessed 11/19/2022

10. Arnold, C. The Non-human Living inside of you Natulus Cold Spring Harbor Laboratory: 2020 Jan 9. https://www.cshl.edu/the-non-human-living-inside-of-you/ Accessed: 22 Feb 2021.

11. Younsuck Koh, Chae-Man Lim, CHAPTER 6 - Role of Changes in Body Temperature in Acute Lung Injury, Editor(s): PETER J. PAPADAKOS, BURKHARD LACHMANN, Laraine Visser-Isles, Mechanical Ventilation, W.B. Saunders, 2008, Pages 51-60, ISBN 9780721601861, https://doi.org/10.1016/B978-0-7216-0186-1.50010-7

12. https://www.ncbi.nlm.nih.gov/pmc/articles/PMC6092479/

13. Shoenfeld Y, Aron-Maor A. Vaccination and autoimmunity-'vaccinosis': a dangerous liaison? J Autoimmun. 2000 Feb;14(1):1-10. doi: 10.1006/jaut.1999.0346. PMID: 10648110

14. D'alò GL, Zorzoli E, Capanna A, et al. Frequently asked questions on seven rare adverse events following immunization. J Prev Med Hyg. 2017;58(1):E13-E26

15. Drago L. Prevotella Copri and Microbiota in Rheumatoid Arthritis: Fully Convincing Evidence?. J Clin Med. 2019;8(11):1837. Published 2019 Nov 1. doi:10.3390/jcm8111837

16. https://www.ncbi.nlm.nih.gov/pmc/articles/PMC3110651/ accessed 05/28/2024

17. van den Elsen LWJ, Garssen J, Burcelin R, Verhasselt V. Shaping the Gut Microbiota by Breastfeeding: The Gateway to Allergy

Prevention?. Front Pediatr. 2019;7:47. Published 2019 Feb 27. doi:10.3389/fped.2019.00047

18. Hesselmar B, Hicke-Roberts A, Lundell AC, et al. Pet-keeping in early life reduces the risk of allergy in a dose-dependent fashion. PLoS One. 2018;13(12):e0208472. Published 2018 Dec 19. doi:10.1371/journal.pone.0208472

19. Chen CC, Chen YN, Liou JM, Wu MS; Taiwan Gastrointestinal Disease and Helicobacter Consortium. From germ theory to germ therapy. Kaohsiung J Med Sci. 2019;35(2):73-82. doi:10.1002/kjm2.12011

20. Langdon, A., Crook, N., & Dantas, G. (2016). The effects of antibiotics on the microbiome throughout development and alternative approaches for therapeutic modulation. Genome medicine, 8(1), 39. https://doi.org/10.1186/s13073-016-0294-z

21. https://phys.org/news/2018-08-giant-monsanto-controversial-chemicals.html accessed 05/28/2024

22. Chappell, Bill (June 24, 2020). "Bayer To Pay More Than $10 Billion To Resolve Cancer Lawsuits Over Weedkiller Roundup". NPR. https://www.npr.org/2020/06/24/882949098/bayer-to-pay-more-than-10-billion-to-resolve-roundup-cancer-lawsuits Retrieved February 5,2021

23. Mills S, Stanton C, Lane JA, Smith GJ, Ross RP. Precision Nutrition and the Microbiome, Part I: Current State of the Science. Nutrients. 2019;11(4):923. Published 2019 Apr 24. doi:10.3390/nu11040923

24. https://www.health.harvard.edu/blog/stool-transplants-are-now-standard-of-care-for-recurrent-c-difficile-infections-2019050916576 accessed 09/20/2023

25. David LA, Maurice CF, Carmody RN, Gootenberg DB, Button JE, Wolfe BE, Ling AV, Devlin AS, Varma Y, Fischbach MA, Biddinger SB, Dutton RJ, Turnbaugh PJ. Diet rapidly and reproducibly alters the human gut microbiome. Nature. 2014 Jan 23;505(7484):559-63

26. Samsel A, Seneff S. Glyphosate, pathways to modern diseases II: Celiac sprue and gluten intolerance. *Interdiscip Toxicol*. 2013;6(4):159-184. doi:10.2478/intox-2013-0026334

27. Kresser, C. (March 9, 2018). "Clinical Utility of Zonulin Testing." https://kresserinstitute.com/clinical-utility-zonulin-testing/ accessed 02/05/2021

28. Fasano A. Zonulin, regulation of tight junctions, and autoimmune diseases. *Ann N Y Acad Sci*. 2012;1258(1):25-33. doi:10.1111/j.1749-6632.2012.06538.x

Timeless Principles of Healthy Traditional Diets. Weston A Price foundation. Published 2000 Jan 1. https://www.westonaprice.org/health-topics/abcs-of-nutrition/principles-of-healthy-diets-2/ Accessed 02/22/2021

Citations From Chapter 8:

1. Lucia Alonso-Pedrero, Ana Ojeda-Rodríguez, Miguel A Martínez-González, Guillermo Zalba, Maira Bes-Rastrollo, Amelia Marti, Ultra-processed food consumption and the risk of short telomeres in an elderly population of the Seguimiento Universidad de Navarra (SUN) Project, The American Journal of Clinical Nutrition, Volume 111, Issue 6, June 2020, Pages 1259–1266, https://doi.org/10.1093/ajcn/nqaa075

2. Hood M. 'Ultra-Processed' Junk Food Linked to Advanced Ageing at Cellular Level, Study Finds 1 September 2020. https://www.sciencealert.com/study-links-ultra-processed-junk-food-to-age-marker-in-chromosomes

3. https://www.ncbi.nlm.nih.gov/pmc/articles/PMC8921009/ Accessed: 06/21/2024

4. https://www.cancer.gov/about-cancer/causes-prevention/risk/diet/acrylamide-fact-sheet Accessed: 04/18/2023

5. https://time.com/5459319/americans-sit-too-much/ Accessed: 6/5/2020.

6. Aladdin H. Shadyab, Caroline A. Macera, Richard A. Shaffer, Sonia Jain, Linda C. Gallo, Michael J. LaMonte, Alexander P. Reiner, Charles Kooperberg, Cara L. Carty, Chongzhi Di, Todd M. Manini, Lifang Hou, Andrea Z. LaCroix, Associations of Accelerometer-Measured and Self-Reported Sedentary Time With Leukocyte Telomere Length in Older Women, American Journal of Epidemiology, Volume 185, Issue 3, 1 February 2017, Pages 172–184, https://doi.org/10.1093/aje/kww196

7. Shorten, Kristin. "Our Grandparents Hold the Secret to Being Skinny." New York Post Online. Oct. 24 2013. https://nypost.com/2013/10/24/our-grandparents-hold-the-secret-to-being-skinny/ accessed. June 5, 2020.

8. https://www.ncbi.nlm.nih.gov/pmc/articles/PMC7014832/ Accessed: 11/12/2021

9. https://www.bmj.com/content/378/bmj-2022-071204 Accessed: 08/02/2021

10. https://foodactive.org.uk/overfed-but-undernourished-the-obesity-paradox-2/ Accessed: 06/21/2024

11. https://pubmed.ncbi.nlm.nih.gov/26745150/ Accessed: 06/21/2024

12. Prescription Cholesterol-lowering Medication Use in Adults Aged 40 and Over: United States, 2003–2012 NCHS Data Brief No. 177, December 2014Qiuping Gu, M.D., Ph.D.; Ryne Paulose-Ram, Ph.D., M.A.; Vicki L. Burt, Sc.M., R.N.; and Brian K. Kit, M.D., M.P.H.

13. https://www.singlecare.com/prescription/lipitor Accessed: 03/25/2021

14. https://doctoraseem.com/the-great-statins-divide/ Accessed: 06/17/2024

15. https://bmjopen.bmj.com/content/5/9/e007118 Accessed: 12/19/2022

16. Obesity alters gut microbial ecology Ruth E. Ley, Fredrik Bäckhed, Peter Turnbaugh, Catherine A. Lozupone, Robin D. Knight, Jeffrey I. GordonProceedings of the National Academy of Sciences Aug 2005, 102 (31) 11070-11075; DOI:10.1073/pnas.0504978102

17. Boulangé, C.L., Neves, A.L., Chilloux, J. et al. Impact of the gut microbiota on inflammation, obesity, and metabolic disease. Genome Med 8, 42 (2016). https://doi.org/10.1186/s13073-016-0303-2

18. Park B, Kim J. Oral Contraceptive Use, Micronutrient Deficiency, and Obesity among Premenopausal Females in Korea: The Necessity of Dietary Supplements and Food Intake Improvement. PLoS One. 2016;11(6):e0158177. Published 2016 Jun 27. doi:10.1371/journal.pone.0158177

19. Seganfredo FB, Blume CA, Moehlecke M, et al. Weight-loss interventions and gut microbiota changes in overweight and obese patients: a systematic review. Obes Rev. 2017;18(8):832-851. doi:10.1111/obr.12541

20. Festi D, Schiumerini R, Eusebi LH, Marasco G, Taddia M, Colecchia A. Gut microbiota and metabolic syndrome. World J Gastroenterol. 2014;20(43):16079-16094. doi:10.3748/wjg.v20.i43.16079

Citations From Chapter 9:

1. Impaired Sensitivity to Thyroid Hormones Is Associated With Diabetes and Metabolic Syndrome Martin Laclaustra, Belen Moreno-Franco, Jose Manuel Lou-Bonafonte, RocioMateo-Gallego, Jose Antonio Casasnovas, Pilar Guallar-Castillon, Ana Cenarro, Fernando Civeira Diabetes Care Feb 2019, 42 (2) 303-310; DOI: 10.2337/dc18-141
2. Hypothyroidism | https://www.niddk.nih.gov/health-information/endocrine-diseases/hypothyroidism Accessed: 06/27/2024
3. Hyperthyroidism | https://www.mayoclinic.org/diseases-conditions/hyperthyroidism/symptoms-causes/syc-20373659 Accessed: 06/27/2024
4. HPA Axis | https://www.ncbi.nlm.nih.gov/pmc/articles/PMC6057754/ Accessed: 06/27/2024
5. Addison's Disease | https://www.mayoclinic.org/diseases-conditions/addisons-disease/symptoms-causes/syc-20350293 Accessed: 06/27/2024
6. Cushing's Syndrome | https://www.niddk.nih.gov/health-information/endocrine-diseases/cushings-syndrome Accessed: 06/27/2024

7. Cortisol and Insulin Resistance | https://pubmed.ncbi.nlm.nih.gov/6348064/ Accessed: 06/27/2024
8. Insulin and Thyroid | https://pubmed.ncbi.nlm.nih.gov/24549605/ Accessed: 06/27/2024
9. SIBO | https://www.ncbi.nlm.nih.gov/pmc/articles/PMC3099351/ Accessed: 06/27/2024

Citations From Chapter 10:

1. Tolkien, J. R. R. 1991. *The Fellowship of the Ring*. The Lord of the Rings 1. London, England: HarperCollins.

2. The Holy Bible, Book of Matthew 11:28 *New International Version* https://www.biblegateway.com/passage/?search=Matthew%2011%3A28-30&version=NIV Accessed 07/02/2024

3. Naviaux RK. Metabolic features of the cell danger response. Mitochondrion. 2014 May;16:7-17. doi: 10.1016/j.mito.2013.08.006. Epub 2013 Aug 24. PMID: 23981537 Cell Danger Response https://pubmed.ncbi.nlm.nih.gov/23981537/ Accessed 07/02/2024

4. Cortisol Awakening Response, https://www.ncbi.nlm.nih.gov/pmc/articles/PMC3527370/ Accessed 07/01/2024

5. Cortisone & Joint Damage, https://archive.niams.nih.gov/newsroom/spotlight-on-research/long-term-benefit-steroid-injections-knee-osteoarthritis-challenged Accessed 07/06/2023

6. Cortisol & Inflammation, https://www.ncbi.nlm.nih.gov/pmc/articles/PMC4263906/ Accessed: 07/11/2024

7. Miller WL. Steroid hormone synthesis in mitochondria. Mol Cell Endocrinol. 2013 Oct 15;379(1-2):62-73. doi: 10.1016/j.mce.2013.04.014. Epub 2013 Apr 28. PMID: 23628605.

8. Duchen MR. Mitochondria and calcium: from cell signaling to cell death. J Physiol. 2000 Nov 15;529 Pt 1(Pt 1):57-68. doi: 10.1111/j.1469-7793.2000.00057.x. PMID: 11080251; PMCID: PMC2270168.

9. Castora FJ. Mitochondrial function and abnormalities implicated in the pathogenesis of ASD. Prog Neuropsychopharmacol Biol Psychiatry. 2019 Jun 8;92:83-108. doi: 10.1016/j.pnpbp.2018.12.015. Epub 2018 Dec 29. PMID: 30599156.

10. Weinberg SE, Sena LA, Chandel NS. Mitochondria in the regulation of innate and adaptive immunity. Immunity. 2015 Mar 17;42(3):406-17. doi: 10.1016/j.immuni.2015.02.002. PMID: 25786173; PMCID: PMC4365295.

11. Firestone, L., & Firestone, L. (2012). Come as you are: The surprising new science of adult attachment and how it can help you find—and keep—love. New Harbinger Publications.

12. Nagoski, E., & Nagoski, A. (2019). Burnout: the secret to unlocking the stress cycle (First edition.). Ballantine Books.

13. Nagoski, E, Nagoski, A. The Answer is not self care. Powel books blog. Published online March 28th, 2019

14. Walker, M. P. (2018). Why we sleep: The new science of sleep and dreams. London, UK: Penguin Books.

15. Otsuka R, Tamakoshi K, Yatsuya H, Murata C, Sekiya A, Wada K, Zhang HM, Matsushita K, Sugiura K, Takefuji S, OuYang P, Nagasawa N, Kondo T, Sasaki S, Toyoshima H. Eating fast leads to obesity: findings based on self-administered questionnaires among middle-aged Japanese men and women. J Epidemiol. 2006 May;16(3):117-24. doi: 10.2188/jea.16.117. PMID: 16710080.

16. Bradford K, Shih W, Videlock EJ, Presson AP, Naliboff BD, Mayer EA, Chang L. Association between early adverse life events and irritable bowel syndrome. Clin Gastroenterol Hepatol. 2012 Apr;10(4):385-90.e1-3. doi: 10.1016/j.cgh.2011.12.018. Epub 2011 Dec 16. PMID: 22178460; PMCID: PMC3311761.

17. Cabeca, A. (2019). The hormone fix: The natural way to balance your hormones and alleviate the symptoms of the perimenopause, the menopause and beyond. London: Quercus.

18. Northwestern University. "'Love hormone' is two-faced: Oxytocin strengthens bad memories and can increase fear and anxiety." ScienceDaily. ScienceDaily, 22 July 2013. www.sciencedaily.com/releases/2013/07/130722123206.htm.

19. Carmichael MS, Warburton VL, Dixen J, Davidson JM. Relationships among cardiovascular, muscular, and oxytocin responses during human sexual

activity. Arch Sex Behav. 1994 Feb;23(1):59-79. doi: 10.1007/BF01541618. PMID: 8135652.

20. Li Q, Becker B, Wernicke J, Chen Y, Zhang Y, Li R, Le J, Kou J, Zhao W, Kendrick KM. Foot massage evokes oxytocin release and activation of orbitofrontal cortex and superior temporal sulcus. Psychoneuroendocrinology. 2019 Mar;101:193-203. doi: 10.1016/j.psyneuen.2018.11.016. Epub 2018 Nov 14. PMID: 30469087.

21. Morhenn V, Beavin LE, Zak PJ. Massage increases oxytocin and reduces adrenocorticotropin hormone in humans. Altern Ther Health Med. 2012 Nov-Dec;18(6):11-8. PMID: 23251939.

22. Love TM. Oxytocin, motivation and the role of dopamine. Pharmacol Biochem Behav. 2014 Apr;119:49-60. doi: 10.1016/j.pbb.2013.06.011. Epub 2013 Jul 9. PMID: 23850525; PMCID: PMC3877159.

23. Kendrick KM, Guastella AJ, Becker B. Overview of Human Oxytocin Research. Curr Top Behav Neurosci. 2018;35:321-348. doi: 10.1007/7854_2017_19. PMID: 28864976.

24. Kosfeld M, Heinrichs M, Zak PJ, Fischbacher U, Fehr E. Oxytocin increases trust in humans. Nature. 2005 Jun 2;435(7042):673-6. doi: 10.1038/nature03701. PMID: 15931222.

25. Carmichael MS, Humbert R, Dixen J, Palmisano G, Greenleaf W, Davidson JM. Plasma oxytocin increases in the human sexual response. J Clin Endocrinol Metab. 1987 Jan;64(1):27-31. doi: 10.1210/jcem-64-1-27. PMID: 3782434.

26. Odendaal JS, Meintjes RA. Neurophysiological correlates of affiliative behaviour between humans

and dogs. Vet J. 2003 May;165(3):296-301. doi: 10.1016/s1090-0233(02)00237-x. PMID: 12672376.

27. Antoni FA, Chadio SE. Essential role of magnesium in oxytocin-receptor affinity and ligand specificity. Biochem J. 1989;257(2):611-614. doi:10.1042/bj2570611

28. Song Z, Hatton GI. Taurine and the control of basal hormone release from rat neurohypophysis. Exp Neurol. 2003 Oct;183(2):330-7. doi: 10.1016/s0014-4886(03)00105-5. PMID: 14552874.

29. Jirikowski GF, Ochs SD, Caldwell JD. Oxytocin and Steroid Actions. Curr Top Behav Neurosci. 2018;35:77-95. doi: 10.1007/7854_2017_9. PMID: 28812264.

30. Luck MR, Jungclas B. Catecholamines and ascorbic acid as stimulators of bovine ovarian oxytocin secretion. J Endocrinol. 1987 Sep;114(3):423-30. doi: 10.1677/joe.0.1140423. PMID: 3668432.

31. The Holy Bible, Psalm 119 *New International Version* https://www.biblegateway.com/passage/?search=Psalm%20119&version=NIV Accessed 07/02/2024

32. Mascaro JS, Darcher A, Negi LT, Raison CL. The neural mediators of kindness-based meditation: a theoretical model. Front Psychol. 2015;6:109. Published 2015 Feb 12. doi:10.3389/fpsyg.2015.00109

33. Uvnäs-Moberg K. Oxytocin - a Possible Mediator of anti Stress Effects Induced by Acupuncture? Acupuncture in Medicine. 2002;20(2-3):109-125. doi:10.1136/aim.20.2-3.109

34. Detillion CE, Craft TK, Glasper ER, Prendergast BJ, DeVries AC. Social facilitation of wound healing. Psychoneuroendocrinology. 2004 Sep;29(8):1004-11. doi: 10.1016/j.psyneuen.2003.10.003. PMID: 15219651.

35. Pruimboom L, Reheis D. Intermittent drinking, oxytocin and human health. Med Hypotheses. 2016 Jul;92:80-3. doi: 10.1016/j.mehy.2016.04.043. Epub 2016 Apr 27. PMID: 27241263.

36. Camerino C, Conte E, Caloiero R, Fonzino A, Carratù M, Lograno MD, Tricarico D. Evaluation of Short and Long Term Cold Stress Challenge of Nerve Grow Factor, Brain-Derived Neurotrophic Factor, Osteocalcin and Oxytocin mRNA Expression in BAT, Brain, Bone and Reproductive Tissue of Male Mice Using Real-Time PCR and Linear Correlation Analysis. Front Physiol. 2018 Jan 11;8:1101. doi: 10.3389/fphys.2017.01101. PMID: 29375393; PMCID: PMC5768886.

37. Ooishi Y, Mukai H, Watanabe K, Kawato S, Kashino M. Increase in salivary oxytocin and decrease in salivary cortisol after listening to relaxing slow-tempo and exciting fast-tempo music. PLoS One. 2017 Dec 6;12(12):e0189075. doi: 10.1371/journal.pone.0189075. PMID: 29211795; PMCID: PMC5718605.

38. Grape C, Sandgren M, Hansson LO, Ericson M, Theorell T. Does singing promote well-being?: An empirical study of professional and amateur singers during a singing lesson. Integr Physiol Behav Sci. 2003 Jan-Mar;38(1):65-74. doi: 10.1007/BF02734261. PMID: 12814197.

39. Tarr B, Launay J, Dunbar RI. Music and social bonding: "self-other" merging and neurohormonal

mechanisms. Front Psychol. 2014;5:1096. Published 2014 Sep 30. doi:10.3389/fpsyg.2014.01096

40. Kaviani M, Maghbool S, Azima S, Tabaei MH. Comparison of the effect of aromatherapy with Jasminum officinale and Salvia officinale on pain severity and labor outcome in nulliparous women. Iran J Nurs Midwifery Res. 2014;19(6):666-672.

41. Tadokoro Y, Horiuchi S, Takahata K, Shuo T, Sawano E, Shinohara K. Changes in salivary oxytocin after inhalation of clary sage essential oil scent in term-pregnant women: a feasibility pilot study. BMC Res Notes. 2017;10(1):717. Published 2017 Dec 8. doi:10.1186/s13104-017-3053-3

42. Bell, R. (2020). Everything is spiritual: who we are and what we're doing here. First U.S. edition. New York, St. Martin's Essentials.

43. Wright KP Jr, McHill AW, Birks BR, Griffin BR, Rusterholz T, Chinoy ED. Entrainment of the human circadian clock to the natural light-dark cycle. Curr Biol. 2013 Aug 19;23(16):1554-8. doi: 10.1016/j.cub.2013.06.039. Epub 2013 Aug 1. PMID: 23910656; PMCID: PMC4020279.

44. Sifferlin, A. The Healing Power of Nature. Time magazine online July 2016. https://time.com/4405827/the-healing-power-of-nature/ Accessed 10-31-2020.

45. Penckofer S, Quinn L, Byrn M, Ferrans C, Miller M, Strange P. Does glycemic variability impact mood and quality of life?. Diabetes Technol Ther. 2012;14(4):303-310. doi:10.1089/dia.2011.0191

46. Voigt RM, Forsyth CB, Keshavarzian A. Circadian rhythms: a regulator of gastrointestinal health and

dysfunction. Expert Rev Gastroenterol Hepatol. 2019;13(5):411-424. doi:10.1080/17474124.2019.1595588

47. Eckel-Mahan K, Sassone-Corsi P. Metabolism and the circadian clock converge. Physiol Rev. 2013;93(1):107-135. doi:10.1152/physrev.00016.2012

Citations From Chapter 11:

1. The Holy Bible, Book of Genesis 3:7 ESV https://www.bibleref.com/Genesis/3/Genesis-3-7.html Accessed 07/25/2024

2. A., V. D. (2015). The Body keeps the score: Brain, mind, and body in the healing of trauma. New York, NY: Penguin Books.

3. Sack V, Murphy D. The Prevalence of Adverse Childhood Experiences, Nationally, by state, and by race or ethnicity. 2018 Feb 20. https://www.childtrends.org/publications/prevalence-adverse-childhood-experiences-nationally-state-race-ethnicity. Accessed: Nov 28, 2020.

4. Dong M, Giles WH, Felitti VJ, Dube SR, Williams JE, Chapman DP, Anda RF. Insights into causal pathways for ischemic heart disease: adverse childhood experiences study. Circulation. 2004 Sep 28;110(13):1761-6. doi: 10.1161/01.CIR.0000143074.54995.7F. Epub 2004 Sep 20. PMID: 15381652.

5. Dube SR, Fairweather D, Pearson WS, Felitti VJ, Anda RF, Croft JB. Cumulative childhood stress and autoimmune diseases in adults. Psychosom Med. 2009;71(2):243-250. doi:10.1097/PSY.0b013e3181907888

6. Kelly-Irving M, Lepage B, Dedieu D, et al. Adverse childhood experiences and premature all-cause mortality. Eur J Epidemiol. 2013;28(9):721-734. doi:10.1007/s10654-013-9832-9

7. Bellis MA, Hughes K, Ford K, Ramos Rodriguez G, Sethi D, Passmore J. Life course health consequences and associated annual costs of adverse childhood experiences across Europe and North America: a systematic review and meta-analysis. Lancet Public Health. 2019 Oct;4(10):e517-e528. doi: 10.1016/S2468-2667(19)30145-8. Epub 2019 Sep 3. PMID: 31492648; PMCID: PMC7098477.

8. https://youtu.be/ypcqSTAzOWs Interview Peter Levine, PHd. "Peter Levine on restoring trauma." Uploaded April 6th, 2020. Neurosci Biobehav Rev. 2013 Sep;37(8):1549-66. doi: 10.1016/j.neubiorev.2013.06.004. Epub 2013 Jun 18. PMID: 23792048

9. Levine, Peter. *In an Unspoken Voice: How the body releases trauma and restores goodness.*

10. https://www.greenbaypressgazette.com/story/news/local/door-co/opinion/2017/02/23/faith-repent-means-change-direction/98269258/# Accessed: 07/24/2024

11. The Holy Bible, Book of Ephesians 5:25 NKJV https://www.biblegateway.com/passage/?search=Ephesians%205%3A25&version=*NKJV* Accessed 07/25/2024

12. Brown, B. (Host). (March 23, 2020). Tarana Burke and Brené on Being Heard and Seen. (3). [Audio podcast episode]. https://brenebrown.com/podcast/brene-tarana-burke-on-empathy/.

13. A., V. D. (2015). The Body keeps the score: Brain, mind, and body in the healing of trauma. New York, NY: Penguin Books.

14. The Holy Bible, Book of Isaiah 41:10-12 NKJV https://www.biblegateway.com/passage/?search=Isaiah%2041%3A10-12&version=NIV Accessed 07/25/2024

15. Ohira H, Winton WM, Oyama M. Effects of Stimulus Valence on Recognition Memory and Endogenous Eyeblinks: Further Evidence for Positive-Negative Asymmetry. Personality and Social Psychology Bulletin. 1998;24(9):986-993. doi:10.1177/0146167298249006

16. Johnson, S. (2011). Hold me tight: Your guide to the most successful approach to building loving relationships. London, UK: Piatkus.

17. Levine, A., & Heller, R. (2010). Attached: The New Science of Adult Attachment and How It Can Help You Find - And Keep - Love. New York, NY: Tarcherperigee.

18. Goleman, D. (1995). Emotional intelligence: Why it can matter more than IQ. New York: Bantam Books.

19. Peck, M. S. 1. (2002). The road less traveled: A new psychology of love, traditional values, and spiritual growth (25th anniversary ed.). New York: Simon & Schuster.

20. Bair MJ., Robinson RL., Katon W., et al. Depression and pain comorbidity: a literature review. Arch Intern Med.

Citations From Chapter 12:

1. The Holy Bible, Book of Jeremiah 9:15 NASB https://www.biblegateway.com/passage/?search=Je

remiah+23%3A15&version=NASB Accessed 07/25/2024

2. Dr. Mehmet Oz, https://www.brainyquote.com/quotes/mehmet_oz_433794 | Accessed 08/01/2024

3. Particulate Pollution, https://www.lung.org/lung-health-diseases/lung-disease-lookup/silicosis/learn-about-silicosis | Accessed 08/01/2024

4. Green River Valley, https://www.nbcnews.com/id/wbna41971686 Accessed 09/22/2023

5. Silica, https://blogs.cdc.gov/niosh-science-blog/2012/05/23/silica-fracking/ Accessed 08/27/2023

6. North Dakota Oil Spills, https://www.propublica.org/article/the-other-fracking-north-dakotas-oil-boom-brings-damage-along-with-prosperi Accessed 08/27/2024

7. Hoffman, J. Teach the Earth Website: Potential Health and Environmental Effects of Hydrofracking in the Williston Basin, Montana. https://serc.carleton.edu/NAGTWorkshops/health/case_studies/hydrofracking_w.html Accessed 12/12/2020.

8. Drinking Water, https://www.epa.gov/archive/epapages/newsroom_archive/newsreleases/f4c64770f0965c35852579cd00668aac.html Accessed 07/13/2023

9. Flint Water Crisis, https://www.nrdc.org/stories/flint-water-crisis-everything-you-need-know Accessed 07/11/2023

10. Environ. Sci. Technol. 2016, 50, 22, 12464–12472 Publication Date:October 4, 2016

https://doi.org/10.1021/acs.est.6b03492 Copyright © 2016 American Chemical Society

11. Valley of the drums, https://bullittcountyhistory.org/bchistory/valleydrum.html Accessed 08/01/2024

12. Ferrey, M., Matinovic, D., Backe, W., Anderews, A. Pharmaceuticals and chemicals of concerns in rivers: Occurrence and biological effects. Minnesota Pollution control agency report. January 2017. https://www.pca.state.mn.us/sites/default/files/tdr-g1-20.pdf. Accessed 2020.

13. [Hermaphrodite frogs, https://eartharchives.org/articles/compound-found-in-contraceptives-might-turn-male-frogs-into-females/index.html](#) Accessed 07/06/2023

14. Hayes TB, Khoury V, Narayan A, Nazir M, Park A, Brown T, Adame L, Chan E, Buchholz D, Stueve T, Gallipeau S. Atrazine induces complete feminization and chemical castration in male African clawed frogs (Xenopus laevis). Proc Natl Acad Sci U S A. 2010 Mar 9;107(10):4612-7. doi: 10.1073/pnas.0909519107. Epub 2010 Mar 1.

15. Lubick N. Drugs in the environment: do pharmaceutical take-back programs make a difference?. Environ Health Perspect. 2010;118(5):A210-A214. doi:10.1289/ehp.118-a210

16. Love Canal, https://en.wikipedia.org/wiki/Love_Canal Accessed 08/01/2024

17. Cobalt Mining, https://www.npr.org/sections/goatsandsoda/2023/02/01/1152893248/red-cobalt-congo-drc-mining-siddharth-kara Accessed 08/01/2024

18. Poverty and pollution, https://www.ncbi.nlm.nih.gov/pmc/articles/PMC1833288/ Accessed 06/03/2024

19. Burning Garbage, https://www.scientificamerican.com/article/burning-trash-bad-for-humans-and-global-warming/ Accessed 06/29/2024

20. Pollution vs GDP, https://ourworldindata.org/grapher/air-pollution-vs-gdp-per-capita Accessed 08/01/2024

21. Epigenetics and toxins, Pivonello, C., Muscogiuri, G., Nardone, A. *et al.* Bisphenol A: an emerging threat to female fertility. *Reprod Biol Endocrinol* 18, 22 (2020). https://doi.org/10.1186/s12958-019-0558-8

22. Mínguez-Alarcón L, Gaskins AJ, Chiu YH, Souter I, Williams PL, Calafat AM, Hauser R, Chavarro JE; EARTH Study team. Dietary folate intake and modification of the association of urinary bisphenol A concentrations with in vitro fertilization outcomes among women from a fertility clinic. Reprod Toxicol. 2016 Oct;65:104-112. doi: 10.1016/j.reprotox.2016.07.012. Epub 2016 Jul 14. PMID: 27423903; PMCID: PMC5067190.

23. D'Angelo S, Scafuro M, Meccariello R. BPA and Nutraceuticals, Simultaneous Effects on Endocrine Functions. Endocr Metab Immune Disord Drug Targets. 2019;19(5):594-604. doi: 10.2174/1871530319666190101120119. PMID: 30621569; PMCID: PMC7360909.

24. Cadmium, https://www.atsdr.cdc.gov/csem/cadmium/Where-Cadmium-Found.html Accessed 06/23/2023

25. Immune Suppression, Nagaraju R, Kalahasthi R, Balachandar R, Bagepally BS. Cadmium exposure

and DNA damage (genotoxicity): a systematic review and meta-analysis. Crit Rev Toxicol. 2022 Nov;52(10):786-798. doi: 10.1080/10408444.2023.2173557. Epub 2023 Feb 21. PMID: 36802997

26. Kim M, Bae M, Na H, Yang M. Environmental toxicants--induced epigenetic alterations and their reversers. J Environ Sci Health C Environ Carcinog Ecotoxicol Rev. 2012;30(4):323-67. doi: 10.1080/10590501.2012.731959. Erratum in: J Environ Sci Health C Environ Carcinog Ecotoxicol Rev. 2013;31(3):285. PMID: 23167630.

27. Fragrances, https://www.ncbi.nlm.nih.gov/pmc/articles/PMC10051690/ Accessed 07/07/2023

28. Seamen, G. Sept. 6, 2017. Top10 plants for removing indoor toxins. https://learn.eartheasy.com/articles/the-top-10-plants-for-removing-indoor-toxins/ Accessed: December 13, 2020.

29. Rustagi N, Pradhan SK, Singh R. Public health impact of plastics: An overview. Indian J Occup Environ Med. 2011;15(3):100-103. doi:10.4103/0019-5278.93198

30. Tran VV, Park D, Lee YC. Indoor Air Pollution, Related Human Diseases, and Recent Trends in the Control and Improvement of Indoor Air Quality. Int J Environ Res Public Health. 2020;17(8):2927. Published 2020 Apr 23. doi:10.3390/ijerph17082927

31. Withworth, J. Food and Safety News Finland assesses heavy metal risk from foods. https://www.foodsafetynews.com/2020/05/finland-assesses-heavy-metals-risk-from-foods/ Accessed: December 16, 2020.

32. Jaishankar M, Tseten T, Anbalagan N, Mathew BB, Beeregowda KN. Toxicity, mechanism and health effects of some heavy metals. Interdiscip Toxicol. 2014;7(2):60-72. doi:10.2478/intox-2014-0009

33. Garbarino, J. R., Hayes, H. C., Roth, D. A., Antweiler, R. C., Brinton, T. I., & Taylor, H. E. (1996). Heavy metals in the Mississippi River. Us geological survey circular usgs circ, 53-72.

34. Daniel T. Sun, Li Peng, Washington S. Reeder, Seyed Mohamad Moosavi, Davide Tiana, David K. Britt, Emad Oveisi, Wendy L. Queen. Rapid, Selective Heavy Metal Removal from Water by a Metal–Organic Framework/Polydopamine Composite. ACS Central Science, 2018; DOI: 10.1021/acscentsci.7b00605

35. Federal Aviation Administration Fact sheet- Leaded Aviation Fuel and the Environment. November 20, 2019. https://www.faa.gov/news/fact_sheets/news_story.cfm?newsId=14754 Accessed December 17, 2020.

36. U.S. Energy Information Administration. The History of Gasoline https://www.eia.gov/energyexplained/gasoline/history-of-gasoline.php Acessed: December 19, 2020.

37. Miranda ML, Anthopolos R, Hastings D. A geospatial analysis of the effects of aviation gasoline on childhood blood lead levels. Environ Health Perspect. 2011;119(10):1513-1516. doi:10.1289/ehp.1003231

38. Ogidi MA, Sridhar MKC, Coker AO (2017) A Follow-Up Study Health Risk Assessment of Heavy Metal Leachability from Household Cookwares. J Food Sci Toxicol Vol.1 No.1:3

39. Zhang, S. Mother Jones Leaded Fuel is a thing of the past unless you fly a private plane. January 10,

2013. https://www.motherjones.com/politics/2013/01/private-planes-still-use-leaded-gasoline/ Accessed: December 17, 2020.

40. Sinclair E, Kim SK, Akinleye HB, Kannan K. Quantitation of gas-phase perfluoroalkyl surfactants and fluorotelomer alcohols released from nonstick cookware and microwave popcorn bags. Environ Sci Technol. 2007 Feb 15;41(4):1180-5. doi: 10.1021/es062377w. PMID: 17593716.

41. EFSA Panel on Contaminants in the Food Chain (EFSA CONTAM Panel), Schrenk D, Bignami M, Bodin L, Chipman JK, Del Mazo J, Grasl-Kraupp B, Hogstrand C, Hoogenboom LR, Leblanc JC, Nebbia CS, Nielsen E, Ntzani E, Petersen A, Sand S, Vleminckx C, Wallace H, Barregård L, Ceccatelli S, Cravedi JP, Halldorsson TI, Haug LS, Johansson N, Knutsen HK, Rose M, Roudot AC, Van Loveren H, Vollmer G, Mackay K, Riolo F, Schwerdtle T. Risk to human health related to the presence of perfluoroalkyl substances in food. EFSA J. 2020 Sep 17;18(9):e06223. doi: 10.2903/j.efsa.2020.6223. PMID: 32994824; PMCID: PMC7507523.

42. Potera C. REPRODUCTIVE TOXICOLOGY: Study Associates PFOS and PFOA with Impaired Fertility. Environ Health Perspect. 2009;117(4):A148.

43. Gupta YK, Meenu M, Peshin SS. Aluminium utensils: Is it a concern? Natl Med J India. 2019 Jan-Feb;32(1):38-40. doi: 10.4103/0970-258X.272116. PMID: 31823940.

44. Bocca B, Pino A, Alimonti A, Forte G. Toxic metals contained in cosmetics: a status report. Regul Toxicol Pharmacol. 2014 Apr;68(3):447-67.

doi: 10.1016/j.yrtph.2014.02.003. Epub 2014 Feb 12. PMID: 24530804.

45. Mandriota SJ. A Case-control Study Adds a New Piece to the Aluminium/Breast Cancer Puzzle. EBioMedicine. 2017;22:22-23. doi:10.1016/j.ebiom.2017.06.025

46. Di Pasquale A, Preiss S, Tavares Da Silva F, Garçon N. Vaccine Adjuvants: from 1920 to 2015 and Beyond. Vaccines (Basel). 2015;3(2):320-343. Published 2015 Apr 16. doi:10.3390/vaccines3020320

47. Thimerosal and Vaccines Centers for Disease Control. https://www.cdc.gov/vaccinesafety/concerns/thimerosal/index.html# Accessed: December 17, 2020.

48. Baker JP. Mercury, vaccines, and autism: one controversy, three histories. Am J Public Health. 2008;98(2):244-253. doi:10.2105/AJPH.2007.113159

49. Muhammad Waqar Ashraf, "Levels of Heavy Metals in Popular Cigarette Brands and Exposure to These Metals via Smoking", The Scientific World Journal, vol. 2012, Article ID 729430, 5 pages, 2012. https://doi.org/10.1100/2012/729430

50. Houghton CA. Sulforaphane: Its "Coming of Age" as a Clinically Relevant Nutraceutical in the Prevention and Treatment of Chronic Disease. Oxid Med Cell Longev. 2019;2019:2716870. Published 2019 Oct 14. doi:10.1155/2019/2716870

51. National Center for Biotechnology Information. PubChem Compound Summary for CID 5280961, Genistein. https://pubchem.ncbi.nlm.nih.gov/compound/Genistein. Accessed Dec. 19, 2020.

Citations From Chapter 13:

1. Dr. Mehmet Oz, https://www.brainyquote.com/quotes/mehmet_oz_433794 | Accessed 08/01/2024

2. Friedrich Miescher, https://www.nature.com/scitable/topicpage/discovery-of-dna-structure-and-function-watson-397/ | Accessed: 09/01/2023

3. Erwin Chargaff, https://www.pbs.org/wgbh/aso/databank/entries/do53dn.html | Accessed 09/15/2023

4. Lynch, B. (2018). Dirty Genes a Breakthrough program to treat the root cause of illness and optimize your health. New York, NY: Harper One.

5. Genome, https://www.genome.gov/genetics-glossary/Single-Nucleotide-Polymorphisms | Accessed 08/15/2024

6. Genetic Diseases, https://www.hopkinsmedicine.org/health/genetic-disorders | Accessed 08/15/2024

7. MTHFR, https://www.ncbi.nlm.nih.gov/books/NBK6561/ | Accessed 08/15/2024

8. Strategene, https://strategene.me/coming-soon.php | Accessed 08/15/2024

9. Opus 23, https://letsgethealthymi.com/index.php/opus-23/ | Accessed 08/15/2024

10. MTHFR Report, https://blog.23andme.com/articles/our-take-on-the-mthfr-gene | Accessed 08/15/2024

11. Voisin S, Eynon N, Yan X, Bishop DJ. Exercise training and DNA methylation in humans. Acta Physiol (Oxf). 2015 Jan;213(1):39-59. doi: 10.1111/apha.12414. Epub 2014 Nov 19. PMID: 25345837.

12. Basu AK. DNA Damage, Mutagenesis and Cancer. Int J Mol Sci. 2018 Mar 23;19(4):970. doi: 10.3390/ijms19040970. PMID: 29570697; PMCID: PMC5979367.

13. Shimizu I, Yoshida Y, Suda M, Minamino T. DNA damage response and metabolic disease. Cell Metab. 2014 Dec 2;20(6):967-77. doi: 10.1016/j.cmet.2014.10.008. Epub 2014 Nov 13. PMID: 25456739.

14. Baccarelli A, Bollati V. Epigenetics and environmental chemicals. *Curr Opin Pediatr.* 2009;21(2):243-251. doi:10.1097/mop.0b013e32832925cc

15. Darkhorse Podcast, https://www.youtube.com/@DarkHorsePod | Accessed 08/15/2024

Citations From Chapter 14:

1. Peterson, J. B., Doidge, N., & Van Sciver, E. (2019). 12 rules for life: an antidote to chaos. [London], Penguin Books.

2. Cuomo takes Ivermectin | https://www.yahoo.com/news/chris-cuomo-makes-ivermectin-face-210453781.html Accessed 09/09/2024

3. JAMA, Medicine & War | https://jamanetwork.com/journals/jamanetworkopen/fullarticle/2809778 Accessed 09/10/2024

4. Obesity in America | https://www.ncbi.nlm.nih.gov/search/research-news/12328/ Accessed 09/10/2024

5. Genesis 1:28, NIV, Holy Bible | https://www.biblegateway.com/passage/?search=Genesis%201%3A28&version=NIV Accessed 09/30/2024

6. Genesis 2:19, NIV, Holy Bible | https://www.biblegateway.com/passage/?search=Genesis%202%3A19&version=NIV Accessed 09/30/2024

7. Organon | https://collections.nlm.nih.gov/catalog/nlm:nlmuid-101305101-bk Accessed 09/24/2024

8. Acupuncture is Effective | https://www.nccih.nih.gov/health/acupuncture-effectiveness-and-safety Accessed 09/17/2024

9. Cold Lasers | https://www.ncbi.nlm.nih.gov/pmc/articles/PMC4126803/ Accessed 09/05/2024

10. Isaiah 61:1, CSB, Holy Bible | https://www.biblegateway.com/passage/?search=Isaiah%2061%3A1&version=CSB Accessed 09/30/2024

11. Angela Duckworth Quote | https://www.goodreads.com/work/quotes/45670634 Accessed 09/30/2024357

www.ingramcontent.com/pod-product-compliance
Lightning Source LLC
Chambersburg PA
CBHW031419150426
43191CB00006B/332